Drug Store
and
Business Management

For Second Year Diploma in Pharmacy & B. Pharm.

Revised as per latest PCI syllabus

Dr. Mohammed Ali
&
Mrs. Jyoti Gupta

Faculty of Pharmacy
Jamia Hamdard (Hamdard University)
Hamdard Nagar, New Delhi-110 062

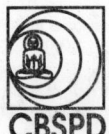

CBSPD

CBS Publishers & Distributors Pvt Ltd

New Delhi • Bengaluru • Chennai • Kochi • Kolkata • Lucknow • Mumbai
Hyderabad • Jharkhand • Nagpur • Patna • Pune • Uttarakhand

Drug Store and
Business
Management

ISBN: 978-81-239-0417-7

First Edition: 1996

Reprint:1999, 2002, 2004, 2005, 2006, 2007, 2008, 2010, 2012, 2014, 2016, 2017, 2018, 2019, 2022, 2024 2025

Published by Satish Kumar Jain and Produced by Varun Jain for

CBS Publishers & Distributors Pvt Ltd

4819/XI Prahlad Street, 24 Ansari Road, Daryaganj, New Delhi 110 002, India.   4819/XI Prahlad Street, 24 Ansari Road, Daryaganj, New Delhi 110 002, India.
Ph: 23289259, 23266861   Website: www.cbspd.com

e-mail: delhi@cbspd.com
Corporate Office: 204 FIE, Industrial Area, Patparganj, Delhi 110 092
Ph: 011-4934 4934   Fax: 011-4934 4935   e-mail: publishing@cbspd.com; publicity@cbspd.com

Branches

- **Bengaluru:** Seema House 2975, 17th Cross, K.R. Road, Banasankari 2nd Stage, Bengaluru 560 070, Karnataka
  Ph: +91-80-26771678/79   Fax: +91-80-26771680   e-mail: bangalore@cbspd.com
- **Chennai:** 7, Subbaraya Street, Shenoy Nagar, Chennai 600 030, Tamil Nadu, India
  Ph: +91-44-26680620/26681266   Fax: +91-44-42032115   e-mail: chennai@cbspd.com
- **Kochi:** 42/1325, 1326, Power House Road, Opp KSEB, Power House, Ernakulam 682 018, Kochi, Kerala, India
  Ph: +91-484-4059061-65, 67   Fax: +91-484-4059065   e-mail: kochi@cbspd.com
- **Kolkata:** 147, Hind Ceramics Compound, 1st Floor, Nilgunj Road, Belghoria, Kolkata-700056, West Bengal, India
  Ph: +033-25633055, 033-25633056   e-mail: kolkata@cbspd.com
- **Lucknow:** Basement, Khushnuma Complex, 7 Meerabai Marg (Behind Jawahar Bhawan), Lucknow-226001, UP, India
  Ph: +91-522-4000032   e-mail: tiwari.lucknow@cbspd.com
- **Mumbai:** PWD Shed, Gala no 25/26, Ramchandra Bhatt Marg, Next to JJ Hospital Gate no. 2, Opp. Union Bank of India Noorbaug, Mumbai-400009, Maharashtra, India
  Ph: 022-66661880/89   e-mail: mumbai@cbspd.com

Representatives

Hyderabad	0-9885175004	**Jharkhand**	0-9811541605	**Nagpur**	0-8692091830
Patna	0-9334159340	**Pune**	0-9664372571	**Uttarakhand**	0-9716462459

Printed at: Mudrak, Noida, UP, India

SYLLABUS

THEORY (75 HOURS)

PART I COMMERCE (50 HOURS)

1. Introduction – Trade, Industry and Commerce, Functions and Subdivision of Commerce, Introduction to Elements of Economics and Management.
2. Forms of Business Organisations.
3. Channels of Distribution.
4. Drug House Management – Selection of Site, Space Lay-out and Legal Requirements.

   Importance and Objectives of Purchasing, Selection of Suppliers, Credit Information, Tenders, Contracts and Price Determination and Legal Requirements thereto.

   Codification, Handling of Drug Stores and other Hospital Supplies.
5. Inventory Control – Objects and Importance, Modern Techniques like ABC, VED Analysis, the Lead Time, Inventory Carrying Cost, Safety Stock, Minimum and Maximum Stock Levels, Economic Order Quantity, Scrap and Surplus Disposal.
6. Sales Promotion, Market Research, Salesmanship, Qualities of a Salesman, Advertising and Window Display.
7. Recruitment, Training, Evaluation and Compensation of the Pharmacist.
8. Banking and Finance - Service and Functions of Bank, Finance Planning and Sources of Finance.

PART II ACCOUNTANCY (25 HOURS)

1. Introduction to the Accounting Concepts and Conventions. Double Entry, Book Keeping, Different Kinds of Accounts.
2. Cash Book.
3. General Ledger and Trial Balance.
4. Profit and Loss Account and Balance Sheet.
5. Simple Techniques of Analysing Financial Statements. Introduction to Budgeting.

   Books Recommended (Latest editions)
   1. Remington Pharmaceutical Sciences.

PREFACE

Management is a universal requirement for making of decision, coordination of activities, handling of people and evaluation of performance. It is an important force for determining objective, taking policy decision, leading towards growth and prosperity and creating resources for economic and special development. Coordination is the essence of management dealing with the task of endless efforts to ensure successful attainment of objectives. Proper channels of communication and personal contacts should be encouraged as they are the most effective means of communication for achieving coordination. The early personal contacts help in exchanging the opinions and ideas in a better way and clarifying the misunderstanding more easily.

A good administrator should have an open mind and be able to foresee the problems. He should have broad interest, balanced temperament, self confidence, try to develop social understanding and be emotionally mature. When monopoly, leg pulling, dictatorship and revenge are principal motives of an administrator, the management process collapses.

The study of 'Drug Store and Business Management' is an integrated part of the course of pharmacy at the undergraduate level. The subject embraces the knowledge of the methods, techniques, principles and practices of an efficient drug store and management of business. Comprehensive understanding of this subject is essential not only for the students, but also for all those who want to enter some line of business and management. The present book is a modest attempt to provide an integrated analysis of various aspects of drug store and management of business.

The basic purpose of the book is to present the subject in a simple language and easily understandable style for the benefit of the student and other readers. It covers the syllabus as prescribed by the Pharmacy Council of India in the Education Regulations-1991, implemented in the year-1993 for Diploma Course, in Pharmacy. The present book is characterized by up to date information about the subject matter, comprehensive treatment and sound observations.

It is impossible to express our indebtedness to those authors of books and articles from which we have gained to much information for writing the book.

Without the encouragement, courtesy and full co-operation of Shri Satish Kumar Jain and Vinod Kumar Jain, CBS Publishers & Distributors, this work might not have reached in its present form. Much of the book's final form and appearance are due to tireless and continuous efforts of Mr. Sunil Kumar Dhir, Super Computers, who has typeset it on a laser printer. Our greatest depth of gratitude is due to Dr. A. Ansari, Dr. M. Altaf Khan and Dr. R. Kumar, Department of Commerce, Jamia Millia Islamia, New Delhi-25, and to Shri Sushil Jain, College Book Store, Nai Sarak, Delhi, for assisting us constantly and providing sufficient literature on the subject. Our family members also deserve special mention for their sustained cooperation in bringing out this book.

We have made every effort to avoid printing errors. However, despite best efforts some might have crept in inadvertently. We shall be obliged if these are brought to our notice.

We are confident that both the students and teachers will find the book useful and rewarding. Constructive and helpful suggestions for improvement of the future editions of the book will be gratefully acknowledged.

Mohammed Ali
Jyoti Gupta

CONTENTS

1

BUSINESS

Business is an economic activity which involves regular production and/or exchange of goods and services with the main purpose of earning profits through the satisfaction of human wants.

Business includes production and exchange of goods with the object of earning profits. All activities concerned with production of goods and services and their distribution are known as business activities. These activities are organised and performed under the framework of an institution known as business organisation/firm/enterprise. Business has been defined in different ways as :

1. Business i. an institution organised and operated to provide goods and services to society under the incentive of private gain.

2. Business is a human activity directed towards producing or acquiring wealth through buying and selling goods.

3. Business is an activity in which different persons exchange something of value (whether goods or services) for mutual gain or profit.

4. Business is a form of activity pursued primarily with the object of earning profit for the benefit of those on whose behalf the activity is conducted. Profit is not the sole objective of the business. It may have other objectives like promotion of welfare of the workers and the general public. Business achieves its objectives by producing and distributing those goods and services which can satisfy human wants.

Thus, business pervades all human activities directed toward earning profits or economic gains. It includes all activities from production to distribution of goods and services. Industry, trade and other activities like bankning, transport, insurance, werehousing, advertising etc. are all parts of the modern business system.

SCOPE OF BUSINESS

The scope of business is very wide. It should not be confused with trade. 'Trade' simply denotes purchase and sale of goods whereas 'business' includes all activities from production to distribution of goods and services. It embraces industry, trade and other activities like banking, transport, insurance, and warehousing which facilitiate production and distribution of goods and services. The whole complex field of commerce and industry, the basic industries, processing and manufacturing industries, the network of ancillary services : distribution, banking, insurance, transport and so on, which serve and interpenetrate the world' of business as a whole are business activities.

The business activities may be grouped under two broad headings, viz., (1) Industry and (2) Commerce. A business undertaking which deals with growing, extracting, manufacturing or construction is called an *industrial enterprise*. On the other hand, a business undertaking which is concerned with exchange (buying and selling) of goods and services or with activities that are incidental to trade like transport, warehousing, banking, insurance and advertising, is called a *commercial enterprise*.

INDUSTRY

The activities of extraction, production, conversion, processing or fabrication of products are described as industry. The products of industry may fall in any one of the following three categories :

(a) **Consumers' Goods :** Goods used by final consumers are called consumers' goods. Edible Oils, Cloth, Jam, Television, Radio, Scooter, Refrigerator, etc. come under this category.

(b) **Producers' Goods :** Goods used for the production of other goods are described as producers' goods. Machine tools and machinery used for manufacturing other products come under this heading. These are also called capital goods.

(c) **Intermediate Goods :** There are certain materials which are the finished products of one industry and become the intermediate products of other industries. A few examples of this kind are the copper industry, aluminium industry, and plastic industry, the finished products of which are used in manufacturing electrical appliances, electricity wires, toys, baskets, containers, and buckets.

Broadly speaking, industrial activities may be classified into *primary* and *secondary* industries. Primary industry may be either extractive or genetic, and secondary industry may be either manufacturing or construction.

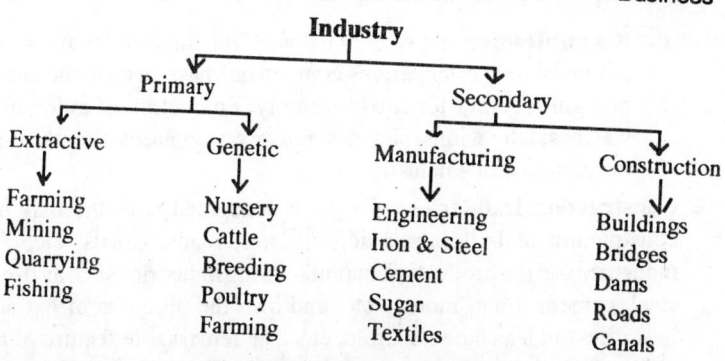

Fig-1. Classification of Industries

1. **Extractive Industries :** They extract or draw out products from natural sources such as earth, sea, air. The products of such industries are generally used by manufacturing and construction industries for producing finished goods. Farming, mining, lumbering hunting, fishing, etc. are some of the examples of extractive industries.

2. **Genetic Industries :** Genetic means parentage or heredity. Genetic industries are engaged in breeding plants and animals for their use in further reproduction. For breeding plants, the nurseries are typical examples of genetic industries. In addition, the activities of cattle-breeding farms, poultry farms and fish hatchery come under the category of genetic industries.

3. **Manufacturing Industries :** These are engaged in producing goods through the creation of utility. Such industries are engaged in the conversion or transformation of raw materials or semi-finished products into finished products. The products of extractive industries generally become the raw materials of manufacturing industries. Factory production is the outcome of manufacturing industry. Manufacturing industries many assume the following forms :

   (a) **Analytical :** The basic material is analysed and separated into a number of products. Petroleum refining is an example of analytical industry. The crude oil is extracted from beneath the earth and is processed and separated into petrol, kerosene, gasoline, lubricating oil, etc.

   (b) **Synthetic :** Two or more materials are mixed together in the manufacturing operations to obtain some new products. Products like soap, cement, paints, fertilisers and cosmetics are produced by synthetic industries.

   (c) **Processing :** In this case, raw materials are processed through a series of manufacturing operations making use of analytical and synthetic methods. Textiles, sugar and steel are example of this category.

(d) **Assembly line :** In assembly industry, the finished products can be produced only after various components have been made and then brought together for final assembly. Production of automobiles, watches, televisions, bicycles, railway wagons, etc. are the typical examples of this industry.

4. **Construction Industries :** They are concerned with the making or construction of buildings, bridges, dams, roads, canals, etc. These industries use the products of manufacturing industries such as iron and steel, cement, lime, mortar, etc. and also the products of extractive industries such as stone, marble, etc. The remarkable feature of these industries is that their products are not sold in the sense of being taken to the markets. They are constructed and fabricated at fixed sites.

COMMERCE

Commercial occupations deal with the buying and selling of goods, the exchange of commodities and distribution of finished products. It may be defined as *an organised system for the exchange of commodities and the distribution of finished products.*

Commerce links producers and consumers. The main object of commerce is to ensure smooth distribution of goods and services to satisfy the wants of consumers. *It is the sum total of all those activities which are concerned with the transfer of goods and services from the producers to the consumers.* Thus, it includes exchange of goods and the services which facilitate exchange of goods. These services are transport, banking, warehousing, insurance and advertising. Both trade as well as aids to trade (i.e., services which facilitate trade) bridge the gap between producers and consumers.

The chief function of commerce is to remove the hindrances of person (through traders), place (through transportation, insurance and packaging), time (through warehousing and storage) and knowledge (through salesmanship, advertising, etc.) arising in connection with the distribution of goods and services until they reach the consumers. By removing these hindrances, commerce ensures a free and smooth flow of goods from producers to consumers or users.

Commerce serves both the producers and the consumers by removing several hindrances exiting between them. The role of commerce in removing these hindrances is discussed below :

1. **Hindrance of Person :** The producers of goods and the consumers of goods are not always situated in the same locality. Thus, the producer is not able to have direct contact with the consumers to sell his products. There is a need of persons who could buy products from the producers and sell them to the ultimate consumers. Traders have emerged to serve as a link between the producers and the consumers. Thus, trade plays an

important role in establishing contacts between the producers and the consumers. Wholesalers, retailers and mercantile agents operate to remove the hindrance of person.

2. **Hindrance of Exchange :** Money removes the hindrance of exchange between the producers and the consumers. It serves as a common denominator of measurement of value. In the modern world, exchange of goods for goods in not always feasible. It is the evolution of money (or currency) which has encouraged national and international trade.

3. **Hindrance of Finance :** This problem is solved by the banks and other financial institutions. Consumers need funds to finance purchase of luxury items such as T.V., refrigerator and car. Businessmen need funds for meeting their working capital requirements. Banks facilitate trade by granting loans, cash credit and overdraft facilities.

4. **Hindrance of Place :** Goods may be produced at a place where advantages of location other than the market are available. The barrier of distance between the place of production and the market where these products can be sold is removed by different means of transport. Besides transport, the services of insurance to cover the risk of loss during transit and storage, and packaging to protect goods against damage and pilferage, are also aimed at removing the hindrance of place.

5. **Hindrance of Time :** Goods, in modern times, are produced in anticipation of demand and as such they are to be stored till the demand for the same comes up. The function of storage and preservation is performed by warehouses which remove the hindrance of time by balancing the time lag between production and consumption, thus creating time utility. During the process of storage, insurance plays its role by providing a cover against the risk of loss or damage through theft or fire.

6. **Hindrance of Knowledge :** A producer may find it difficult to sell his products unless and until he brings to the knowledge of the prospective consumers the utility and the distinctive features of his products. Advertising and salesmanship help to remove the hindrance of knowledge on the part of the prospective buyers by bringing to their notice the utility of the goods and services offered.

7. **Hindrance of Risk :** There are a number of risks in any business activity. These can be covered with the help of insurance companies. Insurance companies undertake to make good the loss by receiving a small amount of premium in advance as consideration.

In brief, commerce is that part of business which seeks to facilitate exchange of goods by removing various hindrances, namely, those of person through trade, of exchange and finance through money and banking, of place through warehousing and storage, and of lack of knowledge through advertising.

Importance of Commerce in Modern Economy

Commerce has gained tremendous importance in the economic system of all countries of the world. The need of commerce is felt because there is generally no direct contact between the producer and the consumer. Moreover, it is of no-use to produce goods unless they could be transferred to the consumers or users. Industry cannot survive if trade, transport, warehousing, insurance, banking and other allied services do not exist. In fact, it is dynamic commerce which has ecouraged the industrialists to produce on a very large scale by ensuring them ready supply of raw materials and other inputs and ready market of their output. With the help of commercial activities, international trade has also been possible.

Modern commerce is dynamic in the sense that it helps the consumers to get want-satisfying products. It does not matter where the consumers live. Commerce works to remove all hindrances between the producers and the consumers. It helps in increasing standard of living of the people by providing them various goods which would not have reached them in the absence of commercial activities. In fact, commerce is the *nerve system* of the economy of a nation. It helps both in production and distribution of want - statisfying products.

SCOPE OF COMMERCE

Numerous activities are necessary to remove the obstacles or hindrances in the way of exchange of goods and services. Each group of activities undertaken to remove a particular obstacle takes the form of a branch of commerce. The branches of commerce can be classified into two broad categories, *viz.*, (i) Trade, and (ii) Aids to trade.

TRADE

Trade refers to the sale, transfer or exchange of goods and services. It constitutes the central activity around which the ancillary functions like banking, transportation, insurance, packaging warehousing and advertising cluster. Trade is actual purchase and sale of goods in a market. It may be a *barter* exchange or a *monetary* exchange. Barter exchange means a system of exchanging goods for goods directly, e.g., wheat for cotton. Monetary exchange means a system of exchanging goods against money. Monetary value of a product is known as its price. Money as a medium of exchange and a common measure of value plays an important role in the modern economies.

Kinds of Trade

Trade may be classified into the following two broad categories :

1. **Internal or Home Trade :** It consists of buying and selling of goods within the boundaries of a country and the payment for the same is made in national currency either directly or through the banking system. Internal trade may be further sub-classified into :

(a) **Wholesale Trade :** It involves purchase and sale of goods belonging to a specific type of variety in bulk. A wholeslaer buys in larger quantities from the producers or manufacturers and sells comparatively in smaller quantities to the retailers. The wholesaler constitutes a link between the producers on the one hand and the retailers on the other.

(b) **Retail Trade :** It refers to the selling of goods by the retailer to the customers, thus acting as a link between the wholesaler and the final consumer. Retail trade is conducted through a variety of forms shops, vendors, pedlars, mail order houses, etc. Retail trade is also conducted in the form of departmental stores, multiple shops, co-operative stores, super bazars and self-service stores.

2. **International or Foreign Trade :** It refers to the exchange of goods and services between two or more countries. International trade involves the use of foreign currency (called foreign exchange). It facilitates the payment of the price of the exported goods and services to the domestic exporter in domestic currency, and for making payment of the imported goods and services to the foreign exporter in that country's national currency (foreign exchange). To facilitate this payment, involving exchange transactions, a highly developed system of international banking under the overall control and supervision of the central bank of the concerned country (Reserve Bank of India in our case) is involved.

International trade may be further sub-classified into :

(a) *Import trade,* involving purchase of foreign goods for use or sale in the domestic market.

(b) *Export trade,* involving supply of domestic goods to foreign buyers or markets; and

(c) *Entrepot or re-export trade,* involving the import of foreign goods with a view to re-exporting them and making a profit in the process.

Auxiliaries to Trade or Aids to Trade

There are certain functions such as banking transportation, insurance, warehousing, advertising, etc. which constitute the main auxiliary functions helping trade. These auxiliary functions have been briefly discussed hereunder :

1. **Transport :** It performs the useful function of carrying goods from producers to wholesalers, to retailers, and finally to customers. Transportation provides the *wheels of commerce.* It has linked all parts of the world with the help of efficient means of transport.

2. **Warehousing :** There is generally a time lag between the production and consumption of goods. This problem can be solved by storing the goods in warehouses. Storage creates *time utility* and removes the

hindrance of time in trade. It performs the useful function of holding the goods for the period they are not demanded. Thus, warehousing discharges the function of storing the goods both for manufactures and traders for such time till they decide to sell the goods.

3. **Insurance :** It provides a cover against the loss of goods in the process of transit and storage. An insurance company performs a useful service of compensating for the loss arising from the damage caused to goods through fire, pilferage, theft, flood and the hazards of sea transportation. It, thus, protects the traders from the fear of loss of goods. It charges a nominal insurance permium for the risks covered.

4. **Banking :** Banks provide a device through which payments of goods bought and sold are made thereby facilitating the purchase and sale of goods on credit. Banks also perform the useful economic function of collecting the savings of the people and business houses and making them available to those who may profitably use them. Thus, banks may be regarded as traders in money and credit.

5. **Advertising :** It performs a useful function of bridging the knowledge or information gap about the availability and uses of goods between traders and consumers. In the absence of advertising, goods would not have been sold to a widely scattered market and customers would not have come to know about many of the new products because of the paucity of time and physical spatial distance between the producers and the consumers.

The terms 'commerce' and 'trade' do not carry the same meaning. The points of distinction between the two are as follows :

1. Commerce includes all activites engaged in distribution of goods and services from producers to consumers. Trade indicates the act of exchange or purchase and sale of goods. Trade helps in passing ownership and possession of goods from seller to buyer.

2. The scope of the term 'commerce' is wider than the term 'trade'. Trade is a part of commerce. Commerce includes trade and various services which facilitate trade.

3. Commerce creates time and place utility whereas trade creates possession utility through buying and selling.

Interrelationship Between Trade, Commerce and Industry

There is a great need of coordination between trade, commerce and industry for the economic development of any nation. Trade, commerce and industry are important segments of the business system. They are interdependent and interrrelated. If any of these is weak, the whole business system will be adversely affected.

Difference between Industry, Commerce and Trade

Industry	Commerce	Trade
1. It means production of goods and services.	It means distribution of goods and services supplied by industry.	It means actual exchange or process of purchase and sale of goods.
2. It represents supply side of goods and services.	It represents demand side of goods and services.	It represents exchange of goods and services.
3. It requires huge fixed and working capital in production.	It requires limited fixed capital, but huge working capital.	It requires limited fixed capital. Limited working capital is enough if turnover is quick.
4. It includes genetic, extractive, manufacturing and construction industries.	It includes trade and auxiliaries to trade.	It includes inland and international trade.
5. It may be carried on at home, workshop, factory or mine.	It involves movement of goods from the place of production to the place of consumption.	It is carried on where buyers and sellers exist.
6. It creates form utility by changing the form or shape of materials.	It creates place utility and time utility through preservation of goods and their movement from one place to another.	It creates possesion utility through exchange of goods and services.

Industry is the backbone of trade and commerce. The problem of distribution of goods and services will arise only when the goods are produced by the industry. Thus, if industry is well developed, there will be a greater need of trading and commercial activities like transport, banking, insurance, storage, packaging, etc. At the same time, it should also be noted that industry depends upon trade and commerce to a great extent. Raw materials, capital and services like transport, banking and storage are almost indispensable for the survival and growth of industry. The goods and services produced by industry are distributed among the customers only with the help of trade and commerce.

Traders help the industry in determining what to produce, when to produce and for whom to produce. They facilitate procurement of raw materials by the industry and marketing of goods and services produced by the industry. Trade is also the nucleus of business since all commercial and industrial activities revolve around exchange of goods and services. Higher the volume of trade, higher will be the need for production of goods and serivces and rendering of allied services such as transport, storage, banking and insurance. The existence of sound industrial base in the country and infra-structural activities also facitlitate trade to a great extent.

Thus, trade, industry and commerce are interdependent and interrelated segments or activities of modern business. None of these can exist in isolation. Each facilitates the other activities of business. For instance, trading and commercial activities help in the growth of industry. Similarly industry stimulates the growth of trade and commercial activities like warehousing, transport and banking.

2

ECONOMICS

Human beings are generally engaged in some activity or the other. Some of the activities are pursued with economic motives and they are called the *economic activities.* The examples are business, profession and employment. many people are also engaged in certain social, cultural and religious activities. Such activities do not generate economic gain. They are termed as *non-economic activities* because they don't have any economic objective.

Economic Activites : *Economic activities are concerned with production, exchange and distribution of products and services.* Human beings undertake to perform economic activities to earn their livelihood and to acquire wealth. A manufacturer, a trader, an agriculturist, an ice cream vendor, a doctor, a teacher and a labourer working in a factory are all doing economic activities. These activities enable people to earn a living and acquire wealth. In other words, these activities satisfy the economic needs of the people.

The essence of an economic activity is production and distribution of goods and services or rendering of some service. The return of economic activities can be expressed in terms of money. A businessman earns profits, a doctor charges fee for his servic and an employee gets wages and salaries from the employer.

Non-economic Activities : Non-economic activities are asumed by human beings because of social, psychological and religious sentiments. There is no place of economic data in the non-ecnomic activities. The examples of non-economic activities are a housewife looking after the household, a person engaged in social work, a person engaged in serving the handicapped pesons, etc. These activities are pursued not to earn any income or profit, but to drive personal activities.

Non-economic activities are pursued by those people who have some social, cultural or religious mission of their life. The element of profit or income and wealth generation is totally absent from the performance of non-economic activities is intagible and it can't be measured in terms of moncy.

Types of Economic Activites

People are engaged in different kinds of economic activites to earn money income. These activites are also called occupations. Human occupations may be classified into three groups as follows :

1. Business
2. Prefession.
3. Emoloyment.

1. **Business :** The term 'business' denotes economic activites pursued primarily with the purpose of earning profits. These involve production and exchange of goods and services on a regular basis and carry an element of risk and uncertainty. Manafacturing, trading, mining, banking, transport, insurance, etc. are business activites.

2. **Profession :** A profession may be defined as *an occupation which involves rendering of personal services of a specialised nature, based on professional knowledge, education and training.* The examples are physicians, lawyers, accountants, etc. The professionals charge professional fee from their clients for the services rendered to them. The important features of a profession are listed below :

   (i) A profession requires *specialised* knowledge and training about the concerned field.

   (ii) The mombership of the *professional body* is compulsory in case of a profession.

   (iii) There is an established *code of conduct* enforced by the professional body.

   (iv) A profossional is responsive to the needs of the society and so enjoys social status.

   (v) Professionals charge fee for their services rendered to their clients.

3. **Employments or Service :** A person is said to be in the employment of an organisation when he undertakes to render personal services under a contract of employment or service. He receives wages or salaries, allowances, bonus and other employment benefit for his services. Employment may be in a Government department or undertaking, or in a private firm. Even professionally qualified person serve as employees of various organisations. The employees perform the duties assigned to them by their employers.

ECONOMIC SYSTEM

An economic system denotes the economic relationships which arise in the community from the organisation or mode of production and distribution. In other words, an economy refers to the system in which peoples organise their acitvities and form institutions whereby the economic resources, namely, land, minerals, power, raw materials, labour, capital, and other inputs of production, are utilised for satisfying the needs of the people living in the society. The fundamental problem for an economy is to provide answers to the following three fundamental questions :

(a) **What things will be produced** : There must be some method of determining the goods which are to be produced.

(b) **How will things be produced** : A primary function which an economic system must perform is to determine the methods of production. The choice of techniques of production is extremely important for any economic sytem.

(c) **For whom will things be produced** : Here the basic problem is to determine how to distribute the total product among the population.

The above question would be decided with refrence to the nature of economy as to whether it is a capitalist economy, or a socielist economy or mixed economy. Each type of economic system would fix certain goals with referece to the given economic structure and the nature and working of particular factots prevalent in that economic system.

An economic system is supposed to exist primarily to create such conditions as to make it easy for human beings to satisfy their wants. However, the exact manner in which the problems like allocation of resources among various alternative uses, fixation of prices, and direction and determination of input and output will be tackled, would depend upon the particular type of economic system which is adopted by a particular country.

TYPES OF ECONOMIC SYSTEM

Different economic systems have prevailed in various countries of the world from time to time. There are two basic economic systems which are prevalent today in different forms. These are *capitalism and socialism*. Some countries also follow the combination of both the systems. For example, in India we have mixed economic system in the sense that both public and private sectors co-exit.

1. Capitalist System

In capitalist system free enterprise, competition and private ownership to the property guided by the profit motive generally prevail. Under capitalism, the means of production and distribution are controlled by private owners who operate them to earn profit. The important features of a capitalist economy are as follows :

(i) **Existence of Private Property** : A capitalist economy is a free enterprise economy or a free market economy in which there is freedom of private ownership of property and means of production. The right to own property also carries with it the right to determine its use.

(ii) **Freedom of Enterprise** : There is a freedom of choice of occupation and free competition in a capitalist economy. The only limitation relates to capacity and efficiency of the sources of supply. The individuals have the right to determine the use to which any unit of productive resources shall be put. People have liberty to decide their own courses of action in various capacities. As borrowers or lenders, as employers and as sellers or buyers, it is open to them to decide how they would behave under given circumstances. Thus, they have got full economic liberty.

(iii) **Profit Motive :** Profit motive acts as the basic incentive for enterprises under capitalism. People invest capital into business to profit. Profit is the guiding force in making decisions regarding use of property. The owners of means of production enter those fields in which property yields maximum profit. Naturally, costs and prices are compared for making business decisions. More resources flow into those channels where profits are higher.

(iv) **Consumer's Sovereignity :** Consumer is king under a capitalist system. The businessman produces the goods and services to satisfy the needs of customers. The customer or consumer has the liberty of buy any commodity. He is free to spend his income in any way he likes.

(v) **Market Mechanism :** Under capitalism, the allocation of economic resources is determined by profit motive in conjunction with the price mechanism. There is a free interplay of the forces of demand and supply. The price mechanism decides the level of consumption and production and distribution. Thus, the whole economic system revolves around the price mechanism. There is no central planning for the allocation of resources and for coordination between production and consumption.

(iv) **Role of Government :** The government is a protector of private property under capitalism. The role of State is limited to the operation of public utilities to avoid unhealthy competition and to provide essential services to the public economically.

2. Collectivist or Socialist System

The socialist system can be defined as a system of economic organisation in which there is public ownership and management of the basic industries and public control of the distribution of income. By public ownership is meant that the large and basic industries are owned and controlled by the Government. Under communism (authoritarian socialism), even the consumption pattern may be controlled by the Government.

3. Mixed Economy

Mixed economy is a term used to describe a compromise between capitalist and socialist economic systems. The idea underlining the policy of mixed economy is to combine the advantages of capitalist system, namely, increased production, improvement in the efficiency of the human progress of science and technology; and the advantages of the socielist system, i.e., reduction of inequality of income, regulation and control of private property, and provision of social security, etc.

The distinctive mark of mixed economy is that a well defined role is allotted to the public sector to assure fast development of the economy and egalitarian distribution of national income. Although the private sector is permitted to base its activities on the profit motive, exploitative character of this motive is effectively curbed by the government. In a fixed economy, the Government has to play an important role in the economic sphere. It must ensure fast economic development and must, to that end, undertake to provide social overheads, industrial climate, and industrial base. It must also ensure that the fruits of economic development are as widely distributed as is fair and possible. It must take adequate steps to make certain that inequalities between man and man, class and class, and region and region are reduced to the minimum.

The Indian economy follows a mixed economic system where both the public and private sectors coexist. The characteristics of a mixed economy are described belew :

(i) **Co-existence of Public and Private Sectors :** In a mixed economy, some field of production are exclusively allotted to the public sector while others are open to the private sector. In India, some sectors like defence, nuclear energy, public utilities, telecommunication, air transport, etc. are reserved for the public sector. In other areas, both the private and public sectors can set up their units.

(ii) **Central Planning :** In a mixed economy, there is a great role of central planning. In India, we have Plannings Commission which is responsible for drafting 'five year plan'. The Planning Commission prepares a plan covering a period of five years. The plan is prepared keeping in view the political ideology, resource constraints and social aspirations of the nation. The plan lays down the socio-economic objectives, set physical targets, specifies the sources of funds for implementing the plan and also prepares specific programes for implementing the plan.

(iii) **Economic Welfare :** The purpose of mixed ecconomic system is fast economic development accompained by a sufficiently rapid increase in opportunities for employment. In addition, the public sector undertakes to reduce inequalities by starting industries in the less developed regions and by opening employment opportunities for backward classes.

(iv) **Market Mechanism :** The output of the public sector has to be sold because there is no question of self-consumption. Even the goods produced in the private sector are largely marketed. A mixed economic systsm is, therefore, known for the market mechanism. Law of demand and supply plays an important role subject to the intervention by the Government.

(v) **Role of Profit Motive :** Profit motive serves a successful stimulus to capital accumulation and rapid industrial expansion in many countries like England and U.S.A. But the progress there has been combined with many undesirable effects. In a mixed economy, profit motive is allowed to play its role within certain limits.

Public sector is mainly guided by social interest. But an element of profit is also there. Social interest, however, continues to be the dominant consideration so that some works may be run even on loss only ensuring that loss incurred is minimum under the circumstances. It is the profit motive which, in combination with the price system, determines the allocation of resources. But profit motive is not allowed unrestricted operation.

In capitalism, profit is the only consideration. In socialism, profit motive is eliminated. In mixed economy, profit motive is permitted to operate to the extent that it serves the social ends.

(vi) **Role of Government ;** In a mixed economy, the government has to play a prominent role in the economic sphere. The public sector covers a substantial field and the government sees to it that it is administered and managed efficiently in the interest of social good. It must step in when and where private enterprise operates against the socio-economic goals of the nation. It must see to it that industrial enterprises, public as well as private, are so located that all regions and classes march forward together on the road to economic development.

The success of mixed economy depends much on the policy of the government demarcating the sectors, co-operation between the private enterprise and the public sector. Sometimes due to a defective policy of the government overlapping and stagnation is introduced in the economic system. It is also possible that the private sector may be so much absorbed with self interest and profit motive that it may completely sacrifice the social interest. A mixed economy, therefore, needs a constant vigilance, on the part of the Government.

3

MANAGEMENT

Management is universal in the modern industrial world. Every institution requires making of decisions, coordinating of activities, handling of people, and evaluation of performance directed towards its objectives. Numerous types of activities have their specific types of management such as business management, farm management, hospital management, school management, public enterprise management, marketing management, production or operations management, and others. All have certain elements in common.

DEFINITION OF MANAGEMENT

The different viewpoints may classify :

1. Management as an art of getting things done.
2. Management as a function.
3. Management as a process.
4. Management as a body of individuals.

1. Management as an Art of Getting Things Done

Management is the art of getting things done through and with people in formally organised groups. It is the art of creating an environment in which people can perform as individuals and yet cooperate towards attainment of group goals. It is the art of removing blocks to such performance, a way of optimizing efficiency in reaching goals.

2. Management as a Function

Management is the fundamental integrating and operating mechanism underlying organised effort. It is the function of working with people and coordinating their efforts so as to accomplish the objectives of the organisation.

3. Management as a Process

Management is a distinct process consisting of planning, organising, actuating, and controlling performed to determine and accomplish stated objectives by the use of human beings and other resources. Management is a process since it comprises a series of functions which lead to the achievement of organisational objective. The functions of management are : planning, organising, staffing, directing and controlling. These functions are inter-dependent and inter-related. There is no specific sequence of their performance. More or less, they are performed simultaneously by the managers.

4. Management as a Group

The term 'management' is frequently used to denote a group of managerial personnel. Management is the body or group of people which performs managerial functions for the accomplishment of certain goals. These people are individually known as 'managers'. In other words, a manager is a person who performs the managerial functions of planning, organising, staffing, directing and controlling.

IMPORTANCE OF MANAGEMENT

Management is an essential activity in every sphere of organised activity. The efficient management of human and material resources is essential for the achievement of objectives of any group. Management pervades virtually every aspect of organised life. It is a process of taking certain decisions and putting them into action. Both these activities, i.e., deciding and doing, are very important in every field of life. The significance of management will be more clear by going through the following points :

1. **Determination of Objectives :** The objectives of any organization are determined by the management. They are put into writing and communicated to all others in the organisation. No organisation can succeed in its operations unless its objectives are identified and well defined.

2. **Achievement of Objectives :** Management is an important force for the accomplishment of the objectives of any group. The perfect coordination and integration of human and non-human resources is brought about by the management or the individuals known as 'managers'.

3. **Brain of Enterprise :** Management is the brain of any enterprise. All the policy decision are taken by it. Management keeps itself in touch with the current environment and supplies foresight to the enterprise.

4. **Efficient use of Resources :** An efficient management can lead a business towards growth and prosperity. It provides leadership to the business and helps in achieving its objectives. It involves scientific thinking, deciding and thoughtful organisation, direction and control to ensure better results.

5. **Economic Development :** Management is the crucial factor in economic and social development. The development of a country is virtually dependent upon the quality of management of its resources.

No amount of capital investment and import of technical know-how and equipment will succeed in further economic development of a country if such wealth producing resources are not managed properly.

FUNCTIONS OF MANAGEMENT

The functions of management are (1) planning (2) organising, (3) directing, (4) staffing (5) coordinating, (6) reporting (7) budgeting. Thus, there is no universally accepted classification of managerial functions.

1. Planning

It involves deciding in advance what to do, when to do it, where to do it, how to do it, who is to do it and how the results are to be evaluated. Thus, planning is the systematic thinking about the ways and the means for the accomplishment of pre-determined objectives.

The process of planning involves the following steps :

  (i) determination of goals or objectives of the enterprise,

  (ii) forecasting,

  (iii) search of alternative courses of action,

  (iv) evaluation of various alternatives and formulation of plans,

  (v) formulation of policies and procedures.

  (vi) preparation of schedules, programmes and budgets.

2. Organising

Organising involves the determination and providing of various resources required to achieve the organisational objectives. In order to put its plan into action, management has to employ people and allocate them the work each has to do. Management has to provide them with material resources like money, materials, machines and equipments to do their jobs well.

Organisation as a function of management involves identification and grouping the activities to be performed and dividing them among the individuals and creating authority and responsibility relationship among them. The process of organisation involves the following steps :

  (i) Determination of objectives and identification of main activities.

  (ii) Division of activities and creation of jobs.

  (iii) Fitting individuals into jobs.

  (iv) Developing relationship in terms of authorities and responsibilities.

3. Staffing

Staffing involves manning the organisational structure through proper and effective selection, appraisal, and development of personel to fill the roles designed into the structure.

The staffing function involves recruitment, selection, training, development and appraisal of personnel. Every manager is continuously engaged in performing the staffing function. He is actively associated with the recruitment, selection, training and appraisal of his subordinates. The Board of Directors of a company undertakes staffing function by selecting, helping develop and appraising a chief executive who in turn performs these functions in relation to the heads of various divisions or departments of the enterprise. The departmental heads also select, train and appraise their assistants and so on. Finally, the first line managers or supervisors perform the staffing function when they participate in selecting, training and appraising their subordinates.

4. Direction

Direction is that part of the management process which actuates the organisational members to work efficiently and effectively for the attainment of organisational objectives. It constitutes the life spark of the enterprise which like electric power, sets it into motion. Planning, organising and staffing are merely preparations for doing the work and the work actually starts when the managers start performing the direction function.

It consists of three sub-functions:

(a) **Communication :** It is the process of passing information and understanding from one person to another. A manager has always to tell the subordinates what to do, how to do it and when to do it. He has to create an understanding in their minds in regard to these things in his department.

(b) **Leadership :** Leadership may be defined as the process by which a manager guides and influences the work of his subordinates or their activities in the desired direction. A manager, as an effective leader, should consult his subordinates.

(c) **Motivation :** Motivation means inspiring the subordinates with a zeal to do work for the accomplishment of organisational objectives. A manager should make appropriate use of motivation to actuate the subordinates to work harmoniously towards the achievement of organisational goals. Different people are motivated by different types of rewards. To some financial incentives like job security, job enlargement, freedom to work, recognition, achievement, etc.

5. Controlling

Control is the process of checking to determine whether or not proper progress is being made towards the objectives and goals and acting, if necessary, to correct any deviation.

Controlling involves the following elements:

1. Setting standards of performance.
2. Measurement of actual performance.
3. Comparing of actual performance with the standards.

4. Taking corrective measures if the performance does not meet the standards of performance.

6. Co-ordination : The Essence of Management

Coordination is a permeating function of management passing through the managerial functions planning, organising, staffing, directing and controlling. It transverses the entire process of managing.

Coordination harmonises, synchronises and unifies individual efforts for better action and for the achievement of the business objectives.

Coordination is the achievement of orderly group efforts and unity of action in the pursuit of a common purpose.

Coordination leads to blending the activities of different individuals and groups of individuals for the achievement of certain objectives. The basic features or characteristics of coordination may be summed up as follows:

1. It is a managerial activity. It is needed at all levels of management.
2. It is an orderly arrangement of group efforts.
3. Its purpose is to secure unity of action towards common objectives.
4. It is a continuous process.

Coordination deals with the task of blending efforts in order to ensure successful attainment of objectives. It is accomplished by means of planning, organising, actuating and controlling.

(a) **Coordination through Planning :** The planning function facilitates coordiination by properly integrating the various plans through mutual discussion, exchange of ideas, etc.

(b) **Coordination through Organising :** Coordination is an essential part of organising, and unless th manager bears in mind how various groups are to function together, the organisation will not be a successful one. The manager must look at it both vertically and horizontally.

(c) **Coordination through staffing :** The right number of executives in various positions with the right type of education and training are taken. This will ensure right persons of right jobs.

(d) **Coordination through Directing :** When a manager directs, he is also performing the function of coordination. The very essence of giving orders, instructing, coaching, and guiding subordinates is coordination of their activities in such a manner that the overall enterprise objectives will be achieved in the most efficient way. Thus, manager's skill in effectively directing his subordinates will bring about coordination.

(e) **Coordination through Controlling :** While performing the function of controlling, the manager comes to know whether or not the current activities are in tune with the desired activities. such frequent evaluation of operations helps to synchronize the efforts of the subordinates. It brings about coordination and leads the organisation to the desired objectives and goals.

Techniques of Effective Coordination

The following steps should be taken for achieving effective coordination :

(i) **Clearly defined Goals :** The goals of the enterprise should be laid down clearly. Every individual in the enterprise should understand the overall objectives and the contribution by his job to these objectives. Unity of purpose is a must for achieving proper coordination.

(ii) **Clear lines of Authority and Responsibility :** The line of authority and responsibility should be clearly defined to achieve coordination. Clear-cut authority relationships help in reducing conflicts among different positions which is essential for sound coordination.

(iii) **Precise and Comprehensive Programmes and Policies :** Laying down well defined programmes and policies is another measure for achieving effective coordination. This brings uniformity of action because everybody understands the programmes and policies in the same sense.

(iv) **Cooperation :** Coordination must be accompanied by cooperation. The individuals in the organisation must be willing to help each other voluntarily. Cooperation can be brought by keeping harmonious relations among the people in the organisation by encouraging informal contacts to supplement formal communication and using committees for exchange of ideas and views at the top level.

(v) **Effective Communication :** Effective communication is the key to proper coordination. The channels of communication used in the enterprise should be reliable so that they are able to create proper understanding in the mind of receiver. Personal contacts should be encouraged as it is the most effective means of communication for achieving coordination.

(vi) **Effective Leadership and Supervision :** Management can achieve better coordination through effective leadership and supervision. Effective leadership ensures coordination both at the planning and the implementation stage. Effective supervision is necessary to guide the activities of individuals in the proper direction.

Principles of Coordination

(i) **Direct Contact :** The activities of different individuals can be coordinated effectively through direct personal contacts. This helps in exchanging the opinions and ideas in a better way and clarifying the misunderstanding more easily.

(ii) **Early Start :** Coordination can be achieved more easily in the early stages of planning and policy making. It becomes difficult to secure coordination at the execution stage.

(iii) **Reciprocal Relationship :** This principle states that all factors in a situation like materials and environment are reciprocally related. For instance, when A works with B, each finds himself influenced by the other and both are influenced by other persons and factors in the total situation.

(iv) **Continuity :** Coordination should be a continuous process starting with planning and running through the other managerial processes. It is something which must go on all the time, it should be viewed as a never-ending process and every manager should strive for it constantly.

LEVELS OF MANAGEMENT

In most of the organisation, there are generally three levels of management, namely, top management, middle management and lower level or first management.

The Management Director or Chief Executive will normally spend more time on planning and organising and less time on staffing, directing and controlling. On the other hand, the foreman representing supervisory level of management on the shop floor will devote less time on planning and organising and more time on directing and controlling. Thus, the time and effort spent on different functions will depend on the level on which a manager is functioning in the managerial hierarchy.

Top Level Management

Top management of a company consists of the Board of Directors and the Chief Executive or the Managing Director. Top management is the ultimate source of authority and it establishes goals and policies for the enterprise. It is accountable to the owners of the business for the overall management. Top management issues orders and instructions and lays down guidelines for the executives at the middle and lower levels.

The top management performs the following functions or activities:

(i)   Top management lays down the objectives of enterprise.

(ii) It prepares strategic plans and policies for the enterprise.

(iii) It issues necessary instructions for the preparation of departmental programmes, budgets, schedules, procedures, etc.

(iv) It appoints the executives for the middle-level positions.

(v)   It reviews the performance and controls the activities of all departments with the help of reports, memoranda, etc.

(vi) It builds and maintains relations with the outside world including general public, government suppliers, chambers of commerce, etc.

Middle Level Management

Middle level management generally consists of heads of functional departments. They are responsible to the top management for the efficient functioning of their departments. They devote more time to the organisation and direction functions of management. In small enterprises, there is only one layer of middle management, but in big enterprises, there may be senior middle level managers and junior middle level managers. The senior level managers include heads of production, finance, marketing and other departments. Junior middle level managers include branch managers, superintendents and heads of various section.

The role played by the middle level executives is stated below :

(i) They execute the plans of the organisation in accordance with the policies and directives of the top management.

(ii) They make plans for the sub-units of the organisation.

(iii) They participate in the employment and training of lower-level managers.

(iv) They evaluate the performance of junior managers.

(v) They attempt to achieve coordination between different departments.

(vi) They send the progress reports and other important data to the top management.

Lower Level Management (Supervisory Level)

Lower level management is also known as supervisory management because it is directly concerned with the control of the performance of the operative employees. Supervisory management refers to those executives whose work has to be largely with personal oversight and direction of operative employees. This level includes supervisors, foremen, accounts officers, sales officers and so on. Lower level managers are more concerned with direction and control functions of management. They devote more time on the supervision of workers.

The important functions of a supervisor or lower level executive are listed below :

(i) To plan and organise the activities of the unit or section.

(ii) To arrange for necessary materials, machines, tools, etc. for workers and to provide them the necessary working environment.

(iii) To provide training to the workers

(iv) To supervise and guide the subordinates and solve their problems.

(v) To communicate workers' problems to the higher level management.

(vi) To maintain good human relations in the unit.

(vii) To send periodical reports about performance to the middle level management.

Qualities of a Good Manager

In order to succeed in managing, a manager should possess the following qualities :

1. **Education** : A manager must be well-educated. In addition to general education, he must have specific education in business management/

administration. Knowledge of business environment is also important to deal with the problem which the organisation may have to face in the future.

2. **Training** : Management skills are not inborn qualities. They are to be acquired through training. Therefore, it is necessary for a good manager to have some sort of training in the branch of management where he is working or going to work.

3. **Intelligence** : A manager should have somewhat higher level of intelligence than the average human beings. He should have the ability to think scientifically, and analyse the problems accurately.

4. **Leadership** : Every manager is supposed to provide guidance and leadership to a number of subordinates. He should be able to channelise the energies of the subordinates for the achievement of organisational objectives. The manager can motivate the subordinates effectively if he has got leadership qualities.

5. **Foresight** : A good manager should have an open mind. He should be receptive to new ideas. He should be able to foresee the problems which might be faced by the business. Only through his foresightedness, he can take good decisions.

6. **Maturity** : A good manager should have broad interest. He should emotionally mature and have balanced temperaments. He should have high frustration tolerance also.

7. **Technical Knowledge** : A manager should have sufficient knowledge of the techniques of production being used in the enterprise. Adequate technical knowledge is necessary so that he may not be befooled by the subordinates.

8. **Human Relations Attitude** : A good manager should try to develop social understanding. He should treat his subordinates as human beings. He should try to maintain good relations with them. He should understand their problems and offer a helping hand to them.

9. **Self Confidence** : A manager should have self confidence. He should take decisions after scientific analysis and implement them with full dedication. He should not shirk taking initiative.

DIFFERENT FIELDS OF MANAGEMENT

1. FINANCIAL MANAGEMENT

Financial management is concerned with managerial activities related to procurement and utilisation of funds for business purposes. It deals with planning, organising, directing and controlling financial activities of the enterprise. Financial activities should not be merely restricted to raising of capital, but also to other aspects of financing like assessing the needs for capital, raising sufficient funds, cost of financing, budgeting, maintaining liquidity, lending and borrowing policies and distribution of profits.

Financial management assesses the needs of the business in advance and then sets itself into motion to procure funds. Procurement of funds is a complex problem as choice of sources of finance is based on complex factors like risk, period, control and cost. Various sources of finance like shares, debentures, banks and other financial institutions, public deposits, etc. have to be compared in the light of these factors. After the funds have been procured, their effective utilisation is another major task of financial management. Funds should be put into those channels which generate an income higher than the costs of procuring them. Safety, soundness and liquidity are three factors which should be taken into consideration before investing funds in any business venture.

Objectives of Financial Management

The objectives of financial management of a big enterprise are stated below:

(a) **Procurement of Funds :** The traditional objective of financial management is procurement of funds. The adequate and regular supply of funds is to be maintained.

(b) **Utilisation of Funds :** The modern concept of financial management emphasises on optimum utilisation of funds. A proper balance of profitability, liquidity and safety is to be achieved.

(c) **Optimum Capital Structure :** The cost of procurement of funds should be minimised by planning optimum capital structure. A sound and economical combination of securities must be achieved.

(d) **Return to Shareholders :** The shareholders return should be maximised. It can be achieved by concentrating on market share price. The market price of shares is largely dependent upon the performance of the company. The market price of shares is a good indicator of net present value or wealth of shareholders. Maximisation of shareholders' wealth is accepted as an important goal of financial management.

(e) **Expansion and Growth :** The surplus should be enough for expansion and growth. Self sufficiency in case of permanent financial requirement by ploughing back of profits is a good indicator of financial health of the company.

(f) **Coordination :** The coordination of activities of the finance department with other departments of the enterprise is necessary. It is also required to match the objectives of financial management with the general objectives of the company.

2. INDUSTRIAL MANAGEMENT

Production is the process by which goods and services are created. In other words, it deals with the conversion of raw materials into semi-finished and finished products with the help of certain production processes. The main aim of any production system is to produce economically the goods and services required by the customers. In order to achieve this aim, it is essential to plan, organise, direct and control the production system. These activities comprise production management. The production manager should have both the technical and managerial qualifications and skills. That is why, generally, technical personnel with managerial skills are appointed as production managers.

Production of goods and services constitutes the point of concentration in all the industrial enterprises. All other activities like purchasing, financing, marketing and storing revolve around this function. It is essential that production function is managed properly so that it may contribute effectively and towards the objectives of the enterprise.

Production management deals with decision making related to production processes, so that resulting goods or service is produced according to the specification, in the amounts and by the schedule demanded and at minimum cost. Production management deals with managerial functions related to the design of the production system and operation and control of the production system, i.e., production planning and control.

Functions or Scope of Production Management

Production management involves a wide range of activities from the plant location to the packaging of products to be distributed by the marketing department of the enterprise. Production management has a very wide scope and it includes the following operations :

(i) **Design of Product :** The product designing deals with form and function. The form design deals with the product's shape and appearance whereas the functional design deals with its working.

(ii) **Design of Production System :** Production system is the framework within which the conversion of inputs into output occurs. There are three basic kinds of production system namely, process production, job production and intermittent production.

(iii) **Production Planning and Control :** It deals with the determination and regulation of production processes. Production control is a process by which actual performance is compared with the predetermined standards. The production manager has to apply control in these important areas : (a) control of inventories, (b) control of flow of raw material into the plant and (c) control of work-in-process.

(iv) **Selection of Location :** Plant should be located at such a place where production and distribution costs are the minimum. Costs which influence the locational decision include cost of land, rental value, transportation costs, labour cost, cost of water and power, etc. Other factors which influence the selection of location are : process inputs, process outputs, process requirements, government policy, availability of site, personal preferences, etc.

(v) **Layout of Plant :** The plant layout represents an arrangement of machines and facilities. The plant layout should be efficient to achieve economy and efficiency in operations of the production department. An efficient layout is one that allows materials to move through the necessary operations rapidly and in the most direct way possible.

(vi) **Selection of Plant and Equipment :** The choice of plant and equipment depends upon technological feasibility constraints, and cost constraints. The quality of output, life of the machine and adaptability of the facilities are also important considerations.

(vii) **Research and Development :** Research means critical investigation in order to acquire new knowledge. Applied research explores information for the practical problems in mind and thus is directed to achieve immediate solutions to practical problem. Development comes after applied research.

3. MATERIALS MANAGEMENT

Materials management is the planning, directing, controlling and coordination of all those activities concerned with material and inventory requirement, from the point of their inception to their introduction into the manufacturing processes.

It generally includes purchasing, storage, traffic, determination and control of inventories, storage, shipping, materials handling, production planning and inspection of materials.

Significance of Materials Management

Efficient management of materials is very important in industrial enterprises. It will help in achieving the following benefits :

(i) Adequate supply of raw materials will be ensured. There will be no stoppage of work because of lack of materials.

(ii) Excessive investment in stocks will be avoided.

(iii) Effective utilisation of materials and other facilities will be ensured.

(iv) Productivity will improve as raw materials of right quality are continuously made available.

(v) Inventory losses will be minimised.

(vi) Reduction in material costs will improve the profitability of the enterprise.

4. SCIENTIFIC MANAGEMENT

Scientific Management is the substitution of exact scientific investigations and knowledge for the old individual judgement or opinion in all matters relating to the work done in the shop. It implies the application of science to the management of a business concern. It aims at replacement of traditional techniques by scientific techniques.

The thread of scientific management runs through operational study of work, the analysis of work into simplest elements and the systematic improvement of the workers' performance of each element.

Scientific management includes finding the most efficient methods of production, scientific selection and training of workers, proper allotment of duties and work and achieving cooperation between workers and management.

In short, scientific management involves :

(i)   scientific study and analysis of work ;

(ii) scientific selection and training of employees ; and

(iii) standardisation of raw materials, working conditions and equipment.

Aims of Scientific Management

The aims of scientific management may be summarised as under :

(a) **Increased Production :** Increase in the rate of production by use of standardised tools, equipment and methods.

(b) **Quality Control :** Improvement in the quality of the output by research, quality control and inspection devices.

(c) **Cost Reduction :** Reduction in the costs of production by rational planning regulation, and cost control techniques.

(d) **Elimination of Wastes :** Elimination of wastes in the use of resources and methods of manufacturing.

(e) **Right Men for Right Work:** Placement of right person on the right job through scientific selection and training.

(f) **Incentive Wages :** Payment of wages to workers according to their efficiency.

5. MARKETING MANAGEMENT

Marketing management is concerned with the direction of purposeful activities towards the attainment of marketing goals. The basic goals of marketing are satisfaction of needs of customers and generation of revenue for the business. Most of the big business enterprises organise the marketing activities separately under the charge of a marketing manager.

Marketing management attempts to contribute to the organisational objectives. Marketing management is the analysis, planning implementation and control of programmes designed to create, build, maintain mutually beneficial exchanges and relationships with target markets for the purpose of achieving organisational objectives. Marketing management deals with planning, organising, directing and controlling the activities related to the marketing of goods and services to satisfy the customers' needs.

Functions of Marketing

In most of the business enterprises, marketing department is set up under supervision of the Marketing Manager. The major purpose of this department is to generate revenue for the business by selling want satisfying goods and services goods and services to the customers. In order to achieve this purpose, the Marketing Manager performs the following functions :

   (i) Marketing research
  (ii) Product planning and development.
 (iii) Buying and assembling.
  (iv) Selling
   (v) Standardisation, grading and branding.
  (vi) Packaging
 (vii) Storage
(viii) Transportation
  (ix) Salesmanship
   (x) Advertising
  (xi) Pricing
 (xii) Insurance

4

BUSINESS ORGANISATION

The term business organisation is very often used in different senses. Firstly, it is used to represent a business enterprise such as Tata Iron & Steel Co., Reliance Industries, Maruti Udyog, Indian Oil Corporation, etc. Secondly, business organisation is a subject of study, consisting of topics concerned with organisation and management of industrial and commercial organisations. Thirdly, the term 'organisation' is used to mean bringing together various elements of business with the object of establishing harmonious relationship and adjustment in their functioning. Taken in this sense, business organisation is the effective coordination of various components or parts of the business enterprise. It embraces planning and control of production, procurement of materials, distribution of products, management of personnel, etc.

Organisation is the harmonious combination of various factors of production for the purpose of acquisition of wealth. It may also be defined as the technique of conducting industrial and commercial activities for the achievement of certain objectives through production and exchange of goods and services.

Organisation is one of the basic functions of management. It involves the determination and provision of whatever capital, materials, equipment and personnel may be required for the achievement of certain predetermined goals. By performing this function, management brings together human and non-human resources to form a manageable unit. Thus, organisation is a process of integrating and coordinating the efforts of manpower and material resources for the accomplishment of certain objectives.

Scope of Business Organisation

The importance of business organisation, has increased so much these days that it has been introduced as a subject of study for the undergraduate students of Commerce and Management in most of the educational institutions. Under this subject, many topics are taught to the students such as scope and objectives of business, functional areas of business, role of government in business, transport, insurance, home and foreign trade, etc. The study of 'Business Organisation' will enable the entrepreneur to organise and run his business successfully.

FUNCTIONAL AREAS OF BUSINESS

In order to achieve its objectives, a business enterprise performs many functions which may be broadly grouped under the following headings: Production, Marketing, Finance and Personnel. In big business organisations, there are separate departments to look after these functional areas. It may be noted that these functions are inter-dependent and inter-related. For instance, production department depends upon marketing department to sell its output and marketing department depends upon production department for the products of required quality to satisfy its customers. Thus, there must be proper integration of various functional areas of business to achieve its objectives. This can be achieved by the management of the enterprise by effective planning, organisation, direction and control.

The important functions of a business are briefly discussed below;

1. **Production Function :** It is concerned with transformation of inputs like manpower, materials, machinery, capital, information and energy into specified outputs as demanded by the society. The production department is entrusted with many activities such as production planning and control, quality control, procurement of materials and storage of materials.

2. **Marketing Function :** It is concerned with distribution of goods and services produced by production department. It can perform this function efficiently only if it is able to satisfy the needs of the customers. For this purpose, the marketing department guides the production department in product planning and development. It fixed the prices of various products produced by the business. It promotes the sale of goods through advertisement and sales promotion devices such as distribution of samples and novelty items, holding contests, organising displays and exhibitions, etc.

3. **Finance Function :** It deals with arrangement of sufficient capital for the smooth running of business. It also tries to ensure that there is proper utilisation of resources. It takes many important decisions such as raising capital from various sources of finance, investment of funds in productive ventures, and levels of inventory of various items.

4. **Personnel Function :** This function is concerned with finding suitable employees, giving them training and fixing their remuneration and motivating them. The quality of human resources working in the enterprise

is a critical factor in the achievement of business objectives. Therefore, it is necessary that the work-force is highly motivated and satisfied with the business.

5. **Purchase Function :** Traditionally, purchasing is considered a part of the production function. But in big organisations, there may be a separate department to perform complicated purchase activities such as inviting tenders, choosing the sources of supply, making transport arrangements and import of raw materials, machines and equipment.

6. **Public Relations Function :** Modern business houses want to be in touch with the public and government through their public relations departments. This department organises publicity campaigns to increase the image and goodwill of the business in the society.

7. **Legal Function :** In a big organisation, the legal department may be organised to ensure that the business house is abiding by the rules and regulations framed by the government. It also gives advice to the management in case of disputes with the customers, suppliers and even government over various commercial matters.

FORMS OF BUSINESS ORGANISATION

A business enterprise may be run by one person or a group of persons. When it is owned by one person, it is known as sole proprietorship. Excepting this form of organisation, all other forms of business organisations come under the category of 'group ownership ' or 'joint ownership '. Group ownership may take the form of Joint Hindu Family business, partnership firm, joint stock company and cooperative organisation. Thus, the important forms of business organisations in the private sector are as follow :

(1) Sole Proprietorship ;
(2) Partnership Firm ;
(3) Joint Hindu Family Firm ;
(4) Joint Stock Company ; and
(5) Cooperative Organisation.

The first three (namely, Sole Proprietorship, Joint Hindu Family business and Partnership Firm) may be categorised as non-corporate and the remaining two (namely, Joint Stock Company and Cooperative Enterprises) as corporate forms of organisation. The essential distinction between these two categories is that a non-corporate form of business may be started without legal formalities while a corporate body can be launched and run only after fulfilling the legal formalities as prescribed under the laws governing their functioning.

Government ownership of business has also gained prominence these days. Government ownership of business is referred to as public enterprise or State enterprise. Public enterprises may be either fully owned by the State (Central Government or State Government or both), or jointly owned by a

Government or Government and by private business houses. Such enterprises may be in the following forms :

(1) Departmental undertaking such as Indian Posts and Telegraph Services, Indian Railways, Defence Establishment, etc.

(2) Government companies such as State Trading Corporation of India Ltd., Bharat Heavy Electricals Ltd., Steel Authority of India Ltd., etc.

(3) Statutory or pubic corporations such as Reserve Bank of India, Industrial Development Bank of India. Air India, International Airlines Corporation. Indian Airlines Corporation, Food Corporation of India, etc.

Ownership is a legal concept and as such is regulated under the laws of the land. Because of this fact, forms of business organisation are also called legal forms of business.

1. SOLE PROPRIETORSHIP

The sole tradership or proprietorship is the oldest form of business organisation. It came into existence when exchange began. It is also known as individual proprietorship or single entrepreneurship. This type of organisation has not lost its utility even today. It can be started by anyone having initiative and aptitude for selling. It can satisfy the ego need of a person who does not want to act under any other person in employment, but wants to have an independent way of life.

Sole tradership is that form of business organisation which is started and run by one person who bears profits and loss of it.

Any person who carries on a business exclusively on his own account and at his own risk is known as a sole trader. The sole trader manages the business himself, bears all risks alone and gets all profits by virtue of the nature of this form of organisation. He may choose to run any line of business without going through the legal formalities excepting those in which licenses may be required from the Health Department, the Municipal Authority, or some other body. The individual may run the business alone with the help of his own skills and intelligence or may employ a few employees for that purpose. It is the simplest and the oldest form of organisation.

Features of Sole Proprietorship

The salient features of sole proprietorship form of organisation are as under:

i. **Single Ownership :** A sole trading concern which is owned by one individual. It is run entirely at his risk of loss. The sole trader provides both capital and management to the business.

ii. **Personal Organisation or Common Identity :** A sole tradership concern has no separate legal entity independent of the owner. The owner and the business concern are one and the same. The owner owns everything the business owns and he owes everything the business owns.

iii. **Capital :** In sole tradership, the capital employed by the owner himself from his personal resources. He may also borrow money from his friends and relatives if he cannot depend solely on his personal resources.

iv. **Unlimited Liability :** The liability of the proprietor for the debts of the business is unlimited. The creditors have the right to recover their dues even from the personal property of the proprietor in case the business assets are not sufficient to pay their debts.

v. **One Man Control :** Sole Tradership is one man show. The sole trader provides management to the business. He takes all the decisions, procures material resources, employs persons and directs and controls the affairs of the enterprise. He is not required to consult anyone case in taking any decision. Though the sole trader may delegate some of his authority to his assistants but the ultimate authority to manage and control rests with him.

vi **Profits and Losses :** The surplus arising in the business of the sole trader entirely belongs to him and similarly all the business losses and risks are to be borne by him alone.

vii. **No Special Legislation :** Sole tradership is not governed by any special legislation. A partnership firm is governed by the Partnership Act, a joint stock company is governed by the Companies Act and a co-operative society by the Co-operative Societies Act. Any person who is competent to contract can start his business as a sole trader. However, he is subject to the common law, the law of contract and the law of insolvency.

2. PARTNERSHIP FIRM

The limitations and deficiencies of sole proprietorship such as limited financial resources, limited, managerial skills and concentrated risk led to the emergence of partnership as a form of organisation. When two or more persons join together in a business with a common ownership and management under and agreement, it is known as partnership.

The proprietor of an expanding business may prefer a partner to appoint a manager because of certain obvious advantages. The manager does not bring capital and he does not share business risks. But a partner generally brings capital to the business and shares the risks of business. As a result, a partner has personal interest in the business of partnership. Sometimes, a partner is admitted into the business who does not offer capital to the business, but brings specialised knowledge into the partnership. In this case also, the new partner will feel fully committed to the business as he has a personal stake in it. Thus, it is advisable for a businessman to find partners to share business responsibilities and risks with him if he wants to increase the scale of business operations.

Definition of Partnership

Partnership means the relation existing between persons who agree to carry on a business in common with a view to private gain. A partnership is an association of two or more persons who carry on business together for the purpose of earning profits. Section 4 of the Indian Partnership Act, 1932 defines partnership as the relation between persons who have agreed to share the profits of a business carried on by all or any of them acting for all. The persons who form a partnership are individually know as 'partners'and collectively 'firm'. The name under which the business is conducted is known as the 'firm name'.

Types of Partners

Partnership firms may have following kind of partners :

(i) **Active or Actual Partners :** Partners who take an active part in the conduct of the partnership business are called "actual" or "ostensible" partners.They are full fledged partners in the real sense of the term. Such a partner must give public notice of his retirement from the firm in order to free himself from liability for acts of the firm after his retirement.

(ii) **Sleeping or Dormant Partners :** Sometimes, there are persons who merely put in their capital (or even without capital they may become partners) and do not take active part in the conduct of the partnership business. They are known as 'sleeping ' or 'dormant ' partners. They do share profits and losses (usually less than proportionately), have a voice in management, but their relationship with the firm is not disclosed to the general public. They are liable to the third parties for all acts of the firm just like an undisclosed principal.

(iii) **Silent Partners :** Those who by agreement with other partners have no voice in the management of the partnership business are called 'silent' partners. They share profits and losses and are fully liable for the debts of the firm.

(iv) **Partner in Profits only :** A partner who has stipulated with other partners that he will be entitled to a certain share of profits without being liable for the losses, is known as 'partner in profits only'. As a rule such a partner has no voice in the management of the business. However, his liability vis-a-vis third parties will be unlimited because in India we cannot have limited partnership.

(v) **Sub-partner :** When a partner agrees to share his share of profits in a partnership firm with an outsider, such an outsider is called a sub-partner. A sub-partner has no rights against the firm nor he is liable for the debts of the firms.

(vi) **Partner by Estoppel or Holding out :** If a person represents to the outside world by words spoken or written or by his conduct or by lending his name, that he is a partner in a certain partnership firm, he is then estopped from denying his being a partner. He is liable as a partner in that firm to any one who has on the faith of such representation granted credit to the firm. Actually such a person is not a partner in that firm (no agreement, no sharing in profits and losses, no say in the management, may not be knowing exact place of business). But as he holds himself out to be a partner, he becomes responsible to outsiders as a partner on the principle of estoppel or holding out. It is for this reason that such a person is called a 'partner by estoppel' or 'partner by holding out'. He may also be called a 'quasi partner'for he is not a partner in the full implications of the term. Only in the eyes if outside world, he is considered a partner. He may also be called a 'nominal partner'.

Rights of Partner

It is advisable to make partnership deed elaborate and clear about all questions which are likely to arise in the course of partnership. In the absence of any agreement on a particular point among the partner, the rights and duties of the partners will be those which have been enumerated in the Partnership Act. The list of important rights of the partners is as follows:

1. Every partner is entitled to participate in the management of the business of the firm.
2. Every partner has a right to be consulted in all matters affecting the business and express his views before the other partners.
3. Every partner has a right to have access to and inspect and copy any of the books of the firm.
4. Every partner has a right to claim interest on capital at a certain rate if it is provided by the partnership agreement.
5. Every partner is entitled to interest at the rate of 6% per annum on the loans advanced to the firm over and above his capital.
6. Every partner is entitled to indemnification in respect of the expenses incurred by him in connection with the business of the firm.
7. Every partner has an equal right with other partners to use the assets of the firm for its business.
8. Every partner has a right to block the introduction of a new partner.
9. Every partner has a right to retire from the firm.
10. Every partner has a right to carry on a competing business after retirement, if not prohibited by the agreement between the partners.

Duties of Partners

Partners have the following duties towards the firm and other partners:

1. Every partner should observe good faith. That means every partner is

bound (a) to carry on the business of the firm to the greatest common advantage, (b) to be just and faithful to each other, and (c) to render true accounts and full information of all things affecting the firm to all partners, and (d) is bound to attend diligently to his duties in conducting the business of the firm.

2. Every partner has a duty to attend diligently to his duties in the conduct of the firm's business.

3. A partner has to indemnify the firm for any loss caused to it through his negligence.

4. A partner has to indemnify the firm for any loss caused to it by his fraud in the conduct of the business.

5. A partner is liable to account for and pay to the firm any private profits derived from the transactions of the firm or from the use of the property or goodwill of the firm.

6. A partner cannot assign his rights in the partnership firm to an outsider without the consent of other partners.

7. Every partner is liable, jointly with all the other partners and also severally, for all the acts of firm done while he is a partner.

8. Unless otherwise agreed, every partner must contribute equally to the losses of the firm.

3. JOINT HINDU FAMILY FIRM

The Joint Hindu Family firm is a form of business organisation in which the family possesses some inherited property and the 'Karta', the head of the family, manages its affairs. It comes into existence by the operation of Hindu Law and not out of contract between the members or co-partners. If the persons who have co-parcenary interest in the ancestral property carry on business, it is a case of Joint Hindu Family firm. Thus, the Joint Hindu Family Business is a business by co-parceners of a Hindu undivided estate.

The Joint Hindu Family Business is confined only to those persons who constitute the co-parcenary interest. Such interest belongs to three successive generations in the male line who can inherit an interest in the ancestral property immediately on their birth in the family. Following the Hindu Succession Act, 1956, a female relative of a deceased male co-parcener will have a share in the co-parenary interest after the death of the co-parcener in question.

Three generations next to the holder in unbroken male line constitute a co-parcenary, and property inherited by a Hindu from his father, father's father and father's grand father is regarded as 'ancestral. A son, grand son and great grand son become joint owners of the property by virtue of their birth in the family. The property is managed and held by the senior male member or the father as the Head of the Family, technically known as 'Karta'. In Hindu law, a family business is taken as a part and parcel of the inheritable property, and therefore, the family business becomes the subject-matter of co-parcenary interest. The rights and liabilities of co-parceners are determined by the general rules of the Hindu Law. It should be noted that joint family firm is created by the operation of law and does not arise out of contract between the co-parceners.

Features of Joint Hindu Family

The Joint Hindu Family Firm possesses the following features:

i. **Status** : The membership of the family business is the result of status arising from birth in the family. There is no question of the members being discriminated in terms of minority and majority on the basis of age.

ii. **Male Members** : Only male persons of the family can claim co-parcenary interest in the Joint Hindu family business firm.

iii. **Karta** : The right to manage the business vests in Karta alone. He has the implied authority to obtain loans through mortgage, etc. or the purpose of the business. Other members have neither any right to manage the affairs of the business nor any right to take loans on mortgage of family assets for the purpose of business.

iv. **Liability** : The liability of all the members of the Joint Hindu Family, except that of the Karta, is limited to the value of their individual interest in the joint property. The liability of the Karta is unlimited and as such extends to all that he owns as his separate and private property.

v. **Fluctuating Share** : The share of each member's interest in the family property and business keeps on fluctuating. The member's interest increases by death of any existing co-parcener and decreases by birth of a new co-parcener.

vi. **Continued Existence** : The existence of the Joint Hindu Family Business is not affected by the death or insolvency of a co-parcener or even that of the Karta.

The sole proprietorship and partnership forms of organisations have failed to meet growing needs of modern industry and commerce. They have many limitations like limited resources, unlimited liability and fear of discontinuity. To get over these drawbacks, joint stock company form of organisation came into existence. Now it is the most widely used form of business organisation not only in the private sector but also in the public sector. This form of organisation is very successful for large scale enterprises. It is also equally good for undertakings doing business on a small scale because of easier access to financial resources, limited liability and continued existence.

4. JOINT STOCK COMPANY

A joint stock company is a voluntary association of individuals for profits, having a capital divided into transferable shares, the ownership of which is the condition of ownership.

A company is defined as a person, artificial, invisible, intangible and existing only in the eyes of law. Being a creation of law, it possesses only those properties which the charter of its creation confers upon its, either expressly or as incidental to its very existence: among the most important of which are immortality and individuality.

Section 566 of the Companies Act, 1956 lays down that a joint stock company limited by shares is "a company having permanent paid up or nominal share capital of fixed amount divided into shares, also of fixed amount, held and transferable as stock and formed on the principles of having as its members only the holders of those shares or stock and no other persons."

A joint stock company represent an incorporated association of persons who contribute money to a common stock known as capital of the company. The capital of the company is divided into shares or stock of fixed amount and every member purchases atleast a minimum number shares in the company. Thus the capital of the company is held jointly by the shareholders. That is why it is known as a 'joint stock company' independent from that of its members. Its shares are transferable and its life is not affected by the incoming and outgoing of its members.

Advantages of Joint Stock Company

Joint stock company has gained popularity throughout the world as a form of business organisation because it is superior to a sole tradership concern and a partnership firm in the following respects:

1. **Vast Financial Resources** : A company can raise huge financial resources. It can issue different types of securities (i.e. equity shares, preference shares, and debentures) to attract different types of investors. A company can also raise finance from the public in the form of public deposits and banks and other financial institutions.

2. **Continued Existence** : A joint stock company is a separate legal entity distinct from those who are its members or who promote it. As an incorporated body, it enjoys perpetual existence. It continues functioning so long it has the minimum number of members required by law. Thus, it is a stable form of organisaion and is best suited for a business which requires a long period to establish and consolidate.

3. **Limited Liability** : The liability of the shareholders of a joint stock company is limited to the face value of the shares held by them. Their private properties are not attachable to recover the debts of the company.

4. **Scattered Risk** : Shares of a company can be held by a large number of people Thus, the risk of loss spread over a large number of persons and the possibility of hardship on a few persons as in case of partnership or on one person as in case of sole tradership is avoided in case of failure of the shares and debentures business.

5. **Transferability of Shares :** The share holders of public companies are entitled to transfer the shares held by them to others. The shares of most companies are listed on the stock exchange and hence can be readily sold. This ensures liqidity of investments and encourages investment of funds in the companies.

6. **Economics :** A company is in a position to raise huge capital and can undertake large scale operations. The increase in the size of the business operations would result in the economies in production, purchase, selling, management, etc. Thus, cost of production will be less and higher efficiency will be achieved as compared to other forms of business organisations.

7. **Expert Management :** Since a company carries business on a large scale and has huge financial resources, it can afford the services of expert personnel. This will lead towards professionalisation of management which is necessary for the efficient management of any business.

8. **Scope for Growth :** The company form of organisation facilitates expansion of business operations because of a sound financial base. Moreover, it employs professional managers who take risks in launching diversification programmes involving huge amount of capital.

9. **Public Confidence :** The formation and running of a company is regulated by the provisions of Companies Act and various other acts. The provisions regarding appointment and remuneration of directors, compulsory audit and publication of accounts, protection of minority shareholders and so on have created greater public confidence in joint stock companies.

10. **Social Advantage :** A joint stock company is also beneficial from the society's point of view. It mobilises the scattered savings of public and invests them in sound industrial and commercial ventures. Because of large scale operations, it provides employment to a large number of people. Economies of large scale operations also lead to economical use of national resources and provision of goods and services to the public at cheaper prices.

Disadvantages of Joint Stock Company

Company form of business organisation suffers from the following limitations:

1. **Difficult Formation :** In order to form a company, a large number of legal formalities have to be complied with. A number of documents have to be drafted and filed with the Registrar of Companies. This requires large amount of expenses to pay for the services of the experts, printing and stationery charges, registration fee and other office and administrative expenses. A public limited company has to go through

additional legal formalities to raise capital and to get certificate of commencement of business. This discourages the formation of new companies.

2. **Government Control :** A company has to follow many provision of different acts. Even the internal working of the company is subjected to statutory restrictions regarding meetings, voting, audit, etc. The existence of so many legal restrictions in running the business might discourage the people to start new companies.

3. **Economic Oligarchy :** The management of a company is supposed to be conducted as per the desires of the shareholder who are owners of the company. But they have practically no say in the affairs of the company. Very often directors tend to mislead the shareholders by their 'window dress' reports. This makes control of shareholders illusory. They also create groups among the shareholders and thus consolidate their hold on the company by manipulation of voting power. Thus, separation of ownership and management results in oligarchic management and it makes control of shareholders illusory.

4. **Fraudulent Practices :** The fraudulent promoters may misuse the capital raised from the public for their personal end. This creates panic among the public. The directors of the company may also manipulate the prices of the shares in the stock exchange by manipulating the books of accounts of the company.

5. **Delayed Decision-making :** The process of decision-making in a company is slow as compared to a sole trader or partnership firm. All the important decisions are to be taken either by the Board of Directors or the shareholders. Calling the meetings of the Board of the shareholders consume a long time. Thus, crucial decisions are delayed in the process.

6. **Neglect of Minority :** All the major issue in case of companies are decided by the shareholders having majority of shares. The majority shareholders may ignore the interest of the minority shareholders. The Companies Act provides measures against the oppression of minority, but the measures are not very effective in actual practice.

7. **Lack of Personal Touch :** This is one of the greatest drawbacks of a company that it is not in a position to maintain personal touch which its workers, customers, suppliers and others. The impersonal management of the company may result in waste and inefficiency.

8. **Difficulty in Winding up :** It is very difficult to wind up a company. A very long and cumberome procedure has to be followed to wind up the affairs of the company.

5. CO-OPERATIVE ORGANISATION

The cooperative fund of organisation is different from the rest insofar as it is not set up with profit as the guiding motive, but with the purpose of rendering service to its members in particular and to the society in general. Co-operative organisations have emerged primarily to protect and safeguard the economic interest of the relatively weaker sections of the society in the face of exploitation by businessmen whose primary motive is profit maximisation. The essential ingredients of a co-operative organisation are service, co-operation and self help. A co-operative organisation rests on the voluntary association of persons joining together on equal basis for the fulfillment of their economic and other interests.

A co-operative organisation is an association of persons, usually of limited means, who have voluntarily joint together to achieve a common economic end, through the formation of a democratically controlled business organisation, making equitable contributions to the capital required and accepting a fair share of risks and benefits of the undertaking.

A co-operative organisation is a voluntary association of individuals, generally belonging to one homogeneous group, who associate together to promote their common interests. The objects of a co-operative organisation are economic in character. It is generally formed and registered under the Co-operative Societies Act, 1912 by the individuals of moderate means to protect their economic interests. This form of organisation can be applied to every conceivable form of economic activity. Thus, the scope of co-operative form or organisation is as wide as the economic life of the members of a community. Today there are a large number of credit societies, retail stores, building societies, marketing societies and producers' societies which are formed and run on the basis of co-operation.

Formation of Co-operative

As stated earlier, a co-operative society enjoys a separate legal entity of its own after getting incorporated. To get a co-operative society incorporated, an application is to be submitted to the Registrar of Co-operative Societies of the concerned state in which the society's registered office is situated. The application contains the following information :

1. The name of the society ;
2. The aims and objectives for which the society is being created ;
3. The amount and division of share capital ;
4. The names and addresses of the members ;
5. Two copies of the bye-laws and
6. Two copies of the rules and regulations of the society.

The Registrar of Co-operative Societies, after getting the application for registration alogwith the copies of the bye-laws and those of rules and regulations of the society, carefully scrutinises them so as to ensure that the two documents do not contain anything which is contrary to the spirit of the

Co-operative Societies Act. In case he is satisfied with regard to these points, the society is registered and a certificate to that effect is issued. After getting the Certificate of Incorporation, the society assumes a separate legal entity of its own and can start its operations.

Management of Co-operatives

The management of a co-operative organisation is vested in the hands of a managing committee which is elected directly by the members in the annual general meeting. The committee meets frequently to lay down general procedures and programmes of the co-operative society and to get the progress report from the office bearers of the society. The co-operative society usually has the following office bearers :

(i) President,   (ii) Vice-President(s),

(iii) Secretary,   (iv) Joint Secretary, if any,

(v) Treasurer.

The office bearers are responsible and accountable to the managing committee initially and to the general body of members ultimately.

On registration, the co-operative society gets corporate status and becomes entitled to certain privileges and subject to certain controls and regulations by the State through the co-operative department. The co-operative organisation must furnish annual reports and return to the Registrar of Co-operatives and must get its accounts audited every year by a qualified auditor.

A co-operative organisation should not be looked upon only as a form of organisation. In the present day context, it has assumed the role of a movement aimed at eliminating the exploitation by private business and ensuring the spirit on self-help on voluntary basis among the members of the society. Thus, it has assumed the role of a socio-economic movement motivated by the ideal of helping and raising the economic status of the weaker sections of the society through collective action.

Types of Co-operatives

On the basis of the nature of services rendered by co-operatives, they may be classified into the following categories :

1. **Produces' Co-operatives :** These co-operative societies are formed to help and strengthen small producers. The Producers' Co-operatives may be organised on either of the following two basis :

   (a) The producer members maintain their separate individual entity. The society supplies them with raw-materials, tools, equipment, etc. The members sell their individual output to the society.

   (b) The member producers produce on behalf of the society as its employees. The member producers are paid wages for their work.

Here again, the society supplies them with raw-materials, tools and equipment, etc.

In either case, the marketing of the products is undertaken by the society.

2. **Consumers' Co-operatives** : These societies are formed for the purpose of making available day to day requirements of goods to their members at cheaper prices. For this purpose they buy their goods from wholesalers at wholesale prices and sell them to members and often to non-members as well at prices slightly lower than the market prices. The difference between the wholesale price and the selling price of the co-operatives represents the surplus which after meeting the operative expenses are distributed among the members as bonus besides transferring a part thereof to general reserve and other kinds of reserves. This form of co-operative has been receiving government's attention and help with a view to check the general problem of price rise.

3. **Marketing Co-operatives** : These societies are set up either for selling manufactured products or agricultural commodities. As such, marketing co-operatives may be classified into two broad categories :

   (a) **Industrial Marketing Co-operatives** : These societies pool the manufactured products of producers such as artisans, weavers, small producers, etc. and sell them at prices which are remunerative to the member producers.

   (b) **Agricultural Marketing Co-operatives** : These are organised by farmers for selling their farm-products and also for obtaining agricultural inputs. Thus, agricultural co-operatives are engaged in a two-way function of selling farm products and buying seeds, manures, implements and many other goods. Since agricultural marketing involves several steps like processing, warehousing, financing etc., these co-operatives are often formed on a multipurpose basis for catering to the needs of agriculturists both as sellers and buyers of products.

4. **Co-operative Credit Societies** : These are formed by members to pool their savings and to invest the resources thus collected for giving loans to members on factorable terms involving interest, security and repayment. Such co-operatives are organised both in rural and urban areas. In rural areas, these are called Primary Credit Societies or Rural Credit Societies. While in urban areas these societies are known as Co-operative Banks.

5. **House Co-operatives** : These societies are formed by those people who strive to own a flat or a plot for constructing their own house. As such, these societies are formed mostly in urban areas and that too in big cities where the problem of housing is acute. These societies are allotted land (developed or undeveloped) by the local authority or by the Urban

Development Authority at concessional prices. The same is true with regard to the allotment of flats. Such societies can also negotiate loans for its members on easy terms from financial institutions. National Housing Bank and other organisations have been established for boosting housing activities. They may also procure building materials in bulk for their members so as to reap the economies of bulk buying.

6. **Co-operative Farming Societies :** In our country, the problem of sub-division and fragmentation of agricultural land-holding is very acute. One of the ways to get over this problem is to organise small land owners and tillers of land into farming societies with a view to reaping the benefits of large scale mechanized farming. The large scale co-operative farming results into raising agricultural output and reducing the cost per unit.

In addition to the types of co-operatives discussed above, there are some other categories of co-operatives which have come up in recent years. The important ones are Processing Co-operatives, (for processing sugar-cane, cotton, jute, paddy, oil-seeds etc.), Labour and Construction Co-operatives comprising skilled, semiskilled and unskilled workers for undertaking the construction of irrigation works, roads, building, etc. They are formed primarily to eliminate the contractors and get honourable and remunerative economic occupation for their members. Other co-operatives are engaged in fisheries, dairying, cold storage, forestry. etc.

To perform the function of overseeing and monitoring of the primary societies, district level, State level and Central level apex federations are also formed. Sometimes, the central apex institution may set up primary unit, at others, primary units themselves may give rise to the federation. In India, the important apex level bodies of co-operatives in different areas of activity are National Federation Industrial Co-operatives, National Federation of Sugar Factories, National Federation Co-operative. spinning Mills, National Federation of Dairy Co-operatives. National Agricultural Co-operative Marketing Federation, Indian Farmers' Fertilizers Co-operative, National Cooperatives union of Indian, etc.

5

CHANNELS OF DISTRIBUTION

Meaning of Channels of Distribution

The term 'channels of distribution' or 'trade channel' signifies various trade links connecting the manufacturers or producers and the ultimate consumers or users. It includes both the producer final user of the product as well as mercantile agents and merchant middlemen engaged in the transfer of title of goods and service. But it does not include concerns such as banks, insurance companies, warehouses, railways and other non-middlemen institutions which render a marketing service but do not play any major role in negotiating purchases and sales.

The simplest channel of distribution is zero stage marketing channel in which there is direct contact between the producer and the ultimate consumer or user. A one stage marketing channel contains one selling intermediary which may be retailer in case of consumer goods and a sales agent or broker in case of industrial goods. A two stage marketing channel contains two intermediaries, namely, wholesaler and retailer. A three-stage marketing channel contains three intermediaries-wholesaler, jobber, and retailer. Further, higher stage marketing channels may also be found in a few cases.

A brief explanation of different channels of distribution is given below

Table 1. Channels of Distribution

Marketing Channels	:	Intermediaries
Zero stage	:	Producer-Consumer
One state	:	Producer-Retailer-Consumer
Two Stage	:	Producer-wholesaler-Agent-Consumer
Three stage	:	Producer-Wholesaler-Jobber-Retailer-Consumer

(i) **Producer and Consumer or Direct Sale :** This is the direct channel of distribution which implies direct sale of goods and services by the producer to the consumers. No middleman is present between the producers and the consumers. The producer creates a link with the consumers directly through door to door salesmen, direct mail or through his own retail shops.

Direct selling is gaining popularity these days because of high costs of distributing the goods and services through middlemen. Direct selling is generally employed to sell industrial goods of high value to the industrial users and to sell consumer goods such as cloth, cosmetics, hosiery products and shoes. Small producers and producers of perishable commodities also sell directly to the local consumers. Big firms adopt direct selling in order to cut distribution cost and because they have sufficient to sell directly to the consumers. Under direct selling, all the marketing activities are performed by the producer or the manufacturer himself.

(ii) **Producer, Retailer and Consumer :** This is one stage distribution channel having one middleman i.e., retailer. Under this, the manufacturer sells to the retailers who in turn sell to the ultimate consumers. This channel of distribution is very popular these days because of the emergence of departmental stores, super markets and other big retail stores. The retailers purchase in large quantities from the manufacturer and perform certain marketing activities in order to sell the product to the ultimate consumers.

(iii) **Producer, Wholesaler, Retailer and Consumer :** This is a 'traditional' channel of distribution for the sale of consumer goods. There are two middlemen in this channel, namely, wholesaler and retailer. This channel is most suitable for the products with widely scattered market.

(iv) **Producer, Wholesaler, Agent, Retailer and Consumer :** This is three stage channel of distribution under which mercantile agents establish a link between the wholesaler and the retailer. This channel is used where the wholesaler is not able to keep contacts with a large number of retailer.

The channels of distribution for consumer goods are generally long, while channels for industrial goods are short. Direct channel (i.e. zero stage) is very popular for selling of industrial goods since industrial users place big orders. However, many producers of industrial raw materials make use of the services of mercantile agents and wholesalers as they want to keep themselves fully away from the problems of distribution or they do not have facilities for the distribution of the products.

CHOICE OF CHANNELS OF DISTRIBUTION

The choice of the appropriate channels of distribution is not a simple job. While taking a decision in this regard, management should carefully consider the following factors :

1. **Market Considerations :** The nature of the market is a key factor influencing the choice of channels of distribution. The following features of the market should be analysed to determine the channels :

   (a) **Consumer or industrial market :** If the product is intended for industrial market or industrial users, the channel of distribution will be a short one. Since industrial users purchase in large quantities, they can purchase directly from the producer or manufacturer. There is no need of retailers. The manufacturer can establish contacts with the industrial users by sending his agents. But in case of goods meant for consumers, retailers may have to be included in the channels of distribution.

   (b) **Number of potential customers :** A large potential market is likely to put weight in favour of the use of middlemen. If the number of customers is relatively small, the manufacturer may be able to sell directly by using his own salesforce.

   (c) **Size of order :** Direct selling is convenient and economical where customers place order in big lots as in case of industrial goods. But where the product is sold in small quantities, middlemen are used to distribute such products. The same manufacturer may adopt different channels to distribute his product. The same manufacturer may adopt diffrent channels to distribute his product. For instance, a manufacturer of food products may sell directly to big retail stores and may use wholesalers to sell to small retailer.

   (d) **Customer buying habits and expectations :** The customer buying habits like the time he is willing to spend, the desire for credit, the preference of personal attention and the preference for one stop shopping significantly affect the choice distribution channels.

2. **Product Considerations :** The type and nature of the product influence the number and type of middlement to be chosen for distributing the product. The important factors with regard to the product are as follows:

   (a) **Unit value :** Usually, if the unit value of the product is lower and the turnover is higher, the channels of distribution will be longer. For instance, products like cosmetics, stationery and small accessory equipments are distributed through agents, wholesalers and retailers. Products of high value like jewellery and industrial machines are sold directly to the users.

   (b) **Product line :** A manufacturer manufacturing several products in the same line will sell directly or through retailers since it is economical. But a manufacturer with only one item may have to appoint the wholesalers and retailers to sell his product.

   (c) **Standardised Product :** Standardised products can be distributed through longer channels because their, brand names are very popular. But custom-make and unstandardised products can more easily be sold directly by the producer to the user.

(d) **Technical nature :** An industrial product which is highly technical is often distributed directly to the industrial users. The manufacturer of such a product can appoint sales engineers who can explain the product to the potential customer and provide pre-sale and after-sale service to them. But cunsumer products of technical nature are generally sold through retailers.

(e) **Bulk and weight :** Bulky and heavy goods are distributed directly to the users in order to minimise the physical handling of the product because transportation of such products involves huge cost.

(f) **Perishability :** The channels of distribution are short in case of products subject to physical or fashion perishability. The producers of perishable products generally sell direct to the consumers or sell through the middlemen who have the special storage facilities. Manufacturers of non-perishable commodities have a wider choice in the channel selection.

3. **Company Considerations :** The nature and size of the business firm have an important impact on the selection of channels of distribution. Following factors are important in this regard :

(a) **Volume of production :** A big manufacturer may find it profitable to sell directly to customers through his sales force. If he is manufacturing a wide range of products, he may sell his products by opening retail outlets in different parts of the country. But a small manufacturer with only a small number of items cannot afford to sell directly because of his small scale operations. He can engage wholesalers and/or retailers to sell his products.

(b) **Financial resources :** A financially strong company can distribute its products itself employing its own sales-force and opening retail outlets. But a weak company which cannot invest money in distribution will have to use middlemen to sell its output.

(c) **Services provided by the sellers :** The choice of a channel of distribution is also influenced by the services provided by the manufacturers. A manufacturer can find good retailers only if he undertakes sufficient advertising. Some manufacturers of technical products undertake to provide after-sale service. Such manufacturers can also get reputed retailers for selling their products.

(d) **Desire for control of channels :** A manufacturer who wants to control the distribution of his product will select a short channel of distribution. He may do so even though the distribution cost is higher if he feels that he can give his product more aggressive promotion.

4. **Middlemen Considerations :** Certain factors related to the middlemen which influence the channel selection are as follows :

(a) **Availability of desired middlemen :** A manufacturer will rely on middlemen if they operate according to his desire. He may not like to entrust his products to a middleman who is handling competitive products. In such a case, he may prefer to open his branches to sell his products.

(b) **Financial ability :** A large manufacturer will generally select those middlemen who are financially strong and can provide credit facilities to the customers and can pay their bills to the manufacturer regularly and promptly.

(c) **Attitude of middlemen :** Sometimes, middlemen are not prepared to carry a manufacturer's products because of the non-acceptability of his marketing policies. For instance, a retailer may want sole selling agency for a particular region or a guarantee against price reduction if he is to handle the products of the manufacturer.

(d) **Sale potential :** A manufacturer will generally select a channel offering the greatest potential sales volume over the long-run. But it is very difficult to forecast which channel will generate the largest sales volume.

(e) **Cost :** The manufacturers also consider the cost of selling through alternative channels. But it does not meant that high cost middlemen are excluded from consideration. A manufacturer may select even a high cost middleman because he provides so many services to the customers which are not provided by other middlemen.

Selection of Middlemen

A manufacturer has to select particular middlemen through whom he will distribute his products. While seleting a particular wholesaler or retailer, the following factors should be taken into consideration :

  (i) location of the middleman's premises ;
 (ii) financial position of the middleman ;
(iii) knowledge and experience of the middleman ;
(iv) capacity of the middleman to promote sale ;
 (v) ability of the middleman to render after-sale service ;
(vi) willingness of the middleman to deal in the products of the manufacturer.

MIDDLEMEN

Middlemen are the persons who provide a link between the manufacturer and the consumer. They facilitate the purchase and sale of goods and services and also perform the marketing functions. They charge for their services and to that extent they are responsible for the increase in the cost of the product to the ultimate consume or user. Despite this, the middlemen constitute an important link in the channels of distribution. They help the manufacturers in selling their products and help the consumers in getting the want-satisfying products.

Middleman may broadly be classified into two categories, namely, (1) mercantile agents or agent middlemen and (2) mrechant middlemen.

1. Mercantile Agents

Mercantile agents are also known as 'agent middlemen' and 'functional middlemen'. They do not handle the goods in the capacity of owners, but they render important services for the exchange of goods. They assist in the buying and selling of goods by taking part in negotiating purchase and sale of goods. Since they do not own the products, they do not earn profits. They take their remuneration for the services rendered in the form of commission or brokerage. Mercantile agents are of the following types :

(i) **Commission Agent :** A commission agent acts on behalf of some other person known as principal for a agreed commission. He undertakes to sell the goods in the name and on the sole risk of the principal. Such an agent may also be employed for the purchase of goods on behalf of the principal. A selling commission agent takes possession of the goods, makes necessary storage arrangements and passes title to the goods to the buyers and gets commission at a fixed percentage on sales.

(ii) **Factor :** A factor is a mercantile agent who keeps the goods of others for sale. He can sell goods in his own name, pledge goods in his possession and do all such acts as can be done by the principal. He receives commission at a fixed percentage on sales from his principal.

(iii) **Auctioneer :** An auctioneer is a mercantile agent who sells the goods on behalf of his principal by undertaking auction of goods. Like commission agent, he takes possession of the goods, displays them to the intending purchasers and receives offers for sale or bids from the intending purchasers. He sells the goods to the highest bidder and transfers the ownership of goods to him. He receives a certain percentage on the sale proceeds of goods as his commission for the services rendered to the principal.

(iv) **Broker :** A broker is a mercantile agent who negotiates purchase or sale of goods on behalf of other parties. He is called selling agent if he is engaged by the seller and buying agent if engaged by the buyer. Brokers obtain neither the possession nor the ownership of goods, but only serve to bring the buyers and sellers together. They get their remuneration in the form of brokerage which is a certain percentage of the value of the transaction involved.

2. Merchant Middlemen

Merchant middlemen, also known as merchants, are the dealers in goods and services who purchase and sell in their own name for a margin of profit. They assume title of ownership to the goods in all cases though physical possession of the goods may be taken place in all cases. They undertake marketing risk and perform many marketing functions. Merchant middlemen may be classified into two categories, viz., wholesalers and retailers.

WHOLESALERS

The term 'wholesaler' applies to all merchant middlemen who purchase and sell in large quantities. A wholesaler provides an important link between the manufacturer or producer and the retailer. He takes title to the goods he handles and assumes marketing risks in the process of distribution of goods. He purchases in bulk and sells in small lots to the retailers or industrial users and is generally away from the ultimate consumers. Wholesalers may be classified into three broad categories :

(a) **Pure Wholesaler :** A pure wholesaler is a merchant who concentrates entirely on buying and selling in large lots and does not engage in manufacturing or retailing operations. He is also known as distribution or wholesaler proper. He purchases goods from one manufacturer or a numbre of manufacturers in large quantities and sells to the retailers in small lots. He generally maintains warehouses for storing the goods and also arranges for transportation for the transfer of goods to the retailer. A pure wholesaler who purchase raw materials from a number of producers for the purpose of selling to the manufacturers is known as a 'mill supply wholesaler'. Some wholesalers specialise in a particular line of product. They are known as 'single line wholesalers'.

(b) **Manufacturer Wholesaler :** A manufacturer wholesaler undertakes the manufacture of goods alongwith distribution to retailers. He may also distribute the goods of other manufacturers. The purpose of combining these two functions is to reduce the overhead expenses per unit of product handled.

(c) **Retailer Wholesaler :** A retailer wholesale combines with his business of wholesale the functions of retail trade. He purchases goods from the manufacturers in large quantities and sells them to retailers and ultimate consumers through his retail outlets.

Functions of Wholesalers

The wholesalers performs the following important functions of marketing in the process of distribution of goods and services :

1. **Buying and assembling :** The wholesalers make an estimate of the demand for the goods and purchase and assemble different varieties of goods from different manufacturers spread throughout the country. They also undertake import of goods from different countries.

2. **Storage :** Wholesalers keep the goods assembled by them in their warehouses to supply them to retailers whenever they require. They relieve

the manufacturers and retailers from the botheration of making storage arrangements.

3. **Transportation :** Wholesalers make trasportation arrangement from the premises of manufacturers to their godowns and from their godowns to the retail stores. They often maintain their own fleet of vehicles for his purpose.

4. **Grading and packaging :** Wholesalers grade the goods according to certain standards which they have purchased from different manufactures. Some manufacturers also give brand names to graded products to convince the consumers or industrial users about the quality of the products they deal in. They also undertake the packaging of goods in convenient lots.

5. **Financing :** Wholesalers provide financial accommodation to both the manufacturers and the retailers. They generally purchase goods on cash basis from the manufacturers and sometimes also give advance to the manufacturers. Thus, the manufacturers need not wait till their products are sold. The wholesalers help the retailers by selling the goods on credit.

6. **Risk-taking :** Wholesalers assume a large number of risks in the process of distribution of goods. These risks may occur on account of changes in prices and demands, spoilage of goods and bad debts. Thus, they undertake many marketing risks which would have been undertaken by the manufacturers and retailers.

7. **Promotion :** The wholesalers job does not end with the selling of goods to the retailers. They also assist in the dispersal of goods by the retailers situated in various markets. They perform advertising and other sales promotion activities in order to promote the sale of their products.

RETAILERS

Retailing includes all activities directly related to the sales of goods or services to the ultimate consumer for personal, non-business use. Retailing or retail trade involves all such activities which are related to direct sale of goods to the ultimate consumer. Retail trade is usually done by the retailers. A retailer may be defined as a dealer in goods and services who purchases from manufacturers and wholesalers and sells to the ultimate consumers.

A retailer is an important link in the channel of distribution. He purchases and collects various kinds of goods from numerous sources and sells them to the consumers in small lots. He is in direct touch with the ultimate consumers. Retailers are generally located near the thickly populated residential areas. Retail stores are mostly organised on proprietorship or partnership basis and their capital investment is small as compared to wholesaling and manufacturing enterprises.

Functions of Retailers

Retail stores or retailers have strategic importance as a channel of distribution. They perform the following functions :

(i) Retailers purchases and assemble goods from a large number of wholesales and manufacturers to meet the needs of the ultimate consumers.

(ii) Retailrs keep a large number of products of different varieties in stock to sell them to the customers whenever they require. Thus, they create time utility.

(iii) Retailers perform transportation function by carrying the goods from the wholesalers and handing them over to the ultimate consumers. Sometimes, they also provide free home delivery of products to the customers. Retailers sell the goods on credit to the customers and they increase their short-term purchasing power. In this process, they undertake the risk of bad debts.

(iv) Retailers educate the customers by informing them about the availability and diverse uses of new products.

(v) Retailers act as agents of customers. They communicate the needs on demands of their customers to the wholesalers and manufacturers. Thus, they help the customers in getting the want-satisfying products and help the manufacturers in purchasing the products which are desired by the customers.

KINDS OF RETAIL DISTRIBUTION

Retailing institutions may broadly be classified, on the basis of their scale of operations, into small scale retailers and large scale retailers. Small-scale retailers include mobile retailers and fixed shopkeepers who operate with small amount of capital. The mobile retailrs do not operate from fixed business premises, but move from place to place for selling their products to consumers. They are also known as 'itinerant retailers'. They include hawkers, pedlars, market traders and pavement sellers. On the other hand, small scale fixed retail shops are located near residential areas. Such retailres generally deal in all types of consumer goods. They may also take the help of their family members or may employ salesmen to sell their products to the customers. They keep personal contacts with their customers and also provide them free home delivery service.

Large-scale retailing has assumed great importance these days. Many types of large-scale retail stores have come into existence to meet the need of urban population. These include departmental stores, multiple shops or chain stores, mail order business houses, co-operative stores and super markets. Now, we shall briefly discuss the various types of retail stores.

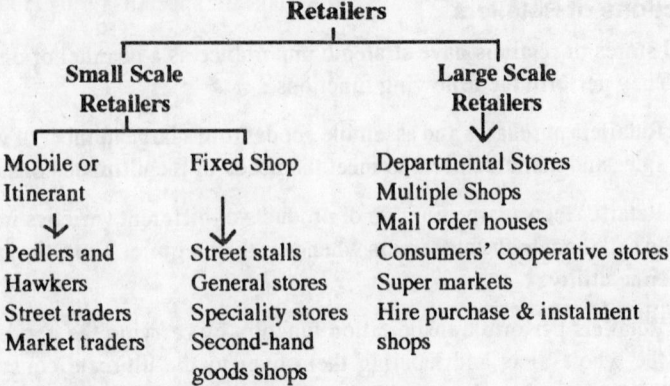

Table 2. Kinds of Retailers

SMALL SCALE RETAILERS

1. **Pedlers and Hawkers :** Sale by pedlers and hawkers is of old origin. They sell almost every article of daily use from house to house on their heads or carrier thelas. They generally keep the limited quantity of goods and sell practically the whole lot during the day. They purchase goods on a day's credit and pay off the next day out of their day's sale. They do not require much capital, and have not to maintain a shop. They do their all works themselves. Inspite of keen competition, they are able to push sales as they deliver the goods at the residence of the customer. The quality of goods is generally inferior. The consumer is attracted to purchase goods from them due to spot delivery.

2. **Street Traders :** Street traders operate near the busy places like railway stations, bus stops, cinema halls, etc. They set up their small shops temporarily. They sell their products at relatively low prices.

3. **Market Traders :** These traders keep on moving from place to place and sell their products at different weekly, fornightly or monthly markets (or bazars) or at annual fairs. They also operate in the vacant front verandahas of fixed shops when the shops are closed.

4. **Street Stalls :** These are located at street crossings or in the busy streets. A stall is an improvised structure - a table or a temporary platform to display the goods for sale. The stall holders, generally, deal in cheaper products like toys, pens, hosiery products, etc.

5. **General Stores :** General stores are set up in residential areas and they stock all kinds of products needed by the local residents for their daily use. A General Store is owned and managed by a sole proprietor who keeps personal contacts with his customers. The general store may be a single line store or a multi-line store. A single line store specialises in selling only products of a single line. For instance, medical stores deal in medicines only and stationery stores deal in stationery items only.

6. **Speciality Stores :** Speciality stores take the specialisation practised by single line stores one step further. If a shop selling ready-made garments (i.e. single line store) deals in children's garments only, it will be called a speciality shop. Speciality shops are generally located at central places only so as to attract a large-number of customers.

7. **Second Hand Goods Shops :** These stores deal in second-hand or used goods like books, clothes, furniture etc. Persons with modest means can make purchases from such stores.

LARGE-SCALE RETAIL SHOPS

Retailing on a large scale brings with it several of the economies associated with large-scale business organisation in general. The more important among them, are better and more effective advertising, better organised selling, increased turnover, lower overheads per unit of commodity sold and improved management of the sales effort under the guidance of experts. All these economies of large-scale retailing place the large retail units in a superior position in the distributive set-up of a country. These units have the advantage of offering convenience of shopping to the customers in various localities and can generally offer more efficient and personalised service to the consumers. Likewise these units can introduce a greater deal of flexibility in their policies than the large-scale organisation. In the distributive set-up, therefore, the large and the small scale retailers are likely to continue to co-exist.

DEPARTMENTAL STORE

The origin of departmental store took place in Frace in 1852. These days, departmental stores have become very popular in many other countries also.

A departmental store may be defined as a retail institution that handles a wide variety of merchandise grouped into well defined departments for purposes of promotion, service, accounting and control. A departmental store is a large scale retail organisation having a number of departments under the same roof. Every department confines its activities to a particular line of business. These departments are centrally organised and controlled to form a single establishment. The management of all the departments is centralised, but the stock of each department is handled separately.

Advantages : The main object of a department store is to satisfy customer's needs at one place. It sells a large number of products through different departments to the customers. It has gained popularity because of the following advantages :

1. A departmental store is generally located at a central place of a city. It is easily accessible to the customers.

2. Customers can purchase almost all the goods they require form a single store. This saves their time and effort as they need not move from one stop to another for the purchase of various products.

3. They provide a number of services to their customers including

recreation, free home delivery and credit facilities. That is why, they attract a large number of customers.

4. A departmental store enjoys the economies of large scale operations. Overhead expenses are spread over a number of departments enabling the stores to keep the prices of products within the reach of customer.

5. A departmental store can make better use of different advertising media than is possible for small retailers. They can also afford window display which serves as a self-advertising medium.

Disadvantages : A departmental store also suffers from the following disadvantages :

1. It offers a number of services to the customers, the cost of which is ultimately borne by the customers.

2. Expensive window dressing, interior decoration and advertising increase overhead expenses.

3. A departmental store is generally located at a central place which creates problems of traffic congestion and parking.

4. There is lack of 'personal touch' with the customers. The paid salesmen may fail to give personal attention to a large number of customers of the store.

5. Huge capital is required to establish a departmental store. The costs of running its operations are also too high. In addition, it also undertake greater risk of loss due to fire, price fluctuation and change in fashion because it keeps huge stocks of various items in one building.

MULTIPLE SHOPS OR CHAIN STORES

A multiple shop system may be defined as a system of branch shops operating under a centralised management and dealing in similar lines of products. The multiple shops or chain stores receive supply from the central office and remit the sales proceeds regularly to the central office. Each shop is allowed to retain a small amount of cash on imprest basis to meet its day-to-day expenses. Purchasing, pricing and advertising are done centrally. There is only decentralisation of selling. The chain stores display goods in an identical manner and sell the same standardised merchandise. Bata, Mafatlal and Raymonds shops are some of the examples of chain stores in India. Unlike departmental stores multiple stores deal only in a limited variety of products. For instance, DCM retail stores deal in textiles only.

Advantages : There are many advantages of multiple shops system :

(i) This system enables a manufacturer to manufacture products on a large-scale and sell directly to the consumers through different retail outlets.

(ii) All branches of a multiple shop are of uniform style and design and are distinctive in appearance. People can easily identify each of them as belonging to a particular manufacturing enterprise. Multiple shops attract the customers in a better way by window display and centralised advertising. They are generally located in different parts of the city and the customers can buy from the nearest shop or branch.

(iii) There is a diversification of risks. Unsold stock of one store can be transferred to others to prevent loss or damage. It is also easier to shift a store from one place to another. Thus, there is a greater flexibility in operation.

(iv) Since multiple shops system provides a direct link between the manufacturer and the consumers, products can be sold to the consumers at lower prices because of less distribution cost.

Disadvantages : The system of multiple shops suffers from a number of drawbacks which are as follows :

(i) It cannot offer a wide variety of products to customers because the range is limited.

(ii) There is lack of free home delivery service and credit facility to customers. This discourages a certain type of people.

(iii) Since products are of standardised nature, they cannot be adjusted to suit the needs of a local market.

(iv) There is a lack of interest on the part of paid employees of the store. There is no motivation for the employees to increase the sales and there is no personal touch between the manufacturer and the employees. The employees are also not able to give personal attention to the customers.

MAIL ORDER HOUSE

Mail order houses are retailing enterprises which carry on business through mail. Mail order business is known as 'selling through post' for the retailer and 'shopping by post' for the consumer. Under this, the retailers contact the prospective customers through some sort of advertising. Advertising is carried through the press or by sending leaflets and catalogues giving the necessary details about the product. Mail order houses maintain mailing lists of potential customers. They send the literature about their products through mail. They also mail reply paid cards to the prospective customers. When they receive orders, they will procure the goods and despatch them to the customers usually by V.P.P. (Value payable post). Sometimes, the goods are sent by railway parcel and the railway receipt is forwarded to the customer by V.P.P.

The main feature of mail order business is that goods are sold without any personal contact between the buyer and the seller. The buyers do not visit the seller business house and thus, do not make any personal examination of the goods before purchase. Mail order selling is popular when (i) goods are identified by brand name and are of standardised quality ; (ii) goods enjoy popular demand by the customer scattered over wide areas ; (iii) goods do not require demonstration or special skills in handling and use ; and (iv) goods are durable and do not get spoiled in the course of transit. Books, drugs, sport articles, and cosmetics are some goods which are sold through mail.

Various factors which have contributed to the growth of mail order house are (i) improvement of postal service and development of railways and other means of transportation ; (ii) increased circulation of newspapers and journals ; and (iii) growing desire of people to have wider varieties and better qualities of goods. But in India, mail order business is not so popular because of poverty and illiteracy among people, lack of effective advertising, lack of standardised products and deceitful practices by the unscrupulous traders.

Advantages : Mail order business offers the following advantages to the seller and the buyer :

  (i) The buyer neet not travel a long distance to reach the retail store to get the delivery of goods.

 (ii) The mail order business houses can be located in less expensive localities.

(iii) Goods can be procured after receiving orders from the customers.

 (iv) The post office acts as the carrier of goods and the collector of sale proceeds. The chances of bad debts are till.

  Disadvantages : There are following demerits of mail order business;

  (i) Thers is no personal contact between the seller and the buyer. The buyer does not get any opportunity to inspect the goods before purchasing them. If goods are sold on sale or return basis, this will result in wastage of cost incurred on postage.

 (ii) Goods mailed by post are costlier because the customers have to pay for postal expenses also.

(iii) The customers are deprived of other services like credit facility from the sellers. Sometimes, there is delay in despatching the goods.

 (iv) Mail order business is not suitable for certain agricultural products.

CONSUMERS' COOPERATIVE STORE

Consumers' cooperative store is organised under the Cooperative Societies Act and is owned and operated by the consumers themselves. The capital of the store is provided by the shareholders. The membership of the store is voluntary. The aim of the store is to provide service to the members and not the maximisation of profit. The establishment of consumers' cooperative store is an attempt to eliminate middlemen who increase the cost of product for the consumers. They buy in large quantities directly from the manufacturers and sell them to the consumers at reasonable prices. Since there are no middlemen, the consumers get products of good quality at cheapre rates. The profits earned by the 'consumers' cooperative store during a year are utilised for strengthening its reserve fund, for declaring moderate rate of dividend and for declaring a bonus to the members according to the purchases made by them. A part of the profit may also be utilised for social purposed.

Merits : The consumers cooperative stores have the following merits:

(i)   It is easier to form a cooperative society. It attracts a large number of members because the value of its shares is nominal.

(ii) The liability of the members of a cooperative store is limited.

(iii) Cooperative societies are democratically managed because every member has one vote irrespective of the number of shares held by him.

(iv) Considerable state patronage is extended to the cooperative societies.

(v)   A cooperative store purchases goods directly from the manufacturers and distributes them on retail basis to the members.

Consumers' Cooperative Societies have not been very much successful because of certain limitations. Firstly, there is lack of initiative among the people to form cooperative societies to protect their interests. They face a shortage of funds since their membership is limited. Due to shortage of funds, small-scale operations, experts and trained personnel cannot be employed. The affairs of the store are managed by the members themselves who may not be able to provide competent management to the store. It has also been seen that members of the store do not patronise them regularly because of which they are not able to operate successfully.

SUPER MARKET

A super market is a large retailing business unit selling mainly food and every items on the basis of low margin appeal, wide variety and assortments, self-service and heavy emphasis on merchandising appeal. It is also known as Self Service store.

A super market deals mostly in food and grocery items. It is generally situated at the main shopping centres. Goods are kept in open racks, and the price and quality are clearly labelled on the goods. A customer can make selection of goods moving from counter to counter and pick up the selected goods and place them in a trolly. After he has completed his selection, the trolly will be carried to the exit where a person computes the total charge and the buyer makes payment to the cashier and then takes delivery of goods. Thus, super market follows the policy of 'self-help' by the customers. The customers are not pressurised by the salesmen. That is why, many people are attracted towards the super market.

Super market is organised on departmental basis and a customer can buy various types of goods under one roof. Super market can be differentiated from departmental store on the main ground that salesmen are not appointed to convince the customers about the quality of the products. The customers are free to choose the commodities of their choice. Moreover, a super market does not offer certain services which are usually provided by a departmental store. For instance, a super market does not allow credit sales and does not provide free home delivery service.

Merits : The following are the merits of a super market :

(i) A super market is a large scale retailing store : It enjoys all the benefits of large scale buying and selling. Its operating costs are lower and it can sell goods at cheaper rates.

(ii) Considerable atention is paid to the packaging of the products since there are no salesmen to convince and pressurise the customers. Many people like this distinct feature of self-service. They are free to compare different brands of a product and make selection without pressure from anybody.

(iii) The customers can make all their purchases under one roof. A super market provides goods to the customers at cheaper rates because of large turnover and absence of sales-force. The administrative over-heads per unit of a product are also lower.

(iv) Since super market sells only on cash basis, there is no chance of bad debts.

Demerits : A super market suffers from the following drawbacks :

(i) There are certain people who give greater weightage to personal attention. Such people do not like shopping through the super market as there are no salesmen.

(ii) Super markets cannot handle commodities that require personal attention by the salesmen.

(iii) Some customers handle the goods carelessly and misuse the opportunity of self-service and selection. This may cause a great cost to the super market.

(iv) In practice, super markets have not been able to create low price appeal among the customers because of higher overhead expenses.

(v) Establishment and running of a super market requires huge investment and its turnover should be very high to keep the overhead expenses under reasonable limits.

HIRE PURCHASE SHOP

Under hire purchase system, the buyer gets the immediate possession of the goods without paying the full price for them. He only pays part of the purchase price at the time of entering into the agreement with the seller and agrees to pay the balance in instalments which may be monthly, quarterly or yearly. An essential feature of hire purchase system selling is that the buyer gets only the possession of the goods, but the ownership of the goods passes to him only after the last instalment has been paid. In other words, the buyer is only the hirer until he pays the final instalment. Instalments paid by him are treated as mere hire charges. However, when the last instalment is paid, all the instalments are adjusted against the sale price of the goods and the interest thereon. If the buyer makes a default in paying any instalment, the seller has the right to take back the goods. Because of this, many people do not show much interest in purchasing goods under the hire purchase system.

One-Price Shops : "One-Price" shops or "Fixed Price Chain Stores" are organised on the same lines as multiple shop retail organisations. Their distinguishing feature is `one price'. They are one-price shops in the sense that almost everything sold at these shops is priced uniformly. Besides, `one price' also implies fixed prices and those stores, therefore, allow no scope for haggling.

6

DRUG HOUSE MANAGEMENT

Every drug store has to deal a number of routine works such as purchase, sell and display of merchandise, cleaning of the store, etc. This chapter is concerned with different aspects of drug store.

SELECTION OF SITE OF A DRUG STORE

From the point of view of drug store, the question of location refers to selection of an area in which the plant is to be located. The selection of the exact site or piece of land is also important. Briefly speaking, the following are the chief considerations which should determine the selection of a site.

  (i) Site is well connected with various modes of transport.

 (ii) The site has good surroundings. There should be no congestion of traffic.

(iii) The size of the plot has a sufficient scope for expansion.

(iv) Municipality rules and regulation allow the construction of building suited to the plant.

 (v) Certain essential service organisations like post office, bank and warehouse exist near the site.

The guiding principle in the fixation of location for the store is that it must result in the lowest unit cost in dispensing and distributing a product. The elements of total cost are transportation costs of material, cost of power and water, cost of plant site and building, rates and taxes, and labour and administrative costs. Besides these economic factors, there are other considerations which are the matter of judgement rather than mathematical calculation. For instance, personal or historical factors may compel a pharmacist to choose a particular site. Sometimes, a sub-optimum site may be chosen because no other site is available.

Urban Vs. Sub-urban Location

While selecting the site of a drug store, an entreprenuer must be clear in his mind about the basic questions, viz., whether the store should be located in an urban area or sub-urban area. Sites at both the places have their relative merits and demerits which are discussed below

Advantages of Urban location of stores are as follows :

1. Better transport and communication facilities.
2. Better supply of skilled labour.
3. Better educational facilities for employees and their children.
4. Better health and medical services.
5. Better publicity.
6. Better technical, financial and commercial facilities.
7. Better facilities for repair and maintenance.

Disadvantages of Urban location of stores are as follows :

1. Higher rates of land.
2. Higher municipal taxes and various restrictions on the use of land.
3. Higher cost of living.
4. Over-crowding and its evils.
5. Higher wages.
6. Extension is usually difficult and expensive.

Advantages of Sub-urban or Country location of stores are as follows :

1. Greater scope of future expansion.
2. Lower rates of land.
3. No congestion and overcrowding.
4. Lower wages.
5. Lower cost of living for the employees.
6. Social benefits arising out of distribution of industries in villages.

Disadvantages of Sub-urban or Country location of stores are as follows :

1. Restricted supply of skilled labour.
2. Difficulties in procurement of materials.
3. Lack of banking facilities.
4. Lack of educational facilities.
5. Lack of transport and communication facilities.

Small Town and Rural areas

For opening a drug store there the Nationalized banks for Rural Development Authorities, can sanction loans, on the premises or for acquiring inventory. The habits and psychology of the community should be studied. The actual site for the store will be in the main market place where people usually go for their shopping. The store should preferably be located near about the nursing home or clinics of the physicians with whom also he will have to build up good and sound professional relationship. A site to be selected is the potential buying power of the community. If it is rural area there will be predominance of farmers. Rural farming area will also be considered whether the potential customers will pay cash for their purchases otherwise the pharmacist will have to be prepared for extending credit, for a period determined by him by having a frank discussions with the community itself.

Selection of Store Site in Industrial Town-ship and Cities

In selecting the site in such areas the considerations is given to a place having industrial houses or industries. The larger number of steady workers will be living there. The viability of the industries and their financial stability is considered because only in such conditions the community member will make reasonably bigger amount of the purchase of articles stored by them. In all such areas a pharmacist will necessarily have to study the normal drugs requirements in order to build up a sound inventory, as well as the population make-up, their buying habits, their standards of living the various age groups of people, since all these factors affect the Store's business its success.

Drug Stores Relation to Other Markets

Neighbouring towns or cities may have many stores. Younger people in rural areas may go out of their houses for visiting theatres etc. If they pass by the store they may purchase drugs, etc. It would therefore, be advantageous to study the position of highway for the site selection. If there are major roads, leading directly to nearby communities and not the pharmacists proposed town, it is difficult to draw rural folks and the transient business.

The other developing trend is to locate drugs stores in the major railway stations, in the vicinity of petrol stations on the national highways, near the towns and villages and the air terminals.

Business Competition

This is a very important aspect of selecting the site of a drug store. In several cities, especially the state capitals, industrial cities, etc. which have lands around them and if newer cooperative housing societies are springing up, they are sure to develop shopping centres and schools etc. Such newly developing areas promise a good future for a drug store if an opportunity is taken well in time, although it may not promise to run well in the beginning.

Means of Determining the Opportunity for Another New Store

The drug purchasing power of the community is estimated for considering such aspects. The number of families is calculated who can buy drugs in the proposed location of the store. Multiply the number of families by a figure representing average family expenditure. This product represents the potential business for all pharmacists in the community. If the income are below or above the national average, adjustments is made to get it corrected.

Sales of existing stores, the number of proprietors and full time sales assistants are estimated. Total wages is approximately equal to one-sixth (1/6) of the total sales figure, and multiply it by six (6) which represents the volume of business. Now deduct family expenditure from the volume of business. The resultant figure indicates how much business will go away from the existing store; should a new owner pharmacist choose to locate the site of a new store in that locality.

Selection of Location in Metropolitan Cities

For establishing a drug store in metropolitan Cities like Delhi, Bombay, Calcutta, and Madras, the factors to consider are (i) nature of community residing, and (ii) their income from industrial or services or business activities sources. These cities are also the centres of wholesale business houses dealing in drugs, which is a distinct advantage to the retail stores. Further such locations have large degree of permanence of the residents, which provide a steady flow of income.

Selection of Store Location on the Outskirts of Big Cities

Here the pharmacist should collect information on such aspects as (1) probable number of customers, (2) their buying capacity which depends on their nature of work and occupation such as office workers, professional classes, casual workers or largely unemployed persons. The purchasing capacity may be determined by studying their income-pattern, the nature of their houses, habits of living, family background, culture, etc.

Newly Developing Areas

Due to population explosion of the country, the building activities are on the rise around such cities establishing newer colonies, cooperative housing societies and even around bigger villages on the fringe of the district headquarters town.

The pharmacist should choose one of these areas for locating his store, to remain away from hard competition.

The location near the traffic signals, should be avoided. In the vicinity of traffic signals there are parking problems for cars, scooters, cycles etc. of the customers. A shop located on that side of the road which takes people to their homes has got better purchasing power potential as majority of the workers prefer to do marketing while returning from their place of work. Thus, there may be a difference in the purchasing power of the two sides of a road.

The potential customers remain away from school premises, campus and the play grounds.

Neighbourhood of Hospitals

It is a good choice provided that the hospital does not maintain a drug store of its own.

Neighbourhood of Physician's Clinics, Dispensaries etc.

It is good if the doctors do not supply all drug to their patients but prefer to write the prescriptions, especially of the factory-made dosage forms. However a dispensing doctor is not helpful. It is rather a servere competition for the drug store.

Neighbourhood of Cinema Houses or Theatres

It is good if the Store has got enough cold storage facilities for serving cooled soft drinks to people, who when they visit for a soft drink after a picture show etc. may buy some drugs as well.

SPACE LAYOUT

Layout problems are fundamental to every type of organisation/enterprise and are experienced in all kinds of undertakings. Housewife must arrange her kitchen, retailer must arrange his counters and display the items in such a manner which facilitates movement and attract the attention of customers.

The adequacy of layout affects the efficiency of subsequent operations. It is an important perquisite for efficient operations and also has a great deal in common with many of the problems.

Impart the layout decisions were based merely on intution, experience, judgement and some sort of improvisation but with increase in the complexities of organisations the layout problems are solved scientifically.

Layout identically involves the allocation of space and the arrangement of equipment in such a manner that overall operating costs are minimised. Planning the layout of a plant is a continuous process as there are always chances of making improvements over the existing arrangement specially with shifts in the policies of management of techniques of production.

A good layout results in comforts convenience, safety, efficiency, compactness and profits. A poor layout results in congestion, waste, frustration and inefficiency. Development of a good layout depends on a series of decisions already taken on location, capacity, facility, manufacturing methods and material handling.

Layout of Stores Section : The layout of the stores section should be conductive to the materials to be stored and equipment etc. There should be enough space for materials handling and labour movement. A good stores layout is characterised by :

  (i) flexibility in arrangement.

 (ii) convenience in physical counting of materials.

(iii) items used sparingly should be easy to locate.

(iv) efficient protection against deterioration and pilferage of materials.

 (v) better stock control but minumum routine work like record maintenance etc.

(vi) efficient use of floor space and height.

(vii) safety from hazards, insurance etc.

(viii) proper illumination and ventillation.

 (ix) proper security arrangement, so that no person other than stores staff can enter the store.

(x)   heavy and bulky items should be stored as low as possible.

(xi) shelves and bins should not be very deep.

(xii) minimum handling and transportation of materials.

OBJECTIVES OF LAYOUT PLAN

1. To attract maximum customers.

2. To increase purchase from each customer.

3. To improve general appearance and professional image.

4. To maximise utilization of space.

5. To reduce pilferage, theft and provide surveillance.

6. To control movement inside the store.

Types of Drug Store and Design

1. **Traditional Drug Store and Design :** The customers are disperse in such a way that all areas of the drug store are exposed to them. Such design has pleasing appearance, professional atmosphere and convenient for workers and customers. It provide opportunity for maximum sales. But there are good chances of theft in such design.

2. **Pharmaceutical Centre :** This type of centre sells medicine, convenience articles, orthopaedic drugs and surgical applications. The store is decorated properly with sufficient floor space. Orthopaedic and surgical appliances are kept in a separate room.

3. **Super Drug Store and Design :** The area is in between 5,000 to 10,000 sq. ft. with a square design. Movement in the store is a major objective. Design is self-service pattern and all items are available in such drug store.

4. **Prescription Oriented Drug Store and Design :** Such drug stores have comfortable waiting area, health related items and drugs, and prescription accessories. These items are displayed near the vicinity. Orthopaedic and surgical appliances are kept in a separate room. Cosmetics and gifts are arranged in a suitable area.

5. **Personal (Clerk) Service Design :** During purchasing process, customer demands an article and a personal or cleric provides the article. This service and design facilitate maximum interchange between drug store persons and the customers. The success of the drug store depends on the convenience and friendly service. An increment of price of the product due to excess service overheads is the drawback of this design. This design can be provided for selected areas.

6. **Self Selection Design :** This Design is preferred for non-prescription drugs, cosmetics, photosupplies, greetings, etc. Customers can inspect, handle and select articles themselves.

7. **Self Service Design :** This service design is utilized in Super Drug Store where the articles are sold in this style. All purchases are controlled by central checkout. All self-service is not possible in a drug store due to prescription department.

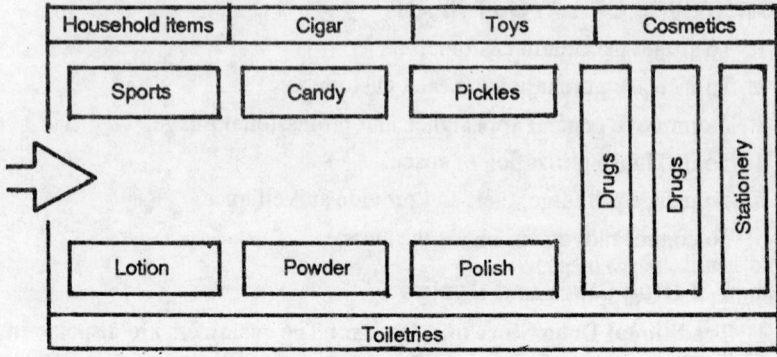

Fig. 1-Central Service Style

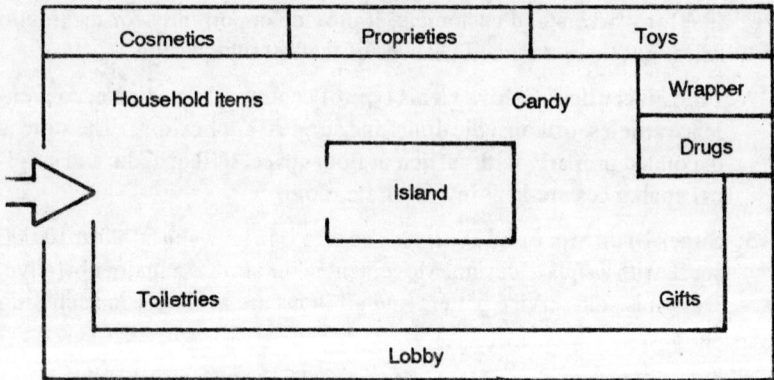

Fig. 2-Lobby Checkout Style

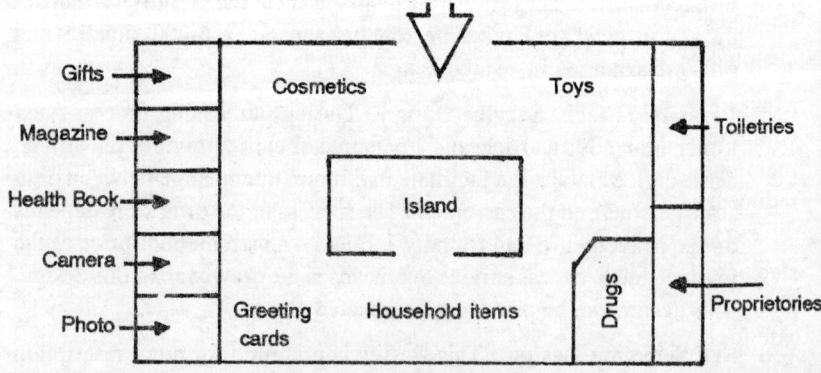

Fig. 3-Off the Wall Style

Styles of Layout Design : The different layout designs are :

(1) Lobby checkout style in which islant is near the gate,

(2) Central service style in which the checkout island is located in the centre,

(3) Right rear service style in which self service is promoted as in super drug stores, and

(4) Off the wall style in which there is a direct entrance from the middle portion and goods are arranged on three sides. This type of arrangement is easy and low costing of installing fixtures.

Characteristics of a Drug Store : The design should accommodate personal service, special selling skill service, cosmetics, gifts, greeting cards, books and health magazines. All the parts of the store should be effective. Cash counter and wrapping counter should be near the gate. The goods should be arranged closely. The dental, toiletries, hygienic, cosmetics and OTC products should be kept near the wrapping counter as they are advertised extensively. Prescription should be arranged as industry-wise, disease wise and alphabetically to facilitate their identification. There should be sufficient waiting space with comfortable chairs and magazines. The items of the special skill department such as photography, imported gifts, jewellery and drugs should be used with special design feature to reflect the profession. Sufficient lightning should be provided which gives cheerful atmosphere for customers and employees. It helps in identifying the goods quickly. Store's name and drug logo in coloured hight attracts the customers very much. The size of a drug store should be 600 sq. ft. to accommodate maximum departments.

There should be convenience to customers and overcrowding should be avoided. Functional areas of a drug store are space for incoming goods, reserve stock and office, counter for customers, resting room and toilet facilities, telephone facility, shutter and flap door entrance for the store personals and important customers, refrigerator and shelves for keeping medicines. Good attractive design layout will improve the sale, attraction of customers and reduction of competition.

Stores Equipments : A good store is equipped with various types of tools/ equipments for handling, measuring and weighing the materials. The equipment should be such that stores investment and operating expenses are reduced.

The various modes of storing are open and closed shelves, cabinets, stacking, pallets and skids, bins, stacking boxes, gravity feed racks, outdoor platforms etc. The facilities can be of wood or steel. Wooden equipment is safe for delicate items and can be installed quickly. It is inexpensive but is rather inflexible. Steel equipment is more flexible with advantages of more strength, fire resistance and easy maintenance.

Material Handling Facilities : These basically depend upon the nature of items as well as the size and shape of the storage space. It also depends on how much frequently an item is used in production operations. The material handling equipments in stores can be trolleys, mobile jigs, cranes, conveyer belts etc.

There should also be proper weighing and measuring instruments at the time of receiving and issuing the materials.

Identification of Materials in Stores : *There should be place for everything and everything should be in its place.* Provision of a good identification system in stores assists those who try to keep everything in place. Depending on the size and nature of the organisation, the store can have a variety of items in stock. It may not be possible to remember and locate these items inside the store simply by their names. The task can be simplified by proper coding of the items as well as their location. Identification can be done by :

(i) tagging some piece of paper or cloth with the items.

(ii) labels may be fixed on the items.

(iii) the coded number or any other identification mark may be embossed on the items (codification).

(iv) painting or colour coding of items.

Advantages of Coding Items

(i) an asset in keeping records.

(ii) facilitates quick identification.

(iii) mechanised accounting is possible.

(iv) eliminates the chances of duplication of items.

Methods of Coding

Generally alphabets, numerals or a combination of the two is used for codification of items. The following methods can be used for code construction:

(a) **Mnemonic Method :** Here alphabets closely associated with the name of the item are used e.g. *MT* can be used for some metallic items. This method is useful when few type of items are to be stored.

(b) **Random Method :** Here both alphabets or numerals can be used randomly. But the method is rather arbitrary.

(c) **Scientific Method :** The items are divided into a number of groups and each group is given some code. Then further sub-grouping is done on the basis of classification of item in any group, its shape, function, etc.

Then complete code of the items is written by combining the sub-codes of groups and sub-groups for that item.

Location Coding : Storeroom is divided in blocks of storage units and each block is identified by lateral block letter and a longitudinal block letter. Within each block every row of shelves is given a number. Each row is divided vertically in to columns and horizontally into shelves. Blocks and Rows are identified by painted signs.

Sometimes items requiring special protection for storages viz. rust/corrison proof space for metal parts are stored in dry areas. It is an asset for easy and quick location of items when the size of the store is very big. Each place is coded by alphabets or numerals. The location can be identified in terms of the number of the warehouse, row number, column number, rack number, shelf or bin number etc. Location of any item inside the store can also be decided in three ways :

(i) **Fixed location :** Here some fixed place is designated to each class of item. The basis can be (i) Supplierwise (ii) Itemwise (iii) Utility of the item, etc.

(ii) **Random location :** Items are places according to the availability of space in store at the time of receiving the items. This method can be applied when the number of items to be stored is few and store-keeper is efficient in remembering the location of each item.

(iii) **Zonal location :** Generally the whole inventory is divided into three Zones, namely (i) Bulk Zone, (ii) Reserve stock and (iii) Indirect material like spares and consumable items. This approach tries to avail full benefit of the space and other storage facilities.

Issue Section : This section handles the issue of materials when required by some department of the enterprise. A storeroom does not always issue a material in the same units in which it is purchased as the materials are purchased in gross and issued in dozen. The standard unit of issue for a material is usually defined as the smallest quantity likely to be issued. Inventory is always recorded in standard units. Materials carry some money value and in order to avoid malpractices and to curb the tendency of waste, the items should be issued against proper requisition. The material requisition is a request to the stockroom to issue materials. It gives details of the type and quantity of the material, the use to be made of them and is duly signed by some authorised person.

The requisition should be properly checked and scruitnised before the issue of the material. The stock clerk puts the identification number of the desired materials on the requisition and passes it to the stock record clerk. The record clerk subtracts the amount of material issued from the record card, calculates the balance in stock and sends it to the accounting department. The accounts clerk subtracts the value of the account for which material is issued.

On the basis of the requisition, the stores staff finally collects the items from the stores and send them to the requisitioning department. All requisitions must be posted daily on the bin cards and the stock control cards. The fresh balance is struck on every receipt or issue.

In some cases due to economy measures and convenience in handling operations the quantity of the material issued from the stores is more than the amount requisitioned from the concerned department. In such cases the charge is made for the actual quantity issued. Similarly when excess materials are returned to stores, a stores debit note or shop credit note is prepared to ensure the proper record and entry of the item in stores.

Handling of Drug Stores

The functions of store keeping are related with receiving, safe custody in stores and issuing the material against authorised requisition at the minimum cost. The main functions of store-keeping can be outlined as :

  (i) receiving, handling and speedy issue of material.

 (ii) custodian of goods in store against damage and pilferage.

(iii) to ensure regular supply of materials.

(iv) effective utilisation of store space.

 (v) to provide service to the organisation in most economical way.

(vi) to keep the details of the items available in store up to date.

(vii) proper identification and easy location of items.

(viii) physical checking of stocks.

Objectives of Store-handling

  (i) easy location of the items in store.

 (ii) proper identification of items.

(iii) speedy issue of material.

(iv) efficient utilisation of space.

 (v) reduction in need of material handling equipment.

Duties of Store-keeper : The following are the main responsibilities of stores controller :

  (i) the items in stores should be placed in such a way that these can be easily located.

 (ii) to maintain the store premises neat and clean.

(iii) efficient and effective service to the customers.

(iv) to ensure that materials are issued against authorised requisition only.

 (v) to keep up-to-date record of materials issued, received and balance in stock.

(vi) planning and executing of stock checking activities.

(vii) communicate the purchase department about its requirements.

(viii) to maintain efficient and effective material handling system.

Receipt System

When a purchase order is placed, a copy of it is sent to the stores department indicating quantity and delivery date. The purchase orders should be arranged choronologically so that total volume of receipt at any time may be estimable.

    Outside Supliers : On despatching items, normally send an advice note to the stores showing date of despatch, carrier details, description of the consignment and the value of items. This ensures quick and easy clearance of bills etc.

The purchase copy, suppliers note and transporter information/consignment note enables the stores manager to organise and plan for expeditious clearance of materials and minimise costly demurrage.

Internal Suppliers : Whenever materials are received from internal divisions or returned from user departments transfer notes and returns to stores documents are usually used for this purpose.

Receiving section in stores department can be centralised, semi-centralised or decentralised. In a centralised receiving department a categories of items are received, checked and inspected at one common place. In semi-centralised light weight items are received, checked and inspected at one common place whereas heavy weight or items of unmanageable size are received, checked and inspected at the place of storage. In both cases the records are maintained in the same stock book. In a decentralised system all items are received, checked and inspected by their respective departments.

The building where receiving section is located should have sufficient space for loading, unloading and inspection of the consignments. Receiving and despatching sections should be at a distance from each other to avoid confusion among incoming and outgoing items.

In case of stores keeping of finished goods, the uptodate position of stocks inside the stores should be regularly communicated to marketing department of the organisation.

Stores Section : This is a place where all materials received by the stores department are kept with protection against deterioation and pilferage. They are stored in such a way that their location is easily indentified as at the time of issue.

Continuous Stock-taking (Perpetual Inventory System) : The store-keeper must always take care to see that the quantity mentioned in the bin card is represented by the actual stock. Many concerns have the practice of checking stocks only annually. Generally, it is found that there is a discrepancy between the figures revealed by the books and the actual stock. If the discrepancy is small, the actual stock figures are accepted and the book figures are adjusted. This is not really proper because this may lead to petty thefts. What should be done is that the storekeeper or somebody else should check about twenty items of stores every day by rotation. In this manner, all the items in a store can be checked up about three or four times in a year. It should be the duty of the storekeeper to explain fully any discrepancy between actual stock and the book figure. In this manner, he will be sure as to whatever the bin card indicates is represented by the physical stock. The management must make it clear to the storekeeper that no unexplained discrepancy will be accepted besides taking care of petty thefts. This practice also has the following advantages :

(a) The annual stock checking will be dispensed with because there will be no difference between actual stock and book figure.

(b) The storekeeper will know if there is any damage occurring to the goods. Such a damage can be stopped in its initial stages.

(c) If any theft has taken place that will be found out at early stages and steps can be taken to catch the culprit.

(d) It acts as moral check on the staff.

Stores Ledger : In a drug store, the stores ledger is of importance because this facilitates the calculation of the value of goods. In a big concern, the maintenance of stores ledger also serves as a check on the storekeeper. There are various methods on the basis of which the issue price can be calculated. These are as follows :

1. **First in first out (FIFO) :** In this case, the price of the earliest consignment lying in stock will be the price at which the issues are to be costed.

2. **Last in first out (LIFO) :** In this case, the price of the latest consignment in stock is used for calculating the value of issues.

3. **Average issue :** In this case, when a new stock of goods is received the total value of goods in stock is divided by the total quantity in hand and this will give the average price. All issues of goods will be made at this price until a new consignment is again received. Then a new price will be calculated.

4. **Market price :** This ignores the cost altogether and the issues are made at the prevailing market price.

5. **Inflated price :** This method is used for those goods which are subject to some wastage. The total amount paid is divided by the quantity expected to be finally available for use and that rate is used for issue of goods.

LEGAL REQUIREMENTS

The drug store may be a rented premises. The rent amount depands on the building in which the shop is located. In bigger cities, there is shortage of space. The store premises are acquired on paying heavy premium and rents. Various terms and agreements concerning rent, length of possession, and actual use of the store premises should be done in writing through a lawyer and the signed agreement should be registered in the office of the government which may be available if the previous copy is lost. The scope of the shop is modified according to need. Usually the store premises rooms are squire or rectangular. The ideal dimensions for suitable rooms area are 7 m width and depth. The shop is occupied after the payment of rent or instalments if the shop is in the shopping centre of a cooperative society. Any damage to the premises, e.g. defacement of walls, broken glass pans, electric supply, etc. should be properly repaired in consultation with the landlord before occupying the store.

The lease should be renewed annually by mutual agreement with the owners. The concellation of the lease agreement may be done by mutual agreement or by taking possession of the vaccant premises. The owner may terminate the lease and take possession of the premise if the tenant does not pay rent, insurance, electric and water charges. The lease agreement may be terminated if the landlord does not fulfil the requirements such as repairing of the premises.

The store may be insured against all exigencies covered by the insurance act such as automobile accidents and public liability.

Legal Aspects to Drug Store

To run a drug store the specific laws imposed are : (1) Drug and Cosmetic Act and Rules (1940 and 1945), (2) Poison Act, 1919; (3) Dangerous Drug Act; (4) Prohibition and excise rule; (5) Pharmacy Act, 1948 and (6) Shop and Establishment Act.

To establish a drug store, The following requirements should be fulfilled :

1. **Minimum Academic Qualification :** A Registered Pharmacist is eligible to establish and run a medical store. This certificate is issued to a person qualifying Diploma or Degree in Pharmacy and has completed a training for 650 hours in a medical store recognized by the State Pharmacy council or usually by a government hospital. The training is not compulsory for the degree students in Pharmacy. The certificatge is issued by the State Pharmacy Council.

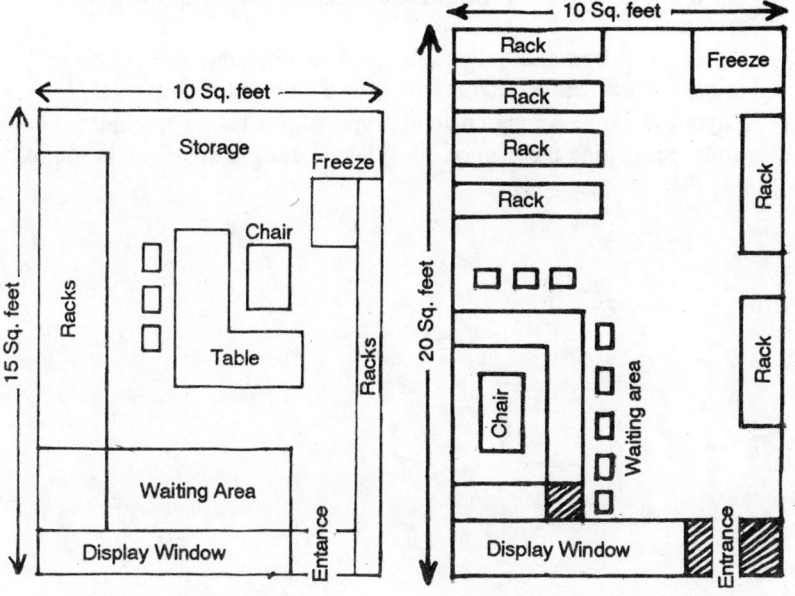

Fig. 4 Drug Store Design

Fig. 5 Wholesale Drug Store Design

For starting a wholesale drug store, sufficient experience in pharmaceutical selling or production in addition to Diploma or Degree Certificate.

A graduate in Science (B.Sc.) with 10 years of medical representative experience can also start the wholesale business.

A retail or wholesale business can be run by appointing a registered pharmacist.

2. **Minimum Space :** Minimum space required to run a drug store is 150 sq. ft. area while an area of 200 sq. ft. is necessary to start a wholesale drug store.

3. **Licence :** A licence is required for running a shop according to shop and establishment act from the labour office situated at district place. The place for the shop should be authorized. For getting a shop act licence, the specified number of people working in organization, weekly holiday, salary paid and attendance register of employees are maintained. Licence is generally issued for 3 years on the basis of ownership proof or rent receipt and renewed for next years.

For selling homoeopathic drugs, the licence can be obtained from FDA. For selling Ayurvedic and Unani drugs, licence is not required. Insecticide and pesticide licences can be obtained from Agriculture College or from the FDA. Central Sales Tax (C.S.T.), State Sales Tax (S.S.T.) and Income Tax numbers can be obtained by applying to the respective office.

All licences are preserved in frames and displayed in the proposed premises.

4. **Other Requirements :** For selling some vitamins, and antibiotics, refrigerator is required. Drugs are placed on wooden or glass shelves.

Layout Design : A rough plan of proposed retail store is submitted in triplet for getting the licence. Ideal layout designs are given in Fig. 4 and Fig. 5.

7

PURCHASING

Purchasing can be defined as that function of a business undertaking which is responsible for the procurement of materials, supplies, tools and implements, machinery and services required to produce certain goods.

Thus purchasing is an operation of market exploration to procure goods and services of desired quality, quantity at lowest price and at the desired time. Supplier who can provide standard items at the competitive price are selected.

Purchasing is a managerial activity that goes beyond the simple act of buying. It includes research and development for the proper selection of materials and sources, followup to ensure timely delivery; inspection to ensure both quantity and quality; to control traffic, receiving, storekeeping and accounting operations related to purchases.

Objectives of Purchasing : The objectives of Purchasing should conform with the overall objectives of the organisation. It is one activity where reasonable economic can be accomplished. The following are the main objectives of purchasing :

(i) **Purchase of satisfactory material :** To procure materials which are most appropriate to the product and are supplied in right quantity and quality at right time and right price.

(ii) **To control the quantity of material :** Purchase of material needs investment. Buying too much or too little quantity may not be in economic interest of the organisation i.e. too much quantity may unnecessary block the capital whereas too little purchase order may affect the regular supply of production. The purchasing department ensures economic capital investment and regular flow of production.

(iii) **Proper negotiations with suppliers :** Search for potential suppliers is an important activity of purchasing. This ensures timely supply of materials in the most economic manner. Wrong selection of supplier may be harmful to the enterprise both in terms of price and delivery time. Purchasing department through its dealing with suppliers creates goodwill and enhances the reputation of the enterprises.

(iv) **Controls proper use of materials :** By analysing the requirement of various departments of the organisation, the purchase department avoids duplication, waste and obsolescence of materials and equipments.

(v) **Co-ordination with other departments :** The purchase department should develop full co-ordination and maintain close relationship between various departments of the organisation.

(vi) **Maintenance of Company's goodwill :** By maintaining the quality standards of the material the purchasing activity is instrumental in generating the confidence of consumer in the product of the company.

(vii) **Other objectives can be :**

(a) exploration to locate new suppliers.

(b) information about new materials and processes which can reduce the cost of production and improve the performance of the product.

(c) to achieve economy and efficiency in the activities of the purchases department by analysing its performance.

Organisation of Purchase Department : The composition of purchase department varies according to the size of the enterprise, its comparative significance towards procurement and the capability of the purchase personnel.

The size of the purchasing departments depends on the nature of products manufactured by the organisation, sizes of the production runs and type of the manufacturing system.

In the organisation, purchase manager occupies an important position. He should be a man of quick decision-making power, pleasing personality, quality of good leadership and farsighted approach should be inherent in him.

In an organisation, where purchasing is recognised as a separate function, a separate department may be set up for the performance of the purchasing activities in the organisation. This is known as centralised purchasing. The central purchase department is organised under the incharge-ship of Purchase Officer or Purchase Manager who is responsible for all the purchasing activities. Centralised purchasing has the following benefits :

(i) **Specialisation :** Specialists can be employed in the purchase department to look after the purchasing activities. Their specialised knowledge will help in achieving the objectives of purchasing discussed above.

(ii) **Economy :** Since purchases are made in large quantities by the expert purchasers, better terms and conditions can be obtained from the suppliers. There are economies in transport also.

(iii) **Better Control** : Centralised purchasing facilitates better control and coordination of activities related to purchasing.

(iv) **No Duplication** : Since purchase is done by one department, there is avoidance of duplication of efforts, correspondence, etc.

(v) **Research** : The purchase department can undertake research of sources óf supplies. It can locate substitutes and novelties for use in the enterprise.

(vi) **Import of Goods** : For importing the goods from foreign countries, centralised purchasing is preferable. Centralisation of authority to purchase will help in specialising in import trade which involves many complicated procedures and regulations.

Centralised purchasing suffers from the following drawbacks :

(i) Centralised purchasing may not be economical because of less than full utilisation of the services of purchase specialists.

(ii) The purchases are not made by the users but by the purchase department. Sometimes, the users are in a position to make better purchases.

(iii) It takes longer time to make purchases through the purchase department.

(iv) It is not suitable when the branches are located at far away places. This will increase transport costs.

Decentralised Purchasing

Under decentralised purchasing, the authority of purchase is delegated to various departments. Every department is responsible for purchasing its own requirements. Decentralised purchasing is better where the various plants of the organisation are quite big, autonomous and located in different territories. This will avoid delay in getting the supplies and local people will be satisfied as they have a say in purchasing. This will increase the efficiency of various departments and will help in maintaining secrecy.

Decentralised purchasing also suffers from certain drawbacks. There will be no uniformity of purchase procedure in the organisation. Some departments may purchase the materials at higher prices because every manager cannot be an expert in purchasing. Moreover, some managers may consider purchasing as an unnecessary botheration. It is advantageous to have centralised purchasing if the various departments require the same types of materials even though they are located at different places. This will facilitate coordination in the purchasing function.

Function of Purchasing Department : The main object of purchase department is to purchase items of specified quality and quantity at lowest price. To accomplish this, the functions of the department are :

1. **Processing the requisition** : The departments of the organisation communicate to the purchase department their requirement for various

items through requisition form. The format of requisition form contains the details of the quality, quantity and other necessary specifications about the item to be purchased. The requisition is to be signed by the competent authority.

The purchase requisition is prepared in duplicate and the original copy is sent to the purchase department. The purchase department processes and scruitinises the requisition and then proceeds to other operations for making purchases.

2. **Selection of suppliers :** The potential vendors are contacted through authorised representatives, their catalogues and sample of the items are inspected and examined either at the purchaser's place or at the vendor's place. On the basis of findings from inspection, examination of samples and analysis of the quoted prices, suppliers are approved for placing the orders. The criterion for the ultimate choice of a vendor is based on following aspects :

   (i) *Reliability of supply :* Past performance specially in the time of crisis as well as sound financial position of a supplier classifies him to be reliable.

   (ii) *Assurance of timely delivery :* The punctuality pattern in observing the delivery schedule provided by the purchaser during past deals ensures the prompt supply by the vendor.

   (iii) *Other considerations :* After sales service, technical assistance, attitude with regard to the goods rejected by the purchaser and co-operation in disposal of waste are some important guiding factors for the choice of suppliers.

   Purchasing agents continually scan the market place in search of potential new suppliers. Continued monitoring and evaluation of the supplier performance is necessary and should be based upon actual results.

3. **Placing of orders :** The purchase department tries to purchase the materials with desired quality and quantity at the most advantageous terms. All purchases should be made through a purchase order in a specified form and duly signed by some authorised person. The purchase order must contain the details about the supplier, description of the items required, corresponding prices and amount required.

   As a rule original copy is sent to the supplier, one copy is retained by the purchase department and one copy is sent to the concerned department requiring the ordered items.

4. **Follow-up or Progressing the purchase orders :** Receiving the ordered material at the right time is most important for an organisation. Late deliveries can close the enterprise. For this follow-up or expediting the purchase order after waiting for some reasonable time is essential. The priority of follow-up operations should be given according to

the importance or classification of items *e.g.* 'A' class items are to be given topmost priority.

It is also necessary to review the outstanding orders at regular intervals.

5. **Invoices received from suppliers are checked and verified with the order specification :** The process includes the following activities :

   (i) the goods supplied are of desired specifications both in quality and quantity.

   (ii) comparison of quoted price and the price charged in the invoice.

   (iii) if some goods supplied does not conform with the specifications or are damaged during transhipment then steps are taken for adjustments on claims.

6. **Some other functions of purchase department can be :**

   (i) to maintain records regarding suppliers, their performance in past, products available with them, probable delivery period for each order etc.

   (ii) to dispose off outdated and scrapped items.

   (iii) control stores operation of receiving the items from vendors and issuing it to concerned departments of the organisation.

   (iv) to evaluate the performance of the department.

   (v) to collect information about trends in market regarding availability of improved goods and services and also about the substitute products in case of emergency.

   (vi) to handle damages and demurrage claims.

Methods of Purchasing : There are a number of methods used by different purchase departments. The methods used depend on the classification of products in the production system, policy of the organisation and behaviour of the market. Following are some popular methods of purchasing :

   (i) **Purchasing according to requirement :** In such cases an order is placed only when there is some need for the product. This method is appropriate for those items which are not of regular and common use in the production process. These items are generally not stored in inventories.

   (ii) **Market Purchasing :** The policy of making the purchases at a time when the fluctuations in price of the items provide advantage to the purchaser is known as market purchasing. This method provides procrument at lower price and saving in purchase expenses. This method is useful in situations where major price variations are prominent.

   (iv) **Speculative purchasing :** Here excessive purchases are made when market is low for the item with the hope of earning profit by selling the items purchased in excess at a higher price. This procedure is most suitable in the case of staple commodities e.g. cotton for textiles. The merits of this method lies in more profits and more protection against shortages. This method involves more financial commitments on the part of the organisation.

(v) **Contract purchasing :** Here the purchase department enters into agreement with various suppliers to supply the items at some future period or periodically. The purchasing under contract is usually formal for the needed material, the delivery of which is frequently spread over a period of time. The organisation tries to enter into the contract when prices are comparatively low.

(vi) **Scheduled purchasing :** It is a scientific method of purchasing. The purchasing is scheduled according to requirements of various departments of the organisation. Vendors know in advance about the future demand of the purchaser. Proper balance is made between amount procured and amount required.

Steps in purchasing procedure : The following is the routine commonly followed by various purchasing departments :

(i) Various departments are requested to send their requirements on a proper requisition form.

(ii) Purchasing department consolidates the requirements from various departments to know the total requirement for each item.

(iii) Market exploration is made to locate the goods and services of desired quality and quantity at the resonable price.

(iv) Potential suppliers are identified from catalogues, quotations and past records.

(v) Purchase order in specified form is prepared and sent to the approved suppliers. Purchase order is the commitment of the buyer to the supplier establishing a contractual relationship between buyer and seller.

(vi) After some time of placing the order, follow-up process starts to get quick delivery of the items.

(vii) The items are received by the purchasing department at the time of delivery and the items received are compared with purchase order. The checking of the delivered goods is done with regard to (a) prices charged and quoted (b) approval of the invoice (c) to ascertain the quality and quantity of the items

Modes of Purchasing : Goods may be purchased in any of the following ways:

(i) by inspection,

(ii) by sample or pattern, and

(iii) by description or brand.

Purchasing by inspection refers to the ordinary method of visiting the premises of the seller for inspection of the whole lot proposed to be purchased. It has limited scope and utility in so far as only consumers living in the local area in which the seller's showrooms are located can really make use of this facility.

"*A sample* is specimen of goods, particularly of raw materials, food-stuffs, etc." It can be regarded as representative of the bulk. Its quality will reflect to a large extent the quality of the whole lot. While purchasing goods, the sample may be carefully examined by the intending purchaser. It will give him a fair idea of the quality of the bulk. Likewise, a pattern is a specimen of standardised manufactured reveals the varieties of shade and texture and provides a convenient way of buying. The code number given on the pattern is all that has to be stated about the type of goods when an order is placed for them. The goods in bulk or bigger lots will be of the same quality as the sample or pattern shown to the buyer.

Yet another method of purchasing is *by description*. Certain products are given brand names which acquired popularity through repetitive advertising. Similarly, certain sellers issue catalogues and price lists which contain the description of goods offered for sale. An intending purchaser may, in these cases, specify a particular brand or particular number in the catalogue to order the goods that he intends to purchase.

Credit Information

An amount entered on the right or credit side is called a credit, or a credit entry. The act of recording of credit is called Crediting the account.

For all sales of merchandise, the terms of payment should be clearly stated, so that buyer and seller can avoid any misunderstandings as to the time and amount of the required payment.

Credit Memoranda

The suppler upon being informed of the return of damage merchandise will issue a credit memorandum as evidence that the account receivable from the purchaser is being credited (reduced) by the supplier.

No business concern wants to sell on credit to a customer who will prove unable or unwilling to pay his or her account. Consequently most business organisations have a credit department which investigates the credit worthiness of each prospective customer. If the prospective customer is a business concern, its financial statements will be obtained and analyzed to determine its financial strength and the trend of operating results. The credit department naturally prefers to rely upon financial statements which have been audited by certified public accountants.

The credit department will probably include the obtaining of a credit report from a local credit agency or from a national credit-rating institution.

A credit agency compiles credit data on individuals and business concerns and distributes this information to its clients. Most companies that make numerous sales on credit find it worthwhile to subscribe to the services of one or more credit agencies.

In pharmaceutical marketing, 45 days credit facility on payment of invoice bill is given from some of the manufacturer's side to the wholesalers. For new wholesale such credit facility is not given initially. He has to take the orders through bank by paying the amount. A wholesaler usually gives the 21 days credits to retailer after established business relationship.

8

TENDERS

A tender or a quotation is a written offer to do a work or to provide a material at a given price within a prescribed period and under certain specific conditions.

Types of Tenders

Following are the four types of tenders :

1. **Single Tender :** When the quality is of extreme importance only a reliable firm will be asked to supply and rates are fixed by mutual acceptance.

2. **Closed Tender :** When material is required, firms which are registered will be invited to tender their rates and the most economic offer will be considered for placing the order.

   In this system, the tenders are invited only from some limited firms. Hence, this system is also called "Limited Tender System".

   The last date to tender, the terms and conditions of supply and payments are mentioned in the tender notice. If the rate quoted by more than one firm are same, the order is placed on a known reliable firm.

3. **Open Tender :** This type of tender system is adopted when quantities to be purchased involve large amount. Here this system is also known as "unlimited tender system". A tender notice in trade newspapers journals etc. is published, so that wide publicity can be given.

   All the interested firms will apply for the tender form, available at certain price. These tender forms contain dates of receiving and opening the tenders, the approximate quantity required, period and place of delivery, specifications and other terms and conditions for supply.

   Any firm is at liberty to quote, without any restriction. Tender forms are supplied on request to parties interested.

4. **Global tender :** Tenders are invited from all parts of the world. These are for large contracts for supplies from foreign countries or when foreign collaboration in proposed projects is considered necessary.

Notice Inviting Tenders

Tenders are invited by the industry when some material is required to be purchased. The tenders are invited from the firms, dealing with the supply of the items to be purchased. The notice should contain the following :

(1) Name of material to be purchased with detailed specification and if necessary drawing must also be enclosed.

(2) Quantity to be purchased.

(3) If the material required is of particular make, it must also be mentioned.

(4) Whether the sample is to be sent with tenders.

(5) Period of delivery.

(6) Earnest money to be deposited.

(7) Terms and conditions of purchase.

(8) Date, time and place for receiving and opening of the tenders.

After receiving the Tender Notice, supplier must send the tenders or quotations so that it may reach before the date and time of opening. While filling up the tenders, conditions mentioned in the notice must be fulfilled. Other conditions, if any must also be mentioned so that no dispute may arise afterward. Following should also be clearly mentioned in the tender :

(1) Whether the rates are F.O.R. or ex-godown.

(2) If rates for items having different specifications are quoted, it must be clearly mentioned.

(3) Guarantee period, if any.

(4) If necessary, drawings must be enclosed.

(5) Whether rates are inclusive of sales tax or not.

(6) Percentage of advance payment, if desired.

(7) Whether packing and forwarding charges are extra or included in the rates.

Opening of Tenders

The tenders are sent by the suppliers in sealed envelope (the word "tender" or "quotation" and its date of opening must be written on the top of the envelope). On the date of opening, at the prescribed time, purchase officer opens all the tenders or quotations received till that time, in the presence of the representatives of the suppliers, if present. At the time of opening the tenders or quotations, the purchase officer writes on each tenders - S.N. of tender/Total No. of tenders received/No. of pages in that particular tender e.g. when he writes on any tender 4/13/3, it means, this tender is IV out of 13 tenders received and it has 3 pages. He also attests the corrections and overwritings if any, at the time of opening the tender.

COMPARATIVE STATEMENT

After opening and numbering of all the tenders or quotation, a comparative statement is prepared. This helps to study the proposals in one sight. Following proforma is generally used for preparing the comparative statement.

Comparative Statement

Date of issue of N.I.T.   Date of receipt of tenders

S.No.	Name of Article with specification	Quantity reqd.	Firm No. 1 Rate in Rs.	Firm No. 2 Rate in Rs.	
			Terms & conditions (1) (2) (3)	(1) (2) (3)	

This statement gives all the details including alternative offers, terms and conditions of delivery, if differs than that required. This statement should be perfectly correct. Purchase Officer studies this statement thoroughly and takes the advise of the experts, if required. It is not always necessary to purchase the items only from the firms quoting lowest rates. For this purpose, sample, specifications, make, guarantee period, period of supply, other expenses like freight, sales tax, packing and forwarding charges etc. are considered.

The person authorised to accept the tenders should be specified. Financial limits are laid down for various levels of management for the purpose of acceptance of tenders so that the value of a tender decides as to who would be the competent person to accept it. For major purchases, other than routine purchases, representatives from the Production Department which is ultimately to use the material are also associated with the opening and acceptance of tenders. Various factors like price, quality, reliability of source, terms of delivery and terms of payment are considered and adjusted to a common denominator and the tender of the firm offering the best advantage is accepted. It is not necessary that the lowest tender would always be the most advantageous and in some cases, higher tenders may be accepted if they offer other compensating benefits like better terms of payment and delivery, superior quality of materials, continuity of supply and improved business relations. Lower tenders may also be discarded on the ground that the quoting firm is found to have resorted to price cutting to eliminate other competitors from the market or that it has failed to deliver goods in time in the past.

Issue of tenders to suppliers : On receipt of the indents from the stores department the next step in purchasing is to issue tenders to the prospective suppliers. Against these tenders, the suppliers quote their prices and terms of delivery for the materials that are required. It is a trade practice that these tenders should be sent out simultaneously to all the suppliers and they are intimated the specific time and date up to which their offers will be received. After the due date for the receipts of quotations is over, the tenders are opened and a comparative statment of the various quotations received is made out. These tenders are prepared in triplicate and the first two copies are sent to the supplier. The supplier returns the original with his quotations and retains the second copy for his record. The third copy is the file copy of the Purchase Department.

In choosing the supplier with whom the order is to be placed, the purchase department must primarily take into consideration the reliability of the supplier. Reliability has to be judged from two angles, viz., quality and timely delivery. The information on this should be readily available from the record of the said supplier's performances against the orders placed with him on earlier occasions. Apart from reliability, the finincial stability and the capacity to deliver the goods should also be ensured. It often happens that a supplier who has quoted a low price, has neither the machinery nor the finances to produce the materials ordered. He invariably buys them from another party or else comes up with a request for advance payment. Both these should be guarded against, as these are likely to affect not only the quality of the material but also the delivery schedule. If a supplier is found satisfactory on these grounds, it will be advisable to place orders with him, even though his price may not be the lowest. The higher price paid will be more than compensated by the comparatively lower percentage of rejections and productions hold-ups.

9

CONTRACTS DETERMINATION

The term "cotnract" stands for a job which is big in size and which requires considerable length of time to complete it. It is normally a type of work which is done outside the premises of the factory. Construction of a building, a road, a bridge are examples of such jobs which can be termed as contracts.

When a job of such a nature is to be performed, then the person who agrees to perform the job is called contractor; the person for whom the job is done is called a contractee ; the job is called a contract ; the price for which it is agreed to be done is called contract price. In order to understand the nature and complexities of contract account it is necessary to know the meaning of some more terms which are given below :

(1) **Work certified :** A contractor, since engaged in a big job which needs heavy investment and long time to complete it, often does not want to wait until the completion of contract for receiving the contract price. It is, therefore, usually agreed that contract price will be paid in instalments. The contractee, before making payment of instalment, wants to be sure that a part of the job for which the payment is being made has been completed according to the specifications. In order to be sure of this, he sends his engineers to verify and certify the value of the job completed. The value of the job so certified by the engineers as complete is called work certified. The payment is made on the basis of the value of the work shown in the certificate. Such payments are known as progress payments.

If the debit side of contract account exceeds its credit side then the difference is termed as loss. If the credit side of contract account exceeds its debit side then difference is called notional profit.

(2) **Work uncertified :** When the contractee's engineers come to certify the work, they often see some work which has not reached a stipulated stage. No certificate is issued for such work and no payment is made for

it. This work is called work uncertified. It is valued at cost price. This figure is similar to closing stock in trading account. The amount of uncertified work is debited to work-in-progress account and credited to contract account.

(3) **Retention money :** The contractee does not make payment of the total amount of the work certified. He often retains some portion of this amount as a guarantee towards any defects which may be located after some time. This retention money is released only after the expiry of the stipulated period.

(4) **Plant :** Depreciation of machine used on the contract is shown on the debit side of the `contract account'. If, however, a machine has been purchased particularly for the contract then it is better to show the book value of the plant in the beginning on the debit side of contract account and its book value at the end (after depreciation) on the credit side of contract account. If this method is followed then depreciation on the machine is not shown in the contract account.

(5) **Work-in-progress :** Work-in-progress for the purpose of balance sheet can be calculated by the following methods :

Method Rs.

Cost of contract incurred   ...
Add : Profit taken   ...

Less : Cash received   ...
Work-in-progress Rs.   ...

(6) **Preparation of contract Account :** Contract account is prepared for calculating the profit or loss on the contract. For each contract a separate contract account is prepared. Like profit and loss account, all expenses relating to the contract, i.e., cost of material, labour and other expenses are shown on the debit side of contract account of contract account. If the debit side of contract account exceeds its credit side then the difference is termed as loss. If the credit side of contract account exceeds its debit side then difference is called notional profit.

Calculation of Profit from the Notional Profit

The difference between the two sides of contract account is either a loss or a notional profit. If there is a loss then the complete amount of loss is to be provided for by debiting the profit and loss account of the business. If there is a profit, which is called notional profit, then only a portion of the notional profit is treated as earned profit. The amount can be calculated as per instructions given hereunder :

(a) **When work on contract has not reasonably advanced :** The work is said to have not reached a reasonably advanced stage when the value of work certified is less than 1/4th of the total contract price. If it is found that contract has not reasonably advanced then the whole of the notional profit is kept in reserve. In other words, no portion of the notional profit is considered as profit earned.

(b) **When work on the contract has reasonably advanced :** When 1/4th or more than 1/4th of the work has been certified as completed work then it is said that work has reasonably advanced. In this case profit earned is calculated by applying the following formula : Notional profit x 2/3 x Cash received/Work certified.

(c) **When the work is almost complete :** When it is seen that work has advanced so much that it is near completion point then it is often advised to calculate the notional profit (termed as total estimated profit) by crediting the contract account with full contract price and debiting the contract account with actual expenses plus estimated expenses for the remaining portion of contract. The 'earned profit', then, is calculated by applying the following formula : Total estimated profit x Value of work certified/Total contract price x Cash received / Work certified.

SPECIFIC ASPECTS OF CONTRACT COSTING

Proper store accounting will be necessary for those materials which are less frequently required and have been stored in the contractor's central store and issued to contracts, whenever required. When materials are specially purchased for a contract, the contract account will be debited and supplier's or cash account will be credited with the value of materials purchased. In case the materials have been issued from stores, the relevant contract account will be debited and stores control account in the General Ledger will be credited with the amount of materials issued. In case certain materials charged to a contract are returned to stores, stores control account will be debited and the contract account will be credited.

Sale of surplus materials at contract sites is also very common. The sale proceeds should be credited to the concerned contract account. In case sale of materials has been made on account of some extraneous reasons, any Profit or Loss on such sale should be transferred directly to the Profit and Loss Account. This also applies not only to materials but also to sale of plant, machinery, tools, etc.

In case the contractee himself has supplied materials for the contract, the value of such materials should not be charged to the contract account. A separate record for such materials should be maintained because the unused materials will have to be returned back to the contractee.

LABOUR

All labour employed at the contract site is regarded as direct irrespective of the nature of job performed by the workers concerned. Salary of the supervisory staff will also be considered as a direct charge against a contract if they have rendered their wholetime attention to it. Wages of workers which cannot be identified with a particular contract, or salary of the supervisory staff looking after two or more contracts, will be considered as an indirect expense. In case the contract has been divided into several sections and it is required to ascertain the labour cost of each section, each worker should be provided with a job card. Where simultaneously a number of contracts are being executed, it will be desirable to maintain a separate wage sheet for each contract as it will facilitate the work of charging wages to individual contracts.

INDIRECT EXPENSES

Where a contractor has a number of contracts-in-process, he may have a common office and common supervisory staff for all contracts. The expenses of the office and the salaries of such supervisory staff will be considered items of indirect expenses. They will be apportioned to different contracts in accordance with any of the methods. Sometimes, the indirect expenses are also apportioned to different contracts on the basis of expenditure incurred on materials, labour and plant for each contract.

Cost-plus Contracts

In certain contracts the contractee agrees to pay to the contractor the cost price (usually prime cost) of the work done on the contract plus an agreed percentage thereof by way of overhead expenses and profit. Such contracts are known as cost-plus contracts. The system of cost-plus contract costing is employed in cases where it is very difficult for the contractor to quote the contract price because there has been no precedent which he may take as a basis. It is also employed where the work to be done is not fixed at the time of placing order for the contract.

Extras

Contractee may require some additions or alterations to be made in the work originally agreed to be done under the contract. The contractor will charge extra money in addition to the contract price for all such extra work. Frequently a charge for extra work is made on the 'cost plus' basis. It, therefore, becomes necessary to maintain separated records for all such extra work done. In case the extra work is not substantial, the cost of such work can be charged to the original contract which may also be credited with the price charged for the extra work. However, separate account should be maintained of extra work if it happens to be quite substantial.

SUB-CONTRACTS

The contactor may entrust some portion of the work to be done under the contract to a sub-contractor. Usually work of a specialised nature, e.g., steel work, special flooring etc., is done by sub-contractors who are responsible to the main contractor. The cost of such sub-contracts is a direct charge against the contract for which the work has been done.

Escalation Clause (or Materials and Labour Variation Clause)

Escalation clause is usually provided in the contract as a safeguard against any likely changes in the price or utilisation of material and labour. The clause provides that in case prices of items of raw materials, labour etc. specified in the contract change during the execution of the contract, beyond a specified limit over the prices prevailing at the time of signing the agreement, the contract price will be suitably adjusted. The terms of the contract specify the procedure for calculating such adjustment in order to avoid all future disputes. Thus such a clause safeguards the interests of both the contractor and the contractee in case of fluctuations in the prices of materials and labour etc.

Work Certified and Payment

In case of small contracts the contractee pays the contract price on the completion of the contract. But in cases of large contracts the system of Progress Payment is adopted. The contractee agrees to pay a part of the contract price from time to time depending upon satisfactory progress of the work. The progress will be judged by the contractee's architect, suveyor or engineer, who will issue a certificate stating the value of work so far done and approved by him. Such work is termed as Work Certified. The contractee usually does not pay 100% of the value of work certified. He may pay only 75% or 80% of the value work certified depending upon the terms of the contract. The balance not paid is called Retention Money.

Work Uncertified

It may be quite possible that at the end of a period a part of the work done may remain unapproved because it has not reached a stipulated stage. Such work which has not been so far approved by the contractee's architect or surveyor is termed as work uncertified. It is valued at cost and credited to the contract account, and debited to the work-in-progress account which will be transferred next year to the debit of the contracting account.

Materials and Stores at Site

If any material or stores remain unutilised at the end of the accounting period, the amount will be debited to the "Materials or stores at Site Account" and credited to the contract account. Next year the Materials or Stores at site account will be transferred to the debit side of the contract account. Alternatively, the amount of materials or stores at the site may be treated as work-in-progress and debited to that account. However, the former method is preferable.

Work-in-progress

The work-in-progress includes the value of work certified and the cost of work uncertified. The work-in-progress account will appear on the assets side of the balance sheet. The amount of cash received from the contractee and reserve for contingencies or unrealised profit will be deducted out of amount.

Profit on Incomplete Contracts

At the end of an accounting period it may be found that certain contracts have been completed while others are still in process and will be comploeted in the coming years. The total profits made on completed contracts may be safely taken to the credit of Profit and Loss Account. But the same can not be done in case of incomplete contracts. These contracts are still in process, and there are possibilities of profits beings turned into losses on account of heavy rise in prices of materials and labour and losses on account of other unforeseen contingencies. At the same time it does not also seem desirable to consider the profits only on completed contracts and ignore altogether incomplete ones because this may result in heavy fluctuation in the figure of profit from year to year. A year in which a large number of contracts have been completed will show an abnormally high figure of profit while reverse may be the case in the year in which a large number of contracts remain incomplete. Therefore, profits or, incomplete contracts should be considered, of course, after providing adequate sums for meeting unknown contingencies.

10

PRICE DETERMINATION AND POLICIES

Definition of Price

The term 'price' denotes money value of a product. It represents the amount of money for which a product can be exchanged. In other words, price represents the money which the buyer pays to the seller for a product. When a person is buying a product, he may buy certain services also alongwith the product. The more the number of services he wants to get, the more price he will have to pay. Thus, in pricing we must consider more than the physical product alone. A seller prices a combination of the physical product plus several other services and benefits alongwith the product including warranty promise, repair facilities, package, free home delivery service and credit facilities. The price a buyer has to pay will depend upon the number of services he requires along with the product.

Some sellers quote a price that includes various services while others price these individual services separately. This point must be taken into consideration while comparing the prices charged by different sellers. We may define price as the amount of money which is needed to acquire in exchange some combined assortment of a product and its accompanying services.

Significance of Pricing

The price structure of a firm is a major determinant of its success. If prices are too high, the business is lost ; if prices are too low, the firm may be in loss. Price structure affects the firm's competitive position and its share of the market. It has an important bearing on the firm's revenue and net profit. With the help of the price, the firm can make an estimate of its revenue and profit. Profit is equal to revenue minus cost. Price also helps in determining the quantum of production which should be carried on by the firm. The management of a firm can make estimates of profits at various levels of production and at different prices and can choose the best possible combination.

The price of a product also affects the other components of the marketing mix of a firm. A firm will improve the quality of a product, increase the number of accompanying services and spend more on promotion and distribution if it feels that it can sell its product at price high enough to cover the cost of these charges. It determines his purchasing power and the standard of living. Goods and service offered by various producers at different prices help the consumer to take buying decisions and satisfy his wants in a better way.

Pricing is the key activity in the economy of a country which permits the system of free enterprise. Pricing influences wages, interest, rent and profit. It regulates production and allocates resources in a better way. High wages attract labour, high interest rates attract capital and so on. The firms which are not able to market their products at good prices cannot survive in the long-run since they are not able to pay for the various factors of production. Thus pricing weeds out the inefficient firms. It compels the existing firms to make better utilisation of economic resources if they want to survive in the long-run.

The pricing objectives should aim at achieving the firm's objectives. Pricing objectives vary from firm to firm. Generally, the firms have multiple pricing objectives. The important pricing objectives followed by various firms are as under :

(1) Target Rate of Return on Investment or Net Sale

This is an important goal of pricing policy of many firms. A firm following this goal tries to build a price structure to provide sufficient return on capital employed. Generally, an estimate is made of return expected rate of return. This leads to cost plus pricing. In other words, the price represents the cost of production and distribution and a margin of profit.

In working towards return on investment objective, pricing decision are made according to cost plus pricing technique so that total sales revenues exceed total costs by enough amount to provide the desired rate of return on the total investment. Let us take the case of a company which anticipates the sales volume of its product to be 10,000 units in an 'average year'. The company's total investment amounts Rs. 10 lakhs and at 10,000 units sales level, total unit cost is Rs. 50. If the targeted return on investment (ROI) is set at 30% before taxes, return of Rs. 3 lakhs is required on an average. The company will calculate the price as under :

Total cost of 10,000 units Rs. 50 per unit	= Rs. 5,00,000
30% before tax ROI on Rs. 10 lakhs investment	= Rs. 3,00,000
Targeted sales amount	= Rs. 8,00,000

$$\text{Price per unit} = \frac{\text{Rs. } 8,00,000}{10,000 \text{ units}} = \text{Rs. } 80$$

Target ROI pricing is commonly used by the firms which are industry leaders because they can set the standards to be followed by the followers. This practice is also common among companies selling in protected markets. Some firms attempt to achieve target return-on net sales, particularly during the short-run. They set a percentage mark-up on sales which is sufficient to cover operating costs and a desired profit. In such cases, the percentage of profit would remain the same, but the quantum of profit will change according to the number of units of a product or service sold.

(2) Price Stabilisation

Many firms have the objective of price stabilisation in the long run. The objective is often found in industries that have a price leader. In oligopolistic situation where there are only a few sellers, each seller will try to maintain stability in his pricing. In such a situation, one seller acts as the price leader and others follow him. Thus, a relationship exists between the leader's price and those charged by other firms. No firm is willing to engage itself in price wars. They may even forego maximising profits in times of prosperity or short supply in order to stabilise the prices. Price stability helps in planned and regular production in the long-run. In order to stabilise prices, many manufacturers follow the policy of re-sale price maintenance by their dealers. In some degree, this goal is collateral to that of a target return on investment.

(3) Meet or Prevent Competition

Same firms adopt the pricing policy to meet or prevent competition. They are ready to fix their prices to meet competition in the market. Sometimes they are prepared to follow 'below cost pricing' in order to fight competition. They charge less than the cost because they feel that it will prevent the new firms to enter the market. This practice is not publicly admitted by the firms even though they follow it while introducing a new product. Sometimes, this practice turns out to be unsuccessful because new firms are attached into the field once the new product becomes popular. It is not possible for a firm to charge less than the cost of a product for a long-term period.

(4) Maintain or Improve Share of Market

This pricing objective is followed by the firm operating in the expanding markets. When the market has a potential for growth, market share is a better indicator of a firm's effectiveness than the target return on investment. A firm might be learning a reasonable rate of return but its share of market may be decreasing. Therefore, a worthwhile pricing objective in times of increasing market should be to maintain or to improve share of the market.

(5) Profit Maximisation

There are many firms which do not care for social responsibilities and follow the pricing policy to maximise their profits. In practice, no firm states explicitly that its pricing objective is to maximise profits because of fear of public criticism. However, in economic theory, there is nothing wrong with the objective of profit maximisation because if profits become unduly high, new entrepreneurs will be attracted into the field. Thus, there will be an automatic balance of demand and supply of the product. But in the recent years, the business philosophy has changed. Most of the businessmen do not attempt to maximise their profits because they realise that they operate in the society and they have certain social obligations.

PRICING POLICIES

Pricing policies provide guidelines within which pricing strategy is formulated and implemented. The following statements will clarify the meaning of pricing policy:

(i) Pricing should aim at maximising profits for the entire product line.

(ii) Prices should be set to promote the long-term welfare of the enterprise, e.g. to discourage competition in the market.

(iii) A predetermined and systematic method of pricing new products should be provided.

(iv) Prices should be adopted and individualised to fit the diverse competitive situations encountered by different products.

A systematic approach to pricing the products of a firm requires that decision of individual pricing situations be generalised and codified into policies covering all the principal pricing policies. Pricing policies should be tailored to meet the various competitive situations. This implies that a firm can follow different pricing policies with regard to different markets or different customers. For instance, full cost pricing may be followed to sell the products to a big buyers like Government, particularly when the plant capacity is lying idle.

PRICING IN PRACTICE

It is very difficult to ascertain precisely the pricing policies and practices followed by a business enterprise because all the policies are not in an explicit form. For instance, a company may follow the practice of charging lower prices to prevent competition in the market, but this may not be admitted publicly. Similarly there are many other pricing policies and practices which may be known by studying the behavior of business enterprises. The major pricing policies which are followed by the business enterprises are as follows:

1. Competitive Pricing

The management of a firm may decide to fix the price at the competitive level during certain situations. This method is most likely to be used when the market is highly competitive and the product is not differentiated significantly from the competitive products. This situation resembles the perfect competition under which prices are determined by the forces of demand and supply. There is no product differentiation, buyers and sellers are well-informed about the market price and market conditions, and the seller has no control over the market price. In such a situation, every firm will follow the price which is in tune with the market conditions.

2. Skimming-the-Cream Pricing

Under this pricing policy, higher prices are charged during the initial stages of the introduction of a new product. The manufacturer fixes higher price of his product in order to recover his initial investment quickly. This policy has been quite successful in many cases because of the following reasons:

(i) Demand is likely to be more inelastic with respect to price in the early stages then it is when the product is fully grown. Promotional elasticity is, quite higher, particularly for the product with high unit price.

(ii) It is an efficient device for dividing the market into segments that differ in price elasticity of demand. The initial high price serves to skim the cream of the market that is relatively insensitive to price. Price may be reduced subsequently to attract successively more elastic segments of the market.

(iii) A manufacturer may charge higher prices in order to restrict the demand to the level which he can easily meet and to avoid the loss resulting from the competition when the entry is quite easy.

(iv) High initial price finances the cost of raising a product family. The manufacturer may charge high prices and plough back the excessive profits into the business for further expansion.

3. Penetration Pricing

Under this pricing policy, prices are fixed below the competitive level to obtain a larger share of the market and to develop popularity of the brand. Unlike skimming price policy, it facilitates higher volume of sales even during the initial stages of a product's life cycle. This method of pricing is usually found at the retail level of distribution. Many retailers offer discount to attract more and more customers. They operate on the principle of low make-up and higher volume.

Penetration pricing may also be used at the time of introduction of a new product to prevent the entry of new firms by keeping the profit margin very low. This policy helps in developing the brand reference of the people and is useful in marketing the products which are expected to have a steady long-term market.

Penetration pricing is an aggressive pricing strategy and is likely to be successful under the following conditions:

(i) the product has a highly elastic demand, i.e., the quantity sold is highly sensitive to price:

(ii) production is carried out on a large scale to achieve low cost of production per unit :

(iii) there is a strong competition in the market : and

(iv) there is an inadequate high income market and, thus, skimming-the-cream price policy cannot be sustained.

4. Keep-out Pricing

It is pre-emptive pricing policy which aims at discouraging the other firms in the market to offer substitutes. Keep out Pricing should be followed for only one product of a firm. It is very risky venture, particularly, when the product is offered to the public at a price which is less than the actual cost of production and distribution. This policy can be followed by big firms with huge resources at their command. But once the price at a low level is fixed, it may not be possible to increase it because of the fear of other firms introducing the substitutes.

5. One Price Versus Variable Price Policy

In case of one-price policy, the seller charges the same price to similar types of customers who purchase similar quantities of the product under essentially the same terms of sale. The price may vary according to the quantity of purchase. However, prices charged for different quantities to different customers are the same. For example, a seller may sell his product Rs. 10.00 per unit if less than one dozen units are purchased and Rs. 9.00 pre unit if one dozen or more units are purchased. On the other hand, a seller may follow a single price policy under which the price per unit of a product remains the same regardless of the number of units being purchased.

In case of variable price policy, the seller sells similar quantities to similar buyers at different prices. For instance, a seller may offer the same quantity of goods to old customers at lower rates. It is also possible that the final price is determined by bargaining and haggling between the buyer and seller. Generally, prices of consumer durable such as refrigerators, automobiles, televisions, etc., are negotiated.

One-price policy builds customer confidence in the seller. It also saves time of the buyer and the seller. Persons who have weak bargaining power prefer the stores offering one price. A variable price policy has its own plus points. It is liked by the customers who have high bargaining power and have sufficient time for bargaining. This policy also offers the seller flexibility in his dealings with different types of customers.

6. Price Lining

Price lining is used extensively by the retailers. The retailers usually offer a good, better and best assortment of merchandise at different price levels. For example, a retailer of ready-made shirts may sell shirts at three prices : Rs. 90. Rs. 160 and Rs. 250. The first price stands for the economy choice, the second for the medium quality and the third for the super-fine quality. Price lining simplifies pricing decisions in the future as retail prices are already set. This helps the retailer to plan his purchases to suit his price lining. It also simplifies buying decisions by the customers.

7. Psychological Pricing

Under this policy, prices are fixed in such a way that they have some kind of psychological influence on the buyers. Customary pricing and price lining are the examples of psychological pricing. Another form of psychological pricing is Odd Pricing i.e., prices are set at odd amount such as Rs. 19, Rs. 49, Rs. 99, etc. For example, a customer may happily Rs.299.95 for a pair of shoes and may not like to buy the same pair if it is priced at Rs.300.Odd pricing is widely used by the publishers of paperbacks.

8. Leader Pricing

A firm may cut prices temporarily on a few in order to attract customers. In other words, 'loss leader' is used to promote higher sales of different products offered by the firm.Leader items are generally well-known i.e.,are highly advertised and purchased frequently. The term 'loss leader' is used because a few popular items are offered at prices below normally expected prices. The rationale of the policy is that customers will come to the store to buy the advertised leader items and then stay to buy other regularly priced merchandise. The net result will be increased total sales volume and profits.

9. Follow the Leader Pricing

This pricing policy is generally used under oligopolistic competition where there are a small number of sellers and any one of them operates on such a scale that an increase or decrease in his turnover will appreciably affect the market price. The commodity produced by the sellers may be standardised or differentiated; the size of each seller's output in relation to the total supply is the major test of oligopolistic pricing. Each seller considers the probable effect of variation in his output upon the price and adjusts his production accordingly. He also considers the probable reaction of his competitors to variations in his pricing. Small firms cannot influence the market significantly. They charge the prices which are charged by the major producers. In such a situation, under-cutting of prices is dangerous because of changed reaction by the other producers. Over charging is not possible in such a situation because it is very difficult to sell the product at a price higher than one charged by other producers. Thus, every firm tries to avoid price competition in its own self-interest and in the interest of the industry. However, it is free to capture a larger share of the market through sales promotion, advertising and other promotional activities.

10. Discriminatory Pricing

Some business enterprises follow the policy of charging different prices from different customers according to their ability to pay. This policy is very popular with the service enterprises, e.g., legal and medical services. Business enterprises marketing tangible products also use the policy of price discrimination successfully if they are able to divide the market in various segments on the basis of the customer's capacity to pay. These days it is not possible to sell the same product at different prices in different market segments because of improved means of transportation and wider communication between the market segments. The manufacturers generally try to differentiate the product through improved packaging and after-sale service. Thus, they charge different prices for the same product by slightly differentiating the features of the product. Price discrimination is successful if the elasticity of demand in one segment of the market is lower than in another.

11. Resale Price Maintenance

Resale price maintenance (RPM) is the policy under which a manufacturer fixes the price of his product below which product would not be sold to the consumers or distributors. Resale price maintenance refers to that price policy under which the manufacturer of a branded product in open competition establishes the price, or the minimum price at which such product shall be resold to the consumers.

Resale price maintenance is possible in case of branded products only. A manufacturer of a popular brand of a product may enter into an agreement with the distributors of his product under which resale price is fixed by the manufacturer and the distributors will not sell the product below that price. The resale price maintenance practice is generally followed by the manufacturers of consumer products such as electric appliances, drugs, cigarettes, liquor and sports goods. The basic purpose of this policy is to protect the interest the manufacturer and to create a good image in the market of the manufacturer and his product.

CONTROL AND REGULATIONS OF PRICES

An important part of the regulatory power of the government impinging on the freedom of private business enterprise is the power of the government to fix, control and regulate prices of materials, semi-finished and finished products.

Drugs Price Control Order 1987 is an order by the Central Government, in exercise of the powers, conferred by sec. 3 of the essential commodities Act 1995.

Its object is to control production, supply, distribution, etc. of essential commodities.

Definitions :

Drug : It means a medicine for use of human beings or animals and all substances intended to be used for diagnosis, treatment, mitigation or prevention of disease.

Bulk Drugs : It means any substance including pharmaceutical, chemical, biological or plant product or medicinal gas confirming to pharmacopoeal or other standards accepted under the Drugs and Cosmetics Act 1940 which is used as such or as an ingredient in any formulations.

Formulation : It means a medicine processed out of, or containing one or more bulk drug(s), with or without the use of any pharmaceutical aids for external or internal use for, or in the diagnosis, treatment, mitigation or prevention of disease in human beings or criminals.

Dealer : It means a person carrying on the business of purchase or sale of drugs, whether as wholesaler or retailer and whether or not in conjunction with any other business and includes agent of a dealer.

Distributor : It means a distributor of drugs or his agent or a stockist appointed by a manufacturer or an importer for stocking his drugs for resale to a dealer.

Free reserve : It means a reserve created by appropriation of profits, but does not includes reserve provided for contingent, liability, disputed claims, goodwill, revaluation, and other similar reserves.

Leader price : It means a price fixed by the Government for formulations specified in category I or category II of the third schedule in accordance with the provisions of the order.

Manufacturer : Any person who manufacturers drugs.

Net-worth : It means share capital of company plus reserve, if any.

Retail price : It means a retail price of a drug arrived at or fixed in accordance with the provision of D.P.C.O. (Drugs Price Control Order) and includes leader price.

Retailer : It means a dealer carrying on the retail business of sale of drugs to customers.

Wholesaler : It means wholesaler of drugs or his agent or a stockist appointed by a manufacturer or an importer for the sale of his drugs to a retailer, hospital, dispensaries, medical, educational or research institutes.

PRICE OF BULK DRUGS

Government has power to fix the maximum sale price of indigenously manufactured bulk drugs, specified in first or second schedule, to fix retention price and common sale price, maximum sale price of new bulk drugs, or imported bulk drugs and also has to fix retention price and pooled price of indigenous or imported bulk drugs specified in first or second schedule.

The Government may take into account the average cost of production of such bulk drug manufactured by an efficient manufacturer whose production of such bulk drug in the country is large or who employs efficient technology in the production of such bulk drug, and allow reasonable return on net-worth.

No person shall sell a bulk drug at a price exceeding the price notified by the Government plus local taxes if any payable.

In case when the price of a bulk drug has not been notified by the Government, the manufacturer shall within 14 days of commencement of the production of such bulk drug make an application to the Government, he may sale the bulk drug at a price not exceeding the price so notified. When a manufacturer produces new bulk drug, within 14 days of commencement of production of such new bulk drug, he shall make an application to the Government in Form-1, and Government may after making such inquiry as it deems fit, decide to include such new bulk drug in this order and by order fix a provisional price at which such new drug shall be sold.

The manufacturer of such new bulk drug, after six months of completion of provisional price, shall apply in Form-1 to the Government. After making such inquiry as the Government deems fit, by notification in the official Gazette fix the price of such bulk drug.

To encourage the manufacturers of new bulk drugs, produced through original research and developmental efforts in the country and have not been produced elsewhere, the provisions of this order shall not apply to such bulk drugs for a period of five years from the date of commencement of production of such new bulk drugs. After expiry of five years the provision of this order shall apply to the new bulk drug.

Power to Direct Manufacturer of Bulk Drugs to Sell Bulk Drugs to Manufacturers of Formulation

The Government may from time to time by order direct any manufacturer of formulations of any bulk drug to sell such bulk drug to such manufacturers of formulation as may be specified in such order.

Calculation of Retail Price of Formulations

The retail price of a formulation shall be calculated in accordance with the following formula, namely

$$R.P. = (M.C. + C.C. + P.M. + P.C.) \times [1+MAPE/100] + E.D.$$

where

R.P. = means retail price

M.C. = material cost and includes the cost of drugs, and other pharmaceutical aids including overages if any and process loss thereon in accordance with such norms as may be specified by the Government from time to time.

C.C. = means conversion cost worked out in accordance with such norms as may be specified by the Government from time -to-time by notification in the official Gazette.

P.M. = means the cost of packing material including process ˡᵒss thereon worked out in accordance with such norms as may be specified by the Government from time-to-time.

P.C. = means packing charges worked out in accordance with such norms as may be specified by Government from time-to-time.

M.A.P.E. = maximum allowable post manufacturing expenses.

M.A.P.E. shall not exceed:

(a) 75% in the case of formulations specified in category I and

(b) 100% in the case of formulations specified in category II.

Combination of the drugs, having one of the drug from category I, will become considered as category I product.

Category I formulations includes drugs required for national health programme and category II formulations includes other essential drugs)

E.D. = means Excise Duty.

The landed cost of imported formulation shall form the basis for fixing its price along with such margin as the Government may allow from time-to-time.

Where an imported formulation is repacked, its landed cost, plus the cost of packing materials land and packing charges as worked out in accordance with the norms as may be specified by the Government from time-to-time are considered to fix the price.

Power to Fix Leader Prices

The Government may from time to time, fix the leader price of a formulation specified in category I or II of the third schedule and such leader price shall operate as ceiling sale price for every manufacturer of such formulation.

The retail price of a formulation once fixed by the Government shall not be increased by any manufacturer without the prior approval of the Government.

Any manufacturer who desires revision of the retail price of a formulation fixed previously shall apply to the Government in Form - 3 or 4 as the case may be, and Government may after calling for such information as it may consider necessary, by order fix a revised price for such formulation.

General Provisions Regarding Prices of Formulation

1. No manufacturer or importer shall market a new formulation or a new pack, or a new dosage form of his existing formation specified in category I or II of the third schedule without obtaining prior approval of its price from the Government.

2. No person shall sell or dispose of any imported formulations specified in category I or II of the third schedule without obtaining prior approval of its price from the Government.

3. For obtaining approval of the Government in respect of the price for any formulations, in category I or II of third schedule, the manufacturer or importer shall make an application to the Government in form 3 and 4 as the case may be and the Government may within a period of 4 months of the receipt of an application accord its approval subject to such modifications as it may consider necessary provided that where approval is not accorded with the said period of four months, the manufacturer or importer as the case may be market the new formulation, or new pack or new dosage form, at the price declared by him in his application, issue the price list and intimate the Government accordingly.

Power to Revise Prices of Formulations

The Government may, if it considers necessary to do so in the public interest, by order revise the retail price of any formulation or bulk drug specified in any of the categories of the third schedule.

Drug Prices Equalisation Account

The Government shall maintain an account, known as the 'Drugs Prices Equalisation Account' in order to maintain overall economic balance. The Government may direct any manufacturer to pay the benefit occurring as a result of purchases of bulk drugs at prices cheaper than those allowed in calculations of retail prices, into the "Drug Prices Equlisation Account".

Sale of Split Quantities of Formulations

No dealer shall sell loose quantity of any formulation drawn from a bottle pack of such formulation at a price which exceeds the retail price of the formulation plus 5% thereof, provided such formulations shall not compounded at the premised of the dealer.

Maintenance of Records and Production thereof for inspection

Every manufacture shall maintain in such forms as may be specified by the Government, records relating to the sales turnover of formulations pack-wise and also such other records as may be directed from time to time by the Government and such records shall be opened for inspection by the Government.

Every dealer or manufacturer shall maintain the cash memo or credit memo, books of account and records of purchase and sale of drugs and shall make available the said records for inspection by the Government.

Price to Wholesaler and Retailer

No manufacturer, importer or distributor shall sell a formulation to a wholesaler unless otherwise permitted under the provisions of this order at a price higher than,

,For Ethical Drugs	:	Retail price minus 20%
For Non Ethical Drugs	:	Retail price minus 18%

No manufacturer, importer, distributor or wholesaler shall sell a formulation to a retailer unless otherwise permitted under the provision of this order at a price higher than :

For Ethical Drugs   :   Retail price minus 17%

For Non Ethical Drugs   :   Retail price minus 15%

For this purpose 'ethical drugs' include all drugs specified in schedule C, C_1, Schedule G and H of the drugs and cosmetics rule 1945 and "non ethical drugs" means all drugs other than ethical drugs.

Government may by general or special order, fix in the public interest the price to the wholesaler or retailer of any formulation the price of which has been fixed already under this order.

Penalties

Any contravention of any of the provision of this order shall be punishable in accordance with the provisions of the Essential Commodities Act.

Power to Exempt

Government may by order in the official Gazette exempt any drug manufacturing unit or a class of such units from the call or any of the provisions of this order and may modify such order, while exempting any such unit Government considers following factors as,

1. Number of workers employed;
2. Amount of capital invested;
3. Range and type of products manufactured; and
4. Sales turnover

THE FIRST SCHEDULE

List of bulk Drugs (including salts, ester and derivatives, if any) required for the following National Health Programmes, used in Category I formulations appearing in Third Schedule.

1. National T.B. Eradication Programme :

   Streptomycin;   Thiacetazone;   Sodium PAS;   Rifampicin;
   Isoniazid;   Ethambutol;   Pyrazinamide;

2. National Leprosy Eradication Programme :

   Dapsone; Clofazamine;   Rifampicin

3. National Trachoma Control Programme and National Programme for Control of Blindness :

   Tetracycline Hydrochoride; Sodium Sulphacetamide;

   Pilocarpine ;   Hydrocortisone ; Indoxouridine ; Timolol ;

   Acetanilide ;   Atropine ;   Homatropin.

4. Programme for prevention of dehydration under ORT-I : oral rehydration salt.

5. National Malaria Eradication Programme :
   Chloroquine;   Amodiaquine;
   Quinoline;   Primetheamine;
   Sulfamethapyrezine;   Paracetamol.

6. National Filaria Eradication Programme :
   Diethyl carbamazine.

THE SECOND SCHEDULE

List of Bulk Drugs (including salts, esters and derivatives, if any) used in Category II formulations appearing in Third Schedule.

Aspirin; Amoxycillin; Ampicillin; Amiloride; Aluminium hydroxide; Amitryptyline; Aminophyline; Baralgan ketone; Bephenium; Benzathine; Benzylpenicillin; Betamethasone; Chlorpheniramine; Cyprocheptadine; Carbamazepine; Chloroquine; Cephalexin; Chloramphenicol; Cloxacillin; Cetrimide; Cemetidine; Carbimazole; Chlorpromazine; Calcium pantothenate; Chlorhexidine; Dextropropoxyphene; Dexamethasone; Diazepam; Dehydroemetine; Diloxanide; Doxycycline; Digoxin; Dihydralazine; Dipyridamole; Dopamine; Dichloro meta xylenol; Diphenoxylate; Epinephrine; Ethosuximide; Erythromycin; Ethionamide; Ergotamine; Ergometrine; Ephedrine; Framycetin; Folic Acid; Frusemide; Furazepam; Furazolidone; Gentamycin; Griseofulvin; Glyceryl trinitrate; Glibenclamide; Hydroxycobalamin/Cynocobalamin; Heparin; Hydralzine; Hydrochlorothiazide; Hydrocortisone; Heptatis-B Vaccine; Ibuprofen; Iodochlorohydroxyquinoline; Iron dextran; Isoprenaline; Isosorbide Dinitrate; Insulin; Imipramine; Ketoprofen; Lidocaine/xylocaine; Levamisole; Loperamide; Lorazepam; Metamizol (Analgin); Mebhydroline; Metronidazole; Methyl Dopa; Metaclopramide; Menthol; Methyl salicylate; Nalidixic acid; Nitrofurantoin; Nitrazepam; Oxytetracycline; Oxethazin; Oxytocin; Oxazepam; Pentazocinel; Piroxicam; Probenecid; Pheniramine; Prednisolone; Prochlorperazine; Phenobarbitone; Phenytoin; Piperazine; Pyrantal; Penicillins; Phenoxymethylpenicillin; Procaine Benzylpenicillin; Protionamide; Pentamidine; Primaquine; Procainamide; Parachloro meta xylenol; Promethazine; Quinidine; Reserpine; Ranitidine; Salazosulfapyridine; Sulphacetamide; Sulphadiazine; Sulphamethizole; Sulphamethoxazole; Sulphaphenazole; Sodium stibogluconate; Sulphadoxine; Sodium nitroprusside; Spironolactone; Sodium nitrate; Salbutamol; Tetramisole; Thiabendazole; Tetracycline; Trimethoprim; Triameterene; Trifluperazine; Triflupromazine; Terbutaline; Triflupromazine; Terbutaline; Theophyline; Valporic Acid; Verapamil; Vitamin A ; Vitamin B_1; Vitamin B_2; Vitamin B_6; Vitamin C; Vitamin D; Vitamin E; Warfarin; Xanthinol.

Note : All Vitamins as Bulk Drugs are exempt from price control as required under paragraph 3.

THE THIRD SCHEDULE
Category I and Category II Formulations
1. Category - I Formulations:

All formulations based on the bulk drugs specified under the first Schedule either individually or in Combination with other bulk drugs.

2. Category - II Formulations:

All formulations based on bulk drugs specified in the Second Schedule either individually or in combination with other bulk drugs except the following :

(i) Single ingredient formulations based on the bulk drugs specified in the Second Schedule and sold under generic name.

(ii) All Single ingredient Vitamin formulations containing individual vitamins specified in the Second schedule sold either in brand name or in generic name.

THE FOURTH SCHEDULE FORMS

1. Form of application for fixation or revision of prices of bulk drugs.
2. Form of application for approval or revision of price of formulation to be submitted in seven copies.
3. Form of application to be submitted for price approval of formulation imported in finished form.
4. Information to be furnished by manufacturer or importer of marketing non-scheduled formulation to be submitted in duplicate.
5. Form of price List.
6. Yearly submission of information.

THE FIFTH SCHEDULE

(Statement showing maximum pre-tax return on sales turn-over or manufacturers or importers of formulations)

Category A:

Large units with turnover exceeding Rs. 6 crores per annum.

1. Having no basic drug manufacturing activity   8%
2. Having basic drug manufacturing activity at 5% or more of turnover but no research activity.   9%
3. Having basic drug manufacturing activity at 5% or more of the turnover and engaged in approved research and development work relating to new drugs.   10%

Category B:

Medium size units with turnover between Rs. 1 crore to Rs. 6 crores per annum.

1. Having no basic drug manufacturing activity nor any research activity. 9%
2. Having basic drug manufacturing activity at 5% or more of turnover but no research activity.   11%
3. Having basic drug manufacturing activity at 5% or more of turnover and engaged in approved research and development work relating to new drug.   13%

Category C:

Other units with turnover of less than Rs. 1 crores per annum.

1. Having only formulation activity.   12%
2. Having basic drug manufacturing activity at 5% or more of turnover.

11

HANDLING OF DRUG STORES

After the drugs have been received and inspected, they are handed over in the custody of the Stores Department. The Store Manager will instruct the store-keeper to record the materials received in the bin card and keep the materials in the proper bin (i.e., a placemeant for storing goods). It is the duty of the Stores Department to hold in custody the raw materials, supplies, etc., in a systematic manner so that they can be issued whenever required. The nature and scope of stores service can be understood easily if we go through the functions of stores department which are as follows :

(i) Issuing requisition on Purchase Department for the most economical quantity of the right kinds of materials for delivery at the most convenient time.

(ii) Receiving materials from suppliers and checking them as to quality and quantity.

(iii) Storing all materials in safe and convenient manner for quick delivery.

(iv) Issuing materials against proper authorisation in right quality, quantity and at right time.

(v) Maintaining proper record of receipts, issues and balance of materials lying in the store.

(vi) Safeguarding the stocks in the stores from breakage, spoilage, deterioration, theft, etc.

In most of the organisations, there is a centralised store which serves as the receiving, storing and distribution centre of all types of materials. However, where the departments are located at places which are far away from the central stores, sub-stores may be set up near these departments in order to keep the transportation costs and handling charges to the minimum level. Each sub-store will draw supplies from the central store and issue to the concerned departments. After the end of a particular period it will again obtain supplies from the central store to replenish the stock of various items. This system of stores is known as 'imprest system' of stores.

Storing Procedure : The store department should be located at a central place in the organisation. The store rooms should have adequate shelves or bins for storing different types of materials. Every store room should be under the charge of a person known as storekeeper. The storekeeper will place the materials in proper order and will lock the room after the working hours to avoid any pilferage of stock. He will issue the materials only after receiving authorised stores requisitions. He will also keep an upto date record of the receipt and issue of every item on separate bin cards. He will also send a purchase requisition to the purchase department when the stock reaches a minimum level determined before hand by the purchase manager.

Storage of Drugs

The function of storage of drugs is performed by the storekeeper. His duties include accepting, identifying, classifying and proper placing of materials. Efficient storage requires the consideration of the following points :

Checking Drugs

The store-keeper should accept drugs after proper checking. He should verify the materials received with the consignment note, inspection report and materials received report. He should send the copy of drugs received report received by him, after verification to the Accounts Department.

Classification and Codification of Drugs

A proper system of classification and codification is necessary to prevent mixing of one type of materials with the other. This also helps in increasing efficiency of the factory on account of instant availability of drugs and supplies in required quantities.

Drugs should be classified according to their nature in appropriate categories. In order to save time in handling of drugs and preparing written documents and to remove ambiguity in description of drugs, it will be better if each store item is given a code number. There are two important methods of codification of materials :

(i) **Alphabetical :** In this method alphabets of letters are used for codification of each category of drugs e.g., Sodium Chloride injection may be coded as SCI or Penicillin tablets may be coded as PT, etc.

(ii) **Numerical method :** Numerical coding should invariably be used where material accounting is to be mechanised by use of punched cards. The first thing to be done in numerical coding is to prepare a list of the various wards and alloting to each of them a number. A list of drugs should also be prepared and each type of drug should also be given a number. The first two digits of the code number may indicate the ward for which the materials are meant and the other two digits may tell the name of drugs as mentioned in the standard list. For example, if the code is 1281 it means material No. 81 (say mild Hydrochloric acid) used in ward No. 12.

A combination of these two methods may also be used for coding. For example, analgin tablets stored in rack No. 15, may be given the code number AT/15. Such a method gives much more exact information than any of the above two methods.

Codification of materials helps in two ways :

(i) In the absence of coding the title of an account may have to be written a number of times. This results in unnecessary clerical work, particularly in case of lengthy account titles.

(ii) Secrecy, about the exact nature of the transaction from the general office employees, can be kept.

Bins and Racks

The store should be divided into several sections, each meant for one particular type of material. Each section should have suitable containers for keeping different varieties of that particular type of drug. Such containers are termed as bins or racks. Each bin or rack should also be appropriately numbered and indexed for each identification. For example, the store may have a separate section for infection. This section may keep injections of different sizes in different bins. To facilitate material handling and easy location of drugs it will be better if floor plans are exhibited at the entrance of each store room exhibiting the location of various sections.

HOSPITAL SUPPLIES

Hospital pharmacist and physicians are the important part of an hospital. They prepare the hospital formulary which is a list of drugs. Medical representatives of different industries make continuous efforts in convincing the pharmacists and physicians for the approval of drugs in the drug formulary. They should provide background information of the drugs, results of formal drugs, cost data, and alternative drug entities to replace currently used drugs. They use educational programmes for hospital staff, report medication errors, and recommended drugs to be stocked for emergency. They describe price of the products, company reputation, dosage forms available, unit-dose packaging, return policy, discount and credit policy, medical information, pharmacokinetic and bioavailability data, stability and compatibility data for injectables and quality control information. The pharmaceutical representative must present uses of the drug as they are required by the physicians and hospitalized patients. The representative should contact teachers, residents and in terms regularly for taking purchase order.

Drugs are ordered by the physician, dispensed by the pharmacist, administered by a nurse and consumed by patients. Quotations are asked by hospitals and the lowest quotation is usually accepted. Generally the products are purchased at economic cost in group purchasing. Such purchasing requires better planning, more cooperation and information sharing. Purchasing pharmacist plays an important role in purchasing process.

Most frequently used drugs are supplied by different industries. Therefore, there is a competition in quality and price of the drugs. Usually for bulk package discounted price and quantity discount is given to hospitals. Packaging and transport costs are always less for bulk packages.

The payment of bills of a hospital supply is very slow from 3 to 12 months. There are few hospitals where the recovery is fast. A medical representative visit many times to recover the payment.

Government purchase system is generally adopted for the drug supply. Pharmacist checks the requirement of drugs before giving to the purchase department. Purchase department asks for quotation. The lowest quotation is accepted for supply. A manufacturer should register himself for government supply. Drugs purchased in bulk are single ingredient I.P. formulations such as chloroquin I.P. 250 mg, pencillin I.P. 500 mg, etc. Hospitals may purchase drugs on the basis of continuous efforts of medical representative.

Both the Department of Defence and the veterans Administration maintain depots and drugs are purchased in bulk amount. Therefore, certain economic advantages for central purchasing, billing and shipping are provided.

For government supply, packaging is different. Price is not quoted but code number to identify the government order is mentioned. Quantity, delivery date, shipping location, description of product, etc. are written in the quotation sheets, which are sent in time, otherwise they would not be considered. Sometimes drugs are purchased from small manufacturers to motivate them.

Hospital supply is considerably large and growing regularly. This kind of supply is made by (1) Director General of Supplies and Disposals, (2) Railway hospitals, (3) Employee's State Insurance Corporation, (4) Armed Forces Medical Stores, (5) Medical Store Depots, (6) Private Hospitals, (7) Primary Health Centres, (8) Hospital attached to medical colleges, (9) Hospitals in Public Sector undertakings like BHEL, BHPV, HAL, etc., (10) Central Government Health Schemes and (11) Government hospitals.

12

INVENTORY CONTROL

INTRODUCTION

Inventory means all the materials, parts, supplies, expense tools and in-process or finished products recorded on the books by an organisation and kept in its stocks, warehouses or plant for some period of time.

Inventory is an essential part of an organisation. Every business/ manufacturing organisation, however, has to maintain some inventory. There are many definitions of inventory in a system explaining various aspects of inventory analysis. Some of these are :

1. Inventories are the piles of raw materials and finished goods in the warehouse.

2. All the materials, parts and in-process or finished products recorded on the books by an organisation and kept in its stores, warehouses and plants are known as inventories.

3. Inventory is a list of names, quantities and/or monetary values of all or any group of items.

4. Inventory is a detailed list of those movable items which are necessary to manufacture a product and to maintain the equipment and machinery in good working order. The quantity and value of every item is also mentioned in the list.

Characteristic of Inventory

From all these definitions it is clear that inventory is stock of raw material, semi-finished and finished goods maintained by an organisation.

The concept of inventory and its relation with performance of any system can be very well explained by the following statements :

1. **Inventories serves as cushions to absorb shocks :** An organisation has to deal with several customers and vendors. There are always fluctua-

tions in demand or supply of the items which disturbs the schedule of an organisation. Inventories absorbs these fluctuations and helps in maintaining undisturbed production and stable employment rates.

2. **Inventory for any organisation is a necessary evil :** Inventories require valuable space and consumes taxation and insurance charges. This leads to considerable investment and causes considerable opportunity loss. This capital invested in inventories remains idle till items present in stocks are not used. On the other hand no organisation can work without maintaining some inventory, i.e. it is a necessity. It is observed that costs of not having inventories are usually greater than the costs of having them. Thus, inventories are necessary evil.

3. Inventories are the result of many interrelated decisions and policies within an organisation. The behaviour of inventories is the direct result of diverse policies and decisions within a company. Marketing, production, finance and purchasing decisions directly influence the level of inventory.

4. Inventory provides production economies. Stocks brings economy in purchase of various inputs due to discounts on bulk purchase. This also minimises ordering, transportation and other costs. They also reduces the number of setups.

Importance of Inventory

The importance of inventory to an organisation can be listed as :

1. provides and maintains good customer service.
2. enables smooth flow of goods through the production process.
3. provides protection against the uncertainties of demand and supply.
4. various production operations can be performed economically and independently. It can allow temporary variations in operating rates.
5. ensures a reasonable utilisation of equipment and labour.
6. with purchases in bulk discount can be availed.

Objectives of Inventory Control

The following are the main objectives of inventory control :

1. **Protection Against Fluctuations in Demand :** The demand forecast of any product can never be exact or accurate. There is likely to be some difference, that too of varying magnitude, in predicted demand and actual demand of the product. If sufficient items are available in the inventory, then the fluctuations in demand can be easily adjusted and the organisation can protect itself from unforeseen economic losses.

2. **Better Use of Men, Machines and Material :** In manufacturing system the production planning can be done with an object to have optimum use of resources namely, men, machines and materials. Here the

resources can remain engaged during slack period of demand and there will be no need of generating additional resources in the boom periods as then the inventory enlarged in slack period can to utilised. This will lead to uniform and proper utilisation of resources available with the enterprise.

3. **Protection Against Fluctuation in Output :** Another important function of inventory is to reduce the gap between actual and scheduled production. In practice, production schedule cannot be adhered due to a number of reasons e.g. sudden breakdown in supply of raw materials, machines, labour strikes, etc. In such cases the difference in actual production and the planned output can be bridged by inventories.

4. **For Production Economies :** The production runs can be planned in economic lot sizes when there is a policy to produce for stocks.

5. **Control of Stock Volume :** Inventory control is concerned with the size and the value of goods present in stock. It is responsible to forecast the value of the stocks at regular intervals, so that

   (a) capital invested in inventories does not exceed the funds available for the purpose.

   (b) the amount invested in inventory is correctly recorded in accounts book.

   (c) protection against theft is ensured.

6. **Control of Stock Distribution :** Stock analysis is done to be sure that it is in balance and that obsolescence and depreciation are kept at the minimum possible level.

   Thus inventory managers try to determine the appropriate size of the inventory keeping in view the interest of the production department as well as of the outside customer and side by side holding down the costs.

Inventory is maintained due to following reasons :

   (i) to carry reserves in order to prevent stock outs or cost sales i.e., never to run out of any thing.

   (ii) never having much of anything on hand.

   (iii) to gain economics in purchase by buying items beyond the desired amount.

   (iv) to maintain reserves in stocks for the period of replenishment.

Thus a well formulated inventory policy of an enterprise is likely to ensure smooth and efficient running of production operations providing optimum utilisation of labour, machine and material.

Factors Affecting Inventory Control Policy

The inventory policy of an organisation has an impact on the whole system.

There are a number of factors which can affect the inventory decisions. These can be broadly divided in the following categories :

(A) **Characteristics of the Manufacturing System :** The nature of the production process, the product design, production planning and plant layout have significant affect on inventory policy.

(B) **Amount of Protection against Shortages :** There is always variation in demand and supply of the product. The protection against such unpredictable variations can be done by means of buffer stocks.

(C) **Organisational Factors :** There are certain factors which are related to the policies, traditions and environment of any enterprise.

Relevant Costs in Inventory-System

The heart of inventory analysis resides in the identification of relevant costs. It is observed that there are many factors whose costs affect the size of inventory directly either advocating to decrease the size of inventory or suggesting an increase in the inventory size, e.g. the risk of the manufacturer for loosing sales decreases with size of the inventory but on the other hand expenditure on storage will increase.

These costs are explained below :

(A) **Costs that encourage to have larger inventories :**

(i) **Set up costs or ordering costs. :** In a production process after each production run, the organisation has to incur expenditure in starting the next production run. This expenditure is independent of the size of the production and is known as set-up cost. This cost can be reduced by planning with fewer setups of large size production run leading to an increase in the size of the inventory.

(ii) **Procurement costs :** An organisation has to incur expenditure on the preparation of purchase order. These costs are related to typing and paper work to place an order, inviting and screening the quotations, making efforts for supply on due date by sending reminders, contacting the supplier and lastly on inspection of the goods after receiving the supply. These costs can be (i) fixed costs, *viz.* salaries of the permanent staff of purchase and inspection departments. This expenditure upto some stage is independent of the size of lots ordered, (ii) variable costs, *viz.* processing an order and dispatching it to the vendor. It is a fact that larger the size of the lots purchased, smaller will be the number of orders and inspection. With decrease in the number of orders, fixed cost remaining constant, the variable cost will decrease. This will reduce average annual cost on procurement.

(iii) **Depreciation Costs :** In every organisation the value of the capital invested decreases with time. Thus there is a tendency among organisations to reduce its capital investment on machines and other equipment. The depreciation costs are thus reduced. Naturally the desired amount of production with reduced number of machines can be obtained by running the machines in slack period, thus increasing the size of inventory.

(iv) **Loss due to non-fullment of demand and delay in production :** If the organisation is not able to meet some demand due to smaller inventory or delay in production then this will adversely affect the profit of the enterprise.

Sometimes, if a company is unable to comply some order then there is some penalty to be paid. This may also imply loss of goodwill. The risk of loosing orders on this count can be minimised by increasing the size of inventory for finished goods. Similarly production delays due to non-availability of raw-materials or spare parts for machines can be avoided by keeping sufficient stocks of these items in inventory. This can also reduce the losses due to unexpected delay in replenishment of the inventory.

(v) **Direct material and labour costs :** It is observed that items are likely to be scrapped during each setup or trial of the equipment. This results in increased costs on material and labour. If the size of lots in each production run is increased then there will be fewer setups and loss on materials and labour costs due to scrapping will be reduced.

(vi) **Costs incurred on overtime, hiring, training and lay-off :** If inventory is not of sufficient size, then the organisation may have to employ additional staff, pay overtime etc. to meet the requirement. Overtime also reduces the efficiency of workers. In such cases the organisation may have to employ more staff in boom periods and rentrench the staff in slack period. Both situations may result in employing untrained staff leading to additional expenditure and adversely affecting the efficiency of production.

The only alternative is to produce more for stock in slack periods. This will lead to efficient and uniform use of resources.

(B) **Costs which encourage smaller inventory :**

(a) **Inventory carrying costs :** For any company inventory is an investment, where the capital is tied up in the form of material and goods. Had this capital been free, it could be utilised elsewhere, e.g. developing a new product or to buy new equipment and an opportunity cost exists. Thus by holding inventory the organisation forgoes the use of invested capital in some alternative way.

Sometimes the inventory investment is made by borrowing money on which interest is to be paid. Furthermore, the inventories for tax purposes are considered to be fixed assets and the amount of tax increases with the size of the inventory. This is generally taken as 10 to 15 per cent.

Since the procurement cost depends on the number of times orders are placed, this cost component behaves in inverse proportions to the level of inventory. This is the only component of the relevent cost which behaves opposite to the rest. There is a trade-off between the procurement cost and the relevant costs of inventory. The other costs are called on the carrying costs or holding costs. If the 'how much' question is answered by a largely amount, the carrying costs increase, whereas the procurement costs decrease. If the 'how much' question is answered by a smaller number, the carrying costs decrease, but the procurement costs will increase.

(b) **Storage costs :** Maintenance of inventory means storage costs. These include expenditure made on inventory staff, expenditure on providing various facilities like heating, lighting, floor space, shelves and racks, bins and containers, material handling equipment and other provisions for safe and proper storage of items. These costs generally depend upon the volume to value ratio of an item. Generally it varies between 1 to 3%.

This advocates smaller size of the inventory.

(c) **Deterioration, obsolescence and pilferage :** Some items are likely to deteriorate in quality with time, e.g. food stuff. If such items are in store for considerable time, then the organisation may decide to dispose them at a loss. This results undue loss to the enterprise. Also, the demand for certain products may fall due to introduction and development of new products. In such cases the manufacturer may decide to scrap the product or sell it at some loss.

These costs may take various forms, *viz.*

 (i) **Outright Spoilage :** The loss is wholly borne at some fixed period of time by the manufacturer.

 (ii) The risk that a particular item will become (a) technologically obsolete or go out of style. Their value in stock decay with life. An exponential decay of value due to obsolescene has been used on occasion in such situations.,

 (iii) The product may become out of date, *viz.* pharmaceutical products.

 (iv) Pilferage, breakage, evaporation, etc. Some goods are subject to theft and misappropriation, breakage or accidental losses, etc. Valuables are more tempting to be stolen and thus be kept under lock.

The costs due to these factors can be quantified as percentage loss. Past write offs and the inventory levels could provide the arithmetic data for such a computation. It varies between 5 to 7 per cent.

(d) **Insurance :** Most of the firms get insurance cover and 1 to 2 per cent may be taken as the representative percentage. Total inventory carrying costs are around 20% of the value of average stock during a year. If the the average stock during a year is Rs. 60,000 and the inventory carrying cost is taken as 20% of the average inventory, then its value will be

60,000 x 20/1000 = Rs. 12,000

The organisation may like to maintain low inventory size to minimise inventory carrying costs.

The general breakup of inventory carrrying costs can be :

METHODS OF INVENTORY CONTROL

The fundamental purpose of inventory analysis is to keep the stock of items at such a level that there is a balance between the costs which increase or decrease with the size of the inventory.

This needs determination of (i) quantities that should be ordered each time and (ii) the time at which this order should be placed so that both inventory carrying costs and the losses arising out of stock-outs are kept at the minimum. These objectives are accomplished by determining :

(i) Economic Lot Size
(ii) Re-ordering level

ECONOMIC LOT SIZE

The amount of material procured or quantity produced during one production run by an enterprise is known as lot size. The quantity to be ordered, whether from inside sources or from outside agencies depends on a number of factors. The size of inventory depends on lot size. Due to increase in inventory size expenditure on storage, deterioration etc. is likely to increase whereas expenditure on setting-up of plant, procurement of materials etc. will decrease. Thus with lot size, there are two set of factors having opposite contributions towards the expenditure, i.e. one encourages the lot size and other discourage.

Thus with lot size, there are two set of factors having opposite contributions towards the expenditure, i.e. one encourages the lot size and other discourage. The total cost associated with particular lot size is a combination of expenditures on all these factors.

These opposing forces exhibit an interesting behaviour towards total costs. It is observed that the factors whose costs decrease with lot size has a tendency to decrease at a faster rate then the rate of increase in cost of those factors whose costs increase with inventory size. Due to this the total cost tend to decrease with lot size. But after certain level of lot size the rate of decreasing costs slows down and the rate of increasing costs steps up. This leads to an increase in the total cost.

Total cost = Purchase price + cost due to factors whose cost increase with lot size + cost due to factors whose costs decreases with lot size.

The lot size Q_E for which the total cost per time period is minimum is known as Economic Lot Size.

The determination of Economic Lot Size is difficult due to problems in the calculation of carrying costs. Carrying cost is related to a number of factors which are difficult to be assessed in practice.

The following assumptions are made in determination of Economic Order Quantity :

(i)   Demand D is assumed to be known with certainty.

(ii)   The size of each order is constant.

(iii)   The procurement cost C_o is assumed to be linearly related to the number of orders.

Replenishment i.e. supply of the items is instantaneous : This is a most ideal system, where the enterprise is not worried about the replenishment of inventory. There is no time lag between the placement of an order and its supply. The items ordered are immediately supplied. It is also assumed that demand remains uniform.

LEAD TIME

This is the time gap between placement of an order and the time of actual supply. It is not necessarily identical to delivery time. It is composed of three components, namely

Lead Time = Servicing time + Delivery time + Receiving time.

Servicing Time : It is the time taken for placing an order. It includes (i) time for obtaining quotations, (ii) time for negotiating price, (iii) time for visiting potential suppliers and (iv) time for 'letting' contracts.

Delivery Time : The time taken by the supplier to comply certain order.

Receiving Time : This includes (i) time for uncrating goods, (ii) time for inspection of goods, (iii) time for movement of goods to store and (iv) time for entering goods in stocks. All these times never remain constant. Thus the determination of Lead Time is a complicated matter. In practice either it is taken to be constant or some reasonable or expected value is assigned to it. Theoreticians recommend that whenever the actual lead time is more than five times the active time, scheduling procedure should be investigated.

SAFETY OR BUFFER STOCK

The demand and supply rates can never be assessed exactly. There is bound to be discrepancy between actual and estimated demand and supply quantities with fair degree of uncertainty. The organisation with a policy of safeguarding their interest against these uncertainties maintain the level of inventory at some desired minimum level. This minimum level of inventory to cover some unforeseen and uncalled for situations is known as Safety or Buffer Stock. Alternately a buffer stock can also be defined as the average stock available in inventory when the fresh supply arrives. It is presumed that this stock will be able to cope with the emergency if and when experienced. Generally, safety stock is maintained at the desired level by discontinuous replenishments at varying intervals of time.

Factors affecting choice of safety stocks are :

    (i) uncertainty in demand

    (ii) degree of insurance for any item

    (iii) uncertainty in lead time, and

    (iv) size of the batch.

Large the uncertainty associated with any factor, larger should be the buffer stock.

Evidently the size of buffer stock mainly depends on two factors, variation in the demand during lead time and the duration of lead time. There are two approaches to determine the safety stock to be left in order to cover demand rate variations, (1) explicit consideration of shortage costs ; and (2) implicit consideration of shortage costs.

1. Since inventory control basically involves the trade-offs between different costs, we may consider (a) the cost of not having the materials in the quantity that may be required and (b) the cost of keeping excess material in stock for fear of demand rate variations. The former cost per unit of the material is called as the "under-stocking cost" or the "shortage cost", the later cost for limit of the material is called as the "over-stocking cost". These two categories of cost are the opportunity costs and a mathematical analysis can be carried out to find the optimal trade-off between these two opposing costs, the stock level at which the total of these two costs is minimum.

2. Instead of speaking in terms of explicit values of the under-stocking and over-stocking costs, one may gauge the uncertain demand rates in terms of a "risk factor" or "risk-level". The safety stock is then determined based on the 'risk' which the organisation is willing to undertake.

Once maximum demand rate is fixed, the calculations of safety stock is easy. Since the safety stock is required for the lead time only, the amount of safety stock will be :

(D maximum - D average) over the lead time.

Material Losses

Material losses do occur in every type of manufacturing organisation. These losses may be in the form of waste, spoilage or defective work. There is no uniformity in the terminology and accounting treatment of these items. The most commonly adopted practice in respect of each of the above items is given below.

Waste

It represents that portion of the basic raw material which has been lost in the manufacturing process and which has no recoverable value, e.g., gases, dust smoke, unsaleable residue, losses on account of shrinkage or evaporation of materials, etc.

Control of waste : Standards or norms should be fixed for each type of waste. The actual percentage of waste should be compared with the standard percentage. Waste Reports should be prepared at regular intervals. Particular care has to be taken to check abnormal waste. This can be done by holding regular meetings with the foreman and his staff.

Accounting treatment : (a) Normal Waste : Waste within the normal limites should be distributed over good output. Thus per unit cost would be increased.

(b) Abnormal Waste : Waste beyond the normal limits should be transferred to costing profit and loss account so as to avoid any fluctuations in the cost of production.

SCRAP DISPOSAL

Scrap is the incidental material residue coming out of certain types of manufacturing processes, usually of small amount and low value, recoverable without further processing. Scrap may arise on account of turnings, borings, trimmings, etc. from metals on which machine operations are carried out. By-products of small value which are sold without further processing are also treated as scrap. It should be noted that 'scrap' is always physically available while waste may or may not be present in the form of a residue.

Control over Scrap : Control over scrap is possible by :

    (i) setting standards for scrap,

    (ii) determining the responsibility for scrap,

    (iii) keeping up proper records of scrap in the form of Scrap Reports.

SURPLUS DISPOSAL

While manufacturing any product or rendering any services, resources in the form of land, labour, capital, material, time, machine, money, energy, transport, etc. are utilized and in this process surplus occurs in every resources. For example, surplus can arise in industry, because of overproduction. It may be due to overspecification and leads to the purchase of costlier than necessary items.

Surplus also occurs because of impulsive buying, wrong identification over-buying, etc. In engineering industries, we often observe, that due to non-availability of the correct size of sheet plates and rods, bigger sizes are used, leaving the remaining difficult as surplus.

Another source is spillage of materials, that are transported in bulk. In case of volatile elements like petrol, surplus or wastage is in the form of evaporation losses. Improper handling leads to breakages thereby results in surplus or wastage. During storage, surplus of materials occurs due to improper warehousing facilities leading to deterioration of quality, corrosion, improper use of preservatives, humidity, excessive heat, cold, and other environmental factors.

DISPOSAL OF SURPLUS

Disposals of surplus, scrap and waste items are indeed a tricky art. One has to deal with a set of hard bargains, who gang themselves into cartels.

Before initiating disposal action, it is essential to segregate the surplus according to metal and size. When costly scrap such as Copper, Aluminium or Tungsten are involved, it is imperative that they are segregated as price differences are huge. Various metallurgical, chemical, magnetic, spectrographic and other tests are available to sort waste by quality, grade size and weight, turnings, cuttings, borings, etc. should be sorted out to avoid getting the price of the cheapest component. Oil scraped lots must be kept separately.

The normal procedure adopted in selling of surplus is either through open auctions or through the commonly used tender system. In some cases organisations also have to pay money to remove the waste occupying huge space in the junkyard. Parties are normally required to inspect the surplus in the scrapyard and deposit requisite earnest money. Very often the finance department insists on a basic price depending upon the category of scrap, which may not always be realisable. The disposal section may usually try to enter into a long term contract with end-users such as steel plants. The collection of scrap may be carried out daily, but the disposal action is usually on a monthly or quaterly basis. Special case must be taken about weighing of these items, so that money is not lost due to short weightments.

MARGIN OF SAFETY

Total sales minus the sales at break-even point is known as the 'margin of safety'. Margin of safety can be expressed as a percentage to total sales also. Thus the formula is :

Margin of Safety = Total sales - Sales at Break-even point

As a percentage = Margin of Safety/Total Sales x 100

If the margin of safety is large, it is sign of soundness of the business since even with a substantial reduction sales, profit shall be earned by the business. If the margin is small, reduction in sales even to a small tune may affect the profit position very adversely and larger reduction of sales value may even result in losses. Thus, margin of safety serves as a guide to the strength of the business.

For rectifying the unsatisfactory margin of safely, the management can take any of the following steps :

(i) Selling prices may be increased but it should not affect the demand adversely otherwise the revenue in sales net shall not be able to cope up with the requirements.

(ii) Fixed or the variable cost may be reduced.

(iii) Production may be enhanced, but it should be at a lower cost.

(iv) Unprofitable products may be substituted by profitable ones.

MAXIMUM AND MINIMUM LEVELS

In order to avoid over under investments in materials, the management should decide the maximum and minimum quantity of materials to be kept in the store. The limits set by the management should be observed by the store-keeper.

Maximum Level

The maximum level is the largest quantity of a particular material which should be kept in the store at any one time. The fixation of maximum level is necessary to avoid unnecessary blocking up of the capital in inventories, losses on account of deterioration and obsolescence of materials, extra overheads (rent etc.) and temptations to thefts. The maximum level of materials should be decided after taking into consideration the following points :

(i) **Storage space** : Large stocks of materials require large storage space, and, therefore, the maximum quantity of a particular type of material will depend upon the total space available, and the space to be allocated or already allocated to other items.

(ii) **Availability of working capital** : stocks require investment of capital and therefore, availability of working capital for investment in a particular type of material should also be considered.

(iii) **Seasonal considerations** : to maintain uninterrupted production larger quantities of material in stores will be required if the materials are available in the market only in certain seasons.

(iv) Rate of consumption of materials and time necessary in obtaining new materials.

(v) Rules framed by Government for import or procurement : If due to these, materials are difficult to obtain and supplies are irregular, the maximum level should be high.

vi) **Economic order quantities** : This has been explained later.

/ii) Cost of storage, insurance, interest on capital invested in stocks are some of the other points to be considered.

ormula

laximum level = Re-order level + Re-order quantity - (Minimum consump-
_n x Minimum Re-order period).

Minimum Level

The minimum level is the lowest quantitative balance of materials which must be maintained in hand at all times so that the assembly line may not be stopped on account of non-availability of materials. It should be decided by taking into account of following factors :

    (i) Average rate of consumption of materials.

    (ii) Average time required to obtain delivery of fresh supplies.

    (iii) Re-order level.

Formula

Minimum level = Re-order level - average rate of consumption x average time required to obtain fresh delivery

RE-ORDERING LEVEL OR ORDERING LEVEL

It is the point at which if the material in store reaches, further supplies must be ordered. The re-order level is fixed somewhere between the maximum and minimum level in such a way that the quantity of materials represented by the difference between the reordering level and the minimum level will be sufficient to meet the demands of production till such time as the order materialises and supplies are received. Re-order level mainly depends on two factors :

    (i) Maximum consumption.

    (ii) Lead time i.e., the anticipated time lag between the dates of issuing orders and the receipt of materials.

Formula

        Re-order level = Maximum re-order period x Maximum usage.

Danger Level

It is the level of stock below which the material stock should never be allowed to fall in normal circumstances. It is slightly less than the minimum level, and at such a point the Purchase Manager should make special efforts to acquire required materials and stores.

     In some concerns danger level is fixed above the minimum level but below the re-order level. In case the order has been placed for materials on reaching the re-order level, the only significance of such a level is to check up with the Purchase Department that materials will be received in time. Thus fixation of danger level below the minimum level is meant for taking corrective action, while its fixation above the minimum level is an indicator for preventive action.

ECONOMIC ORDERING QUANTITY

It refers to the size of the order which gives maximum economy in purchasing any material. It is also referred as optimum or standard ordering quantity. It is fixed mainly after taking into consideration the following costs :

(i) **Ordering cost :** It is the cost of placing an order and securing the supplies. It varies from time to time depending upon the number of orders placed and the number of items ordered. The more frequently the orders are placed, and fewer the quantities purchased on each order, the greater will be the ordering cost and vice versa.

(ii) **Inadequate inventory or stock out cost :** The precise ascertainment of such cost is virtually impossible. It includes the cost of expending purchases, obtaining rush deliveries, keeping rack of back orders etc., all associated with carrying too little inventory. Besides that loss of sales, customers' goodwill etc., arising from non-fulfilment of delivery promises are also covered by this category.

(iii) **Inventory carrying cost :** It is the cost of keeping items in stock. It includes interest on investment, obsolescence losses, store keeping cost, insurance premium etc. The larger the volume of inventory, the higher will be the inventory carrying cost and vice versa.

The first two costs may be referred as the "cost of acquiring" while the last as "cost of holding" inventory. The cost of acquiring decreases while the cost of holding increases with every increase in the quantity of purchase lot. A balance is, therefore, struck between the two opposing factors and the economic ordering quantity is determined at a level for which the aggregate of two costs is the minimum.

Formula

$$Q = \sqrt{2U \times p / S}$$

where,

Q = Economic ordering quantity

U = Quantity (units) purchased or used in a year

P = Cost of placing an order

S = Annual cost of storage of one unit

Re-ordering Quantity

The term re-ordering quantity refers to the standard quantity of material which is normally placed on order when the stock reaches the re-order level. The term is used generally in synonymous with the economic ordering quantity since order should be placed only in such size which will be economical for the enterprise in all respects.

Average Stock Level

The level indicates the average stock held by the concern. It is calculated with the help of following formula :

Average stock level = 1/2 (Maximum level + Minimum level)

A more refined method of measuring average stock level is one involving re-order quantity. The formula is :

Average stock level = Minimum stock level + 1/2 (Re-ordering quantity)

ABC (Always Better Control) Analysis

It is based on the concept 'Thick on the best and thin on the rest'. It is observed that any organisation have to stock and keep track of large numbr of items of different kinds. These can be service parts of products no longer available, supplies of law materials for general use, maintenance items and items for various other purposes. The investment in such items is substantial and record keeping is expensive.

In practive it is experienced that a bulk of items in an inventory have low usage value.

Annual usage value = (Annual requirement)   ×   per unit cost.

Thus for better and more economic control of items in inventory the items should be classified according to their significance or priority for reordering. The production manager should recognise the unequal contribution of different items in the inventory and the fact that equal effort should not be sent on improving the inventory policy of the items. On the other hand, the inventory should not run out of items whose usage value is low but which are of great importance in production process, e.g. washer of some component has low cost but if it is out of stock then the machine may become out of order.

Economy in control can be obtained by paying little attention on those items which usually costs less to absorb the loss due to waste than to keep a record, e.g. paper clips, rubber bands etc. which are generally kept on hand and people help themselves.

So for effective inventory control, a decision has to be made that which items are little things and which need more careful control. The items of an inventory can be categorised as :

  (i) Items which are functionally critical to the operations; no matter how little they cost.
 (ii) Items that are important because their usage value is high.
(iii) Items having average usage value.
 (iv) Items which have low usage value.

One such way of classifying the items of an inventory is ABC analysis. It focusses attention on those items where more savings can be expected. A few high usage value items constitute a major part of the capital invested in inventories whereas bulk of inventory items having low usage value constitute insignificant part of the capital. The concept is based upon selective control, when there are large number of items to be analysed then sampling may be done for ABC analysis.

In ABC analysis the items are categorised in three main categories on the basis of their usage value :

(i) More costly and valuable items are classified as A. These are large investment items but not much in number, i.e. vital few say 10% of the items account for 75% of total capital invested in inventory. These items need more closer and careful control.

The requirement for A class items should be ascertained ahead of time according to the period of use and their production of purchase should be scheduled such that these arrive just before needed. These items should be ordered frequently but in smaller size. A periodic review policy should be followed to minimise the stock out percentage of such items and top inventory staff should control these items.

These items have high inventory cost and frequent orders of smaller size for these items can result in enormous savings.

(ii) Average usage value items are classified as B. About 15% of the items in an inventory account for 15% of the total investment. These items are less important than A class items but are costly enough to have more attention on their use. These items cannot be overlooked but need lesser degree of control than those in class A. Statistical sampling is generally applied in their control.

(iii) Low usage value items are put in class C. About 75% of the inventory items account for only 10% of the invested capital. These items can be stored at an operative place where people can help themselves without any requisition formality. These can be charged to an overhead account. No doubt loose control of 'C' items will increase their investment cost and expenditure on shelfwear, obsolescence and wasteful use but this will not be so much to offset the savings in recording costs.

ABC analysis focuses the attention of management where it is needed in due proportion.

An objective of such classification is to separate out the group C which is large in number and which may potentially require a large amount of record keeping and attention but which is relatively unimportant from the point of view of keeping inventory investment at reasonable levels. Here the items are classified in terms of their usage value. Usage value is not the price of an item but it is the product of usage over a period generally a year and its unit price.

The items in A, B and C classes can be compared in the following tabular form :

Class of Items

	A	B	C
1.	Maintains close control	Maintains moderate control	Maintains loose control
2.	Size of order based on calculated requirement	Size of order based on usage	Size of order based on the level of inventory
3.	Procured from many sources	Procured from two or three sources	Procured from two sources
4.	Keeps records of receipt and use	Keeps records of receipt and use	No records are kept
5.	More effort to reduce lead time	Moderate effort	Minimum effort
6.	Close checks on schedule revision	Some checks on changes in need	No checks against need
7.	Frequent ordering	Less frequent ordering	Bulk ordering
8.	Continual expediting	Expediting for prospective shortages	No expediting
9.	Accurate forecasts	Less accurate forecasts	Approximate forecasts
10.	Low safety stock for less than 2 weeks	Large safety stock upto 2 to 3 months	Large safety stock for more than 3 months
11.	High consumption value	Average consumption value	Low consumption value

The following points should be kept in mind for ABC analysis :

(i) Where items can be substituted for each other, they should be preferably treated as one item.

(ii) More emphasis should be given to the value of consumption and not to price per unit of the item.

(iii) All the items consumed by an organisation should be conisdered together for classifying as A,B or C instead of taking them as spares, raw materials, semi-finished and finished items and then classifying as A,B or C.

(iv) There can be more than three classes and the period of consumption need not necessarily be one year.

The following are the steps for classification of items as A,B or C.

(i) Take a representative sample of stock items.

(ii) The annual usage value is calculated for each item to be classified by multiplying the quantity used with the unit price of the item.

(iii) The usage values in step (ii) are arranged in descending order.

(iv) Calculate the cumulative total of the number of items and the usage value obtained in step (iii).

(v) Find the percentage of the values obtained in step (iv) w.r.t. the grand total of the corresponding columns.

(vi) Percentage of items are taken on X axis and the corresponding usage value percentage on Y arises to plot various points on graph paper and to draw a smooth curve.

(vii) Mark the points X and Y where the slope of the curve changes sharply (points of inflexion). The usage value and the percentage of items corresponding to these points will determine the items to be classified as A, B or C.

Application of ABC Analysis

ABC analysis can be effectively used in Material Management.

The various stages where it can be applied are :

(i) Information of items which require higher degree of control.

(ii) To evolve useful re-ordering strategy.

(iii) Stock records.

(iv) Priority treatment to defferent items.

(v) Determination of safety stock limits.

(vi) Stores layout.

(vii) Value analysis.

Vital Essential Desirable (V.E.D.) Analysis

This analysis is applied to old brands which have greater requirement. The past trends are not useful in the analysis of these brands. The important criteria are the availability and price. When there are six brands of the same formulation, the formulations are classified as vital, essential and desirable. For example, quinine is available as quinine sulphate, quinine hydrochloride, quinine ethyl carbonate, and quinine bisulphate. Then quinine sulphate is vital (more demand), quinine hydrochloride is essential (less demand) and quinine ethyl carbonate is desirable (very less prescriptions). Therefore, maximum inventory of quinine sulphate should be kept.

13

SALES PROMOTION

Sales promotion is an important method of promotion which has been developed in recent years to supplement and coordinate personal selling and advertising efforts. Sales promotion includes those marketing activities, other than personal selling, advertising, and publicity, that stimulate consumer purchasing and dealer effectiveness, such as displays, shows and expositions, demonstration, and various non-recurrent selling efforts not in the ordinary routine. Sales promotion includes free sample, premium on sale, sales and dealer incentives, contesting, fairs and exhibitions, public relations activities, etc.

Sales promotion has a distinct field of operation. It is different from personal selling which is persuasion of customers by the sales persons to buy certain products. It is also different from advertising. Except for direct mail, advertising deals with media owned and controlled by the firm itself. Usually, sales promotion deals with non-recurring and non-routine methods in contrast to personnel selling or advertising.

Sales promotion techniques are used for the following purposes :

   (i) Introduction of new products .

   (ii) Winning new customers.

   (iii) Increasing sales during slack season.

   (iv) Increasing the public image of the firm.

Techniques or Devices of Sales Promotion

A wide variety of sales promotion devices are used by different business undertakings. Some of the important devices are discussed below :

1. **Distribution of Samples :** Distribution of samples is an expensive but a powerful tool of sales promotion. Many big businessmen offer free samples of their products to the selected people in order to popularize their products. Regular size packages or special sample size packages

may be used. The sample may be delivered door to door, offered in retail stores or fairs. This device is suitable for introducing new products such as soaps, drugs, cosmetics, perfumes, tea, etc. Since the distribution of samples is very costly, this device is confined to those products which are likely to create repeated sales.

2. **Coupons :** Coupon is a certificate that entitles its holder to a specified saving on the the purchase of a specified product. Coupons may be issued by the manufacturers either directly by mail or through the dealers. The holders of coupons can go to the retailers and get the product at a cheaper price. The retailers are reimbursed by the manufacturer for the value of coupon redeemed and also paid a small percentage to cover handling cost. But many retailers do not patronise this because it involves financial and accounting problems for them.

3. **Premium or Bonus Offer :** It is an offer of a certain amount of product at no cost to the customers who buy a specified quantity of a product or a special pack there of. There are three types of premium offers : (i) with-pack premium, (ii) a reusable container, and (iii) a free in the mail premium. A with-pack premium is included either inside or outside the packet. For example one silver spoon inside the economy size Horlick Bottle. A reusable container is a container that has utility to the consumer after the product is consumed, such as a detergent powder is offered in a plastic bucket. A free in the mail premium is an item that the company will send by mail to the customer who makes a request for it, enclosing a proof of purchase (cash memo or wrapper).

4. **Trading Stamps :** Trading stamps are quite popular in the western countries. Even in India, they are used in a few big cities. Trading stamps (Ramon Bonus Stamps) are issued to customer through the retailers in proportion to their purchases (2.5 % of the amount of sale in the form of Ramon Bonus stamps). The customer collects the stamps until he has a sufficient number of stamps to obtain a desired product in exchange of the stamps from the stamp redemption centres. The customer can choose the premium article from the premium catalogue supplied by the dealers.

5. **Contests :** There may be customers' contest, salesmen contest, and dealers contest. Contests for salesmen and dealers are intended for inducing them to devote greater efforts and/or for obtaining new sales ideas in the task of sales promotion. Contest for consumers is held on the subject of writing a slogan on the product. Such slogan centres around the questions as to the likings of a customer for the product, or formulation of new advertising idea for the product. Such contests are held through radio, T.V., newspapers, magazines, etc.

6. **Public Relations :** Public Relations activities strive for creating a good image of the enterprise in the eyes to the customers and the society.

These activities are not aimed at immediate demand creation. It is very common that big business enterprises convey their greetings and thanks to the people through newspapers and other published media. Space donated by the business houses in the published media in spreading some noble ideas is also a public relations activity.

7. **Fairs and Exhibitions :** Fairs and exhibitions provide an important avenue of sales promotion to the businessmen. Businessmen can demonstrate their products explaining their special features and usefulness. They can also distribute free literature to introduce their firm and products to the public.

ENTREPRENEURIAL DECISIONS IN PROMOTION

(Problems in Establishment of a business)

A business enterprise cannot come into existence without the pioneering efforts of a person or a group of persons known as entrepreneurs or promoters. A promoter conceives the idea of a business enterprise, analyses its prospects, works out the tentative scheme of organizations, brings together the requisite men, materials, machines, money and 'managerial ability and floats the new enterprise. The decisions which an entrepreneur or promoter takes to bring a business into existence are known as entrepreneurs decisions. Entrepreneurial decisions are taken to tackle the problems in setting up a new enterprise business who wants to launch a new business enterprise has to take decisions with regard to the following factors :

1. **Selection of Business Activity :** The process of launching a new business enterprise begins when the businessman has some idea which can be implemented to earn profits. The businessman will analyse the proposed idea to find out whether the business would be profitable or not including the analysis or risks involved and the probable amount of capital required for this purpose. He will conduct a survey of various business opportunities in order to know the various lines of business which he can take up. For this purpose, he has to determine the market demands for the various products which he wants to produce or manufacture and the costs which he would incur for procuring different factors of production. He will prepare a systematic report of the exercise he undertakes. This is known as 'feasibility report' or 'project report'. The project report will show the data collected, estimates of cost and income, opinions of experts in different fields, etc. What is intended to arrive at by the project report is whether the estimated income will be large enough to take care of the estimated operational costs, interest on borrowings and return to owners for the capital invested and the risk undertaken.

The availability of technical and other specialised knowledge required for running a business is another important factor for its selection.

2. **Choice of Form of Ownership :** The choice of the form of organisation will determine the authority of the entrepreneur starting the business. However, in certain lines of business, there is no choice left in the selection of the form of organisation. For instance, insurance and banking business can be done only by the joint stock companies. Size of the business will also determine the form of organisation. Company form of organisation is more suitable in case of large scale operations. Sole tradership or partnership are suitable for small scale and medium scale operations. The other factors which affect the choice of form of ownership are capital requirements, managerial skills requirement, limit of liability, tax liability, legal formalities, etc.

3. **Financing the proposition :** The promoters or the entrepreneurs have to make available sufficient amount of capital for the initiation and continuation of the business enterprise. Capital is required for investment in fixed assets like land, buildings, machines and equipment and in current assets like materials, supplies and book debts. Capital is also needed for meeting day-to-day expenses of the business. In case of small enterprises, the promoters can provide funds from their own savings. But in case of large enterprises; funds have to be raised from various sources like general public, commercial banks, financial institutions, etc. It is of utmost importance to have adequate capital for meeting the initial need and future requirements of the business.

4. **Location of Business :** the location of a business enterprise is an important problem which its promoters have to tackle. The promoters have to take extra care while selecting the location at which the organisation will have easy access to raw materials, labour, power, markets and certain services like banking, transportation, communications, insurance and warehousing. As far as possible, the location must be optimum so that the cost of production and distribution are the lowest possible. If the location of a plant is not suitable, it will cause many problems. The cost of production may increase and the growth of the firm may be restricted. Once the site is selected for the business operations, it is very difficult to change it.

5. **Size of Unit :** Size of the firm is influenced by various forces like technical, managerial, financial and marketing. Some forces favour the larger size while other forces operate to restrict the scale of operations. Where the entrepreneurs are confident that they will be able to market their products and raise sufficient amount of capital, they will start their operations on a large scale. Usually, the businessmen start their operations at small or medium scale. If new ideas are to be tried out, it is preferable to start with a small scale operation. This will help in adapting to changes without much loss. Moreover, huge investment will not be blocked in permanent assets. Forces of risks and uncertainty

compel the business to restrict the scale of their operations. A good businessman should always consider the impact of various forces which determine the scale of operation. The basic purpose of the optimum size is to achieve maximum output at minimum cost.

6. **Machines and Equipment :** The choice of machines and equipment is a delicate problem before starting a new business. It will depend upon various factors like availability of funds, size of production, and the nature of production process. The benefits to be derived from the machine and equipment must justify the amount of investment made on them. Greater mechanisation should not be resorted to look modern, but to have higher productivity. There is no use of installing a plant unless right types of workers are available. Availability of repair and maintenance services and spare parts is also an important consideration while selecting a particular machine or equipment. Special purpose machine should be installed only when the scale of operations is very large..

7. **Plant Layout :** Plant layout should be efficient to achieve economy and efficiency in operations. An efficient plant layout is one that allows materials to move through necessary operation rapidly and in the most direct way possible. It takes care of intensity of in-process and tries to shorten all heavily travelled routes. This reduces transport, materials handling, clerical and other costs and increases inventory turnover. It also minimises the space required.

8. **Labour Force :** The entrepreneur cannot run the business himself along. He has to take the help of a large number of persons including skilled and un-skilled workers and managerial staff. The employment of right type of person for the enterprise is necessary, otherwise, there will be huge wastage of time, money and effort. After the placement of personnel, they have to be given the necessary training. Motivation of the personnel is another area which deserves attention of the entrepreneur. The work-force must be motivated to contribute effectively for the achievement of the objectives of the enterprise.

9. **Procedural formalities :** In almost every type of business, some procedural formalities have to be observed while starting a new enterprise. In case of a sole proprietorship or a partnership, there are practically no procedural formalities. Only permission from the municipality is to be taken to start the specified line of business. Registration of a partnership firm is not compulsory. Government regulation is the minimum possible if the partnership firm operates on a small or medium scale. But a joint stock company is exposed to greater procedural formalities both at the time of incorporation and during its life. Incorporation of a company is compulsory. For this purpose, many documents have to be prepared and fee deposited with the Registrar of companies. A public company has also to secure a certificate to commence business before

it starts its operations. After this, the company is require to send periodical returns to the Registrar of Companies and stock exchange authorities.

10. **Launching the Enterprise :** At this stage, the promoter arranges for the acquisition of necessary men, materials, machinery, money and managerial ability. After getting these resources, he will develop an organisation structure and divide work among the personnel. After this, the production will start taking into consideration the needs of the customers. Various departments like production, financing, marketing, personnel, etc. are created to accomplish the objectives of the enterprise. Management coordinates the working of these departments and communicates the availability of the products to the prospective customers through advertising and sales promotion activities.

11. **Tax planning :** Tax planning has become an essential task these days because of a number of tax laws prevailing in the country. The promoter of the business has to visualise well in advance the various taxes which the enterprise will have to pay. Of all the taxes, income tax is the most important factor which determines the type of ownership organisation.

Companies are subjected to uniform rate of taxation. The rate of tax remains the same irrespective of the volume of profits. Profits earned by a sole proprietorship or a partnership firm are subjected to a progressive rate of taxation. The rate of tax goes on increasing with the increase in the volume of profits.

Requisite of Success in Business

Business has become a very complex activity in the modern era of change. A business does not operate in vacuum ; it is constantly under the pressure of a large number of environmental forces. These forces create difficulties for any business enterprise. A successful business enterprise is one which has appropriate interaction with the environmental forces and which is able to manage the achievement of its objectives effectively and efficiently. Such an enterprise not only survives in the market, but is also able to proceed towards growth and prosperity.

Growth is an important objective of business enterprises. They seek to become bigger each year in earnings, assets, market size or influence. The growth objective can be achieved if a business enterprise takes care of the following requisites :

(i) **Clear-cut Objectives :** The objectives of a business enterprise must be well-defined. The primary as well as the secondary objectives should be laid down separately. Objectives should also laid down in various areas of business on which its survival and growth depends. These areas include production, marketing, financing, purchasing, research and development, etc. The objectives in these areas should be in harmony with the overall business objectives. The objectives should be capable of being achieved during a specified period.

(ii) **Location, Layout and Size :** These factors also influence the success of a business enterprise to a great extent. Proper location will reduce the cost of operation. Proper layout will increase efficiency and avoid wastage of various kinds. Optimum size will lead to lowest average cost of production. Any mistake committed in regard to these factors may prove to be fatal or for the survival of the enterprise.

(iii) **Effective Business Planning :** Efficient business planning is based on sales forecasting. The entrepreneur must make an accurate forecast of sales in the forthcoming year if he wants to make sound plans. Separate plans should be prepared for every department of the enterprise. The departmental plans should be coordinated with the master plans of the enterprise. Sound planning aims at running the business enterprises smoothly and dealing with the future contingencies efficiently and effectively.

(iv) **Sound Organisation :** Sound organisation is necessary for the accomplishment of business objectives. Organisation deals with division of work among the personnel of the enterprise in such a way that proper coordination of their operations and other factors of production is facilitated. A clear-cut organisational structure should be laid down to show authority and responsibility relationships throughout the enterprise. Everybody should also know relevance of his job for the achievement of the business objectives. The management of the business should also make available machines and equipment, tools, raw materials, etc. of proper type to the workers.

(v) **Financial Planning :** Finance is the life-blood of a modern business. The finance function of the business should be efficiently managed. Business requires funds for long-term and short-term capital. It is also the responsibility of financial management to see that funds are invested in worth-while projects and ventures. The capital structure should also be a balanced one. It should contain various types of securities, namely, equity shares, preferential shares and debentures in a proper proportion.

(vi) **Efficient Marketing :** The survival of a business depends upon the acceptability of its goods and services by the customers. Therefore, approach to marketing should be customer oriented. The marketing department should conduct market survey to understand the needs of the customers and convey them to the production department so that goods and services of right specifications and quality are produced. It should be the endeavor of every business to produce and sell those goods and services which will satisfy the needs of the customers.

(vii) **Dynamic Management :** The management is an agency which can help a business enterprise to achieve its objectives or goals. It is of utmost importance that the business is managed by competent managers who are efficient and have dynamic outlook. Good management will get the desired results from the people working in the enterprise and will coordinate the working of various segments of the enterprise.

(viii) **Human Relations :** There should always be good relations in the enterprise. An effective two-way communication system between the management and the workers should be installed so that reactions, suggestions and grievances of the workers are known immediately. Management should treat the workers as human beings and should take steps for their welfare. It should motivate the employees by providing them financial as well as non-financial incentives. These steps would lead to building a work-force which will co-operate with the management for the realisation of business objectives.

(ix) **Research and Innovation :** Every business must spend a part of its earnings on research and innovation activities so that it may offer better products to the customers at reasonable prices. This will raise the standard of living of the society. It is also essential for the business to engage in research and development activities. This will lead to finding of new production processes which are cheaper than the existing ones.

Qualities of a Successful Entrepreneur of Promoter

A man who has once mastered the business of being a businessman, who has learnt the fundamentals of organisation of financial management, of accounting, of working with and commanding men, of buying or selling, can therefore, quickly master and succeed in new business. A businessman who is going to provide leadership to his business should possess the following qualities :

1. **Wide knowledge :** A businessman must have wide knowledge of the economic and non-economic environment of the business. He must be well-known about the latest technological developments and marketing conditions. In the absence of wide knowledge, the decisions taken by him will be poor and will not contribute to the well-being of his business in the long-run.

2. **Foresight :** Business is full of risks and uncertainties. In order to deal with various kinds of risks and uncertainties efficiently, the businessman should be intelligent and have far-sightedness to make good forecasts for the business. The quality of forecasting will determine the quality of business planning.

3. **Dynamic Outlook :** A good businessman is dynamic in nature. He has the capacity to take quick and sound decisions on various problems of the business. He is always prepared to take initiative whenever an opportunity arises.

4. **Adaptability :** A good businessman knows how to change with the changed circumstances. He can adapt himself to the changed environ-

ment. He does not put resistance to change. He his an open mind towards new developments in technology and marketing.

5. **Business Morality and Social Responsibility :** A good businessman does not indulge in unethical business practices. He is honest towards consumers, workers, suppliers, Government and society. He works sincerely to satisfy certain demands of the society and to raise the standard of living of the people. He is not tempted by unfair trade practices to maximise his profit. He understands his social obligations and takes steps to perform these obligations.

6. **Consistency in Behavior :** The behavior of the businessman should be consistent and dependable. He should take firm decisions and should not change his policies quite often. He should create confidence among workers, suppliers and consumers. If a businessman is dependable, the various groups of the society dealing with him will cooperate with him in expanding the scale of operations of his business.

7. **Aptitude for Research :** A businessman should have aptitude for innovation and research for the benefit of the society. He should understand the utility of his products from the point of view of the society and take steps to help the people to derive greater utility from his products.

8. **Self-Confidence :** A good businessman should have self-confidence. Self-confidence is created only if the businessman is honest and dependable and has the capacity to take initiative. He should not lose heart if he does not achieve success in a particular project.

9. **Business Connections and Goodwill :** The success of a business depends to a great extent on its connection with other business undertakings and its goodwill in the market. A good businessman should try to build up the reputation of his business and keep good relations an other business enterprises. He should be co-operative in nature.

10. **Winning Personality :** A businessman should possess the minimum qualities required of a good leader. He should have self-discipline, presence of mind, sense of justice, honour and dignity, and above all a high moral character. He should have constructive imagination and ability to take quick decisions.

14

MARKETING RESEARCH

Marketing research is the intelligence service of a business enterprise. It means the careful and objective study of product design, markets, and such transfer activities as physical distribution and warehousing, advertising and sale management. American Marketing Association defined marketing research as "the gathering, recording and analysing of all facts about problems relating to the transfer and sale of goods and services from producer to consumer."

Marketing research is a systematic and intensive investigation of all phases of marketing on a continuous basis with a view to have a better understanding and knowledge about the present and future marketing problems in the direction of satisfaction of the needs of the customer. Marketing research is a wider term and includes market research. Market research merely deals with the discovery of the capacity of the market to absorb a particular product. Other areas covered by marketing research include location of the market, nature of the market, product analysis, sales analysis, time, place and media of advertising, personal selling and channels of distribution.

Objectives of Marketing Research

Marketing research is usually conducted to achieve the following objectives:

1. **To know about the persons buy the firm's products :** Marketing research tries to reveal the number of persons who buy, the frequency of their buying and the sources of their buying. It also includes the social status and the regional location of the customers.

2. **To find out the impact of promotional efforts :** Marketing research facilitates appraising and improving the methods of sales promotion. It also leads to measure the effectiveness of advertising, pricing policies and channels of distribution.

3. **To know customer response to a new product :** This is also known as product testing. Marketing research is frequently used to know the opinion of the consumers about the satisfaction given by a new product. This helps in knowing the desired improvements in quality, design, size, packing, distribution method, etc.

4. **To forecast sales :** Marketing research helps in sales forecasting and market planning. The researchers make sales forecast on the basis of the response from the customers and the distribution media.

5. **To study the goodwill of the firm in comparison with the competing firms :** This helps in revealing the important information regarding the moves of the competitors, new products and substitutes entering the market and their impact over the firm's product.

Significance of Marketing Research

Marketing is one of the most important areas of any business enterprise. Making of right type of decisions in the areas determines the success of the enterprise. Correct and sound marketing decision can be made only if right type of information is available to the management. The required information can be made available by conducting marketing research. The significance of marketing research has increased because of severe competition in the market, frequent technological changes and the emergency of buyers' market. Marketing research is also the corner stone of the marketing concept. No business enterprise can claim to be customers centered without the performance of the marketing research function. Marketing research is an invaluable tool of management to implement the marketing concept and to take various decisions to satisfy the demands of the customers.

There is generally a time lag between production and consumption due to large scale production. The greater the time lag, the greater is the need for marketing research. The taste and behavior of the consumers change very fast. It is always necessary to have information about such changes and adjust production accordingly. If it is not done, the product manufactured by the firm may not be sold in the market.

The gap between the manufacturers and the consumers has increased these days because of the existence of a large chain of middleman. There is virtually no communication between the manufacturers and the consumers in order to fill up this communication gap, marketing research is necessary. It will help in knowing the needs, opinions and reactions of the customers. This will enable the management to take appropriate decision to supply the kinds of goods and services demanded by the customers. Marketing research will also facilitate in catching up with the new developments brought about by science and technology.

Advantages of Marketing Research

A business enterprise can derive the following benefits by conducting market research :

1. Marketing research facilitates forecasting of demand for the products of the firm. This will help in adjusting the production schedules accordingly.

2. Marketing research helps in knowing the probability of acceptance of the product in its present form. Such type of research may lead to alterations in design, colour and other features of the product to make it more acceptable by the consumers.

3. Marketing research reduces wasteful expenditure on production and advertisement. It tells in advance the products and services which are required by the customers.

4. Marketing research helps in discovering new markets and in understanding the behaviour of various types of customers.

5. Marketing research can be used to study the effectiveness of existing channels of distribution, advertising, sales promotion activities and other marketing activities.

6. Marketing research provides invaluable information which not only affects the working of the Marketing Department but has also an important impact on the functioning of other departments of the enterprise, particularly production and purchase departments.

7. Marketing research helps in knowing the reaction of the middlemen in regard to the company's marketing politics. This may lead to the discovery of the new lines of production which can be taken up alongwith the existing products.

Limitation of Marketing Research

Marketing research suffers from the following limitations :

1. Marketing research involves huge expenditure of money, efforts and time on the collection and analysis of data. Small firms cannot afford marketing research.

2. The effectiveness of marketing research depends largely on the type of data or information collected. The business or subjectivity of the investigators may have adverse effect on the effectiveness of the marketing research.

3. Marketing research is mainly a study of the behaviour of human beings. The individuals may not always give adequate and accurate data. Thus, the results of the marketing research are not cent per cent accurate.

4. Marketing research is not an end in itself. It is a means to decision making. It requires competent and experienced managers to use the results of marketing research.

Market Research

Market research is the gathering, recording and analysis of market data to identify the present and potential customers and their motives and buying habits. It is the discovery of the capacity of the market to absorb the products of a firm. Marketing research is the systematic, objective and exhaustive search for and study of the facts relevant to any problem in the field of marketing. Market research is restricted to the study of actual and potential buyers, their location, their actual and potential value of purchases and their motives and habits.

Market research may be conducted for the following reasons :

1. To identify the present and potential customers and their needs.
2. To forecast the demand of a product.
3. To determine customers' preference with regard to packaging, design, size, price and other features of a product.
4. To locate the demand for products with regard to time and place such as festival demand.
5. To explore new markets for existing products.

Marketing Research Procedure

A systematic procedure of marketing research involves the following steps :

1. **Identification of area or kind of research :** It is essential to identify the area in which the research is to be conducted. This will help in determining the problem of marketing research. Marketing research may be conducted in any field of marketing. But generally, it may take any or all of the following forms :

    (a) Research on products, i.e., determining needs and demands of customers for development of the product of right type.

    (b) Research on markets, i.e., investigation into the size and character of markets, territorial sale opportunities and economic factors operating on markets.

    (c) Research on promotional activities, i.e., evaluation of advertisement media, personal selling and other techniques of informing and persuading the customers.

    (d) Research on marketing policies, i.e., effectiveness of marketing policies in the field of pricing, distribution channel, advertisement, sales promotion, public relations, credit and so on.

2. **Collecting necessary information :** The marketing research department may collect information from various sources which may be either primary or secondary. The primary sources of data refer to the first hand original data collected by the investigators through observations, interview, questionnaire, and an field survey. The information may be collected directly from the customers dealers and salesmen. The secondary data include facts and figures which are already collected by other individuals and institutions. The sources of secondary data include publications of Government, private institutions like Trade

Association and Chambers of Commerce, international institutions like the International Monetary Fund and the World Bank, and data collected by other researches.

3. **Analysing information :** The information collected by the marketing research department is compiled and tabulated for the purpose of analysis of the problem. The data are studied minutely to discover the fundamental issues and answers to them. Analysis of data is the process of determining what the data mean. The generalisations derived from the analysis of data are helpful in taking the right course of action.

4. **Making recommendations :** Conclusions are drawn after the analysis of the data and recommendations are made to the management for taking steps in various areas of marketing. The findings and recommendations should take the form of a report and they should be presented separately in the report. The report should be written in unambiguous language so that it may be understood properly.

Sources of Data

The data for marketing research can be obtain from (a) internal sources, and (b) external sources.

(a) **Internal Sources :** The management of a business enterprise should not ignore the uses of internal data for marketing research. In many cases, internal data are very much relevant and useful, and without their help it is not possible to get the desired results. Internal data have the advantage of being easily available. Moreover, it does involve any extra expenditure as it is already available with the enterprise. The illustration of internal data are - Salesmen's reports, Figures of turnover, Expenditure on advertisements, Obsolete stocks, Commission paid to salesmen, etc.

(b) **External Sources :** External sources of information are to be tapped for getting more data to make a more detailed study of a marketing problem. The sources can be sub-classified into two categories, namely, primary data and secondary data.

Primary Data

The primary data refer to the first-hand original data collected by the investigator through interview, mail survey, field survey, or any other method. It is collected for a specific objective. It is not a published source of data, but has to be collect by the researcher. This data can be collected slowly at a huge cost. But it is very useful as it is collected for a specific objective. The sources of primary data include : Salesmen, Dealers and Consumers.

Salesmen : Salesmen are an important source of data. They are in close touch with the customers. They can be of great help in knowing data about the buying habits of the customers, changing tastes of the customers, and the preferences of the customers for the products of the competitors. The marketing manager should ask the salesmen to prepare periodical reports about such things and submit to him. He can also lay down the guidelines for the salesmen for preparing the report.

The salesmen provide the first-hand information of the conditions in the market. They provide the information within a short period. Salesmen can appraise the market manager of the opinions and reactions of the consumers. This has also the effect of motivating the salesmen because they feel that information provided by them is being used in framing marketing policy of the firm. But, sometimes, the reports submitted by salesmen suffer from business. The information provided by them may not be accurate because they feel that giving an accurate information will affect their interest adversely.

Dealers : The Incharge of marketing research can also collect first hand information from the dealers in goods and services of the firm. Investigations may be sent to contact the dealers or distributors personally to know the popularity of the firm's product, the share of firm in the market, acceptability by the consumer and so on. The dealers may also be requested to provide information about the marketing policies of the competitors. Dealers may not always provide cent per cent accurate information. They may not like to leak out the secrets of their arrangements with other manufacturers and they may not even take interest in the products of the firm in question.

Consumers : Consumers are an invaluable source of primary data. A representative sample of the consumers may be selected and information may be obtained from them regarding the prices, quality, packaging, etc. of the products of the firm. By having direct contacts with the consumers, the reliability of the information provided by the salesmen and dealers can also be checked. The firm can also use this opportunity of inviting suggestions from the customers regarding the importance of the characteristics of the products. Some firm follow the practice of regularly knowing the opinion of ultimate consumers from the panel called 'consumers panel'. Such a panel is formed to know the fashion, taste and attitudes of the consumers. The members of the panel are interviewed personally for obtaining the necessary information.

Secondary Data

Secondary data consists of data which have already been collected by some other persons and have passed through the statistical machine atleast once. Primary data are in the shape of raw materials to which statistical methods are applied for the purposed of analysis and interpretation. But secondary data are usually in the shape of finished products as it has already been treated statistically. The task of gathering secondary data is the task of compilation of data from various published or unpublished sources. In other words, secondary data include data which have already been collected by some individuals or institutions. The significance of secondary data lies in the fact that it is available at a very low cost. It can be collected within a short period of time. However, the effectiveness of the results based on secondary data will depend upon its reliability, completeness and right choice. Therefore, the secondary data should be used with great care. There are a number of sources of secondary data which are discussed below :

1. **Press :** Data about various aspects of business appear in newspapers and business magazines. This can be used for the purpose of conducting marketing research.

2. **Publications of Trade Associations :** Various associations of business men (Trade Association, Chambers of Commerce, Associations of Manufacturers, etc.) publish useful data for the benefit of their members. The data can be very useful in conducting marketing research in specific areas of business.

3. **Government Publications :** Various departments of the Central Government and State Governments publish regularly certain bulletins, periodicals, journals and magazines which contain very useful data relating to various aspects of business. For instance Census Reports, Yojana, Company News, Import Policy, etc. reveal useful data for various undertakings. In addition, Government also appoint various work groups and committees whose reports can be used for marketing research.

4. **Publications of Reserve Bank of India and Financial Institutions :** The Reserve Bank of India, Commercial banks and other financial institutions publish much useful information. For instance, the monthly bulletin of the Reserve Bank of India contains statistical data concerning monetary and fiscal aspects of the economic functioning of the Indian economy.

5. **Publications of Private Individuals, Companies and Research Institutes :** These are very useful sources of information. In particular, research institutes like Institute of Applied Manpower Research, Indian Law Institute, Institute of Foreign Trade, etc. undertake various studies and publish many types of data helpful for the business undertakings.

6. **Foreign Government and International Agencies :** Publications of foreign governments and the international agencies like UNO, ILO, World Bank and IMF also provide data which many be helpful in making a comparison with the Indian conditions and exploring markets in other countries.

Collection of Primary Data for Marketing Research

The quality of marketing research findings mainly depend on the quality of data available. Therefore, many firms collect the necessary data by using more than one method. The data regarding a particular problem collected with the help of various methods can be compared to examine the reliability of various methods. Important methods used for the collection of primary data or first-hand information are discussed below :

1. **Observation Method :** By observation we mean the process of recognising and noting facts or occurrences. Under this method, the researcher arranges to observe the behaviour of consumers rather than asking them to describe the various aspects of their behaviour. The observer takes notes of things as they happen and does not ask any question from the people observed by him. Observation method can be used to determine the effectiveness of sales techniques, response of consumers towards a particular product, utility of an advertising medium, etc. Researcher records the facts and then tries to interpret the pattern of behavior of different types of customers. This method of research is very much used by the Traffic Department. Similarly, departmental stores can use this method to improve the store display. The difficulty with this method is that it simply narrates the facts and it does not give the reasons of the behaviour of the persons observed.

2. **Experimentation Method :** Experimentation is the process of noting reaction of a phenomenon under controlled conditions. It refers to the act of doing something to test a theory. An experiment is conducted and observations are recorded. Such observations are properly classified, tabulated and analysed with a view to use them for preparing the report. Experimentation can be done to test the effectiveness of an advertisement campaign before undertaking it on a large scale. Similarly, a company can test its new product in a local market before introducing it in the national used for future managerial decisions. However, this is a costly and time confusing device. It may delay the introduction of a marketing programme.

3. **Survey Method :** A survey is a detailed inquiry and examination in order to collect information from the respondents. The survey method of collecting information from the respondents or information is frequently used for collecting necessary information. A survey can be conducted either of the entire universe or a part of it. When all the units of information connected with the problem are taken into account, it is known as census enquiry or survey. But when only some selected representative units are studied, it is known as sample inquiry or survey. Generally, sampling technique is adopted where the number of respondents is very large and it is very costly and time consuming to contact each one of them. However, if sufficient time and money are available and the highest possible degree of accuracy is desired, census method of inquiry may be adopted.

Survey method secures both quantitative as well as qualitative information directly from the respondents. It is flexible in terms of type of data to be collected. Census or sampling can be used depending upon the time and money available and the objectives of the survey. It can be used for motivation or why research which will probe into the feelings, emotions, motives, attitudes, etc. of the informants. Survey method can be used to obtain the opinion of the respondents about a particular issue. Such type of survey is known as opinion survey.

Types of Survey

Survey method uses questionnaire for the collection of data. Surveys with the help of a questionnaire can be conducted in the following ways:

1. **Personal Interview :** It involves face to face communication between the investigator and the respondent. The investigator is given a list of questions (known as questionnaire or schedule) which he has to put to the persons concerned. However, the investigator is given some freedom to put the questions in different styles to suit the needs of a particular situation. Thus, it is a flexible form of data collection. This interview can also be held without a questionnaire. Personal interview helps in asking complex and probing questions to secure more information. The investigator can also observe certain factors related to income, occupation, standard of living, etc. of the respondent.

   Personal interview helps in contacting only those respondents from whom the required information can be obtained. It helps in getting detailed and accurate information. Literacy of the respondent is no problem. But this method is an expensive one, particularly when a large number of respondents are to be covered. A long time is required to collect data. The interviewers must be competent, trained and experienced. They must be honest and free from any business. Otherwise data collected will not be accurate and reliable.

2. **Mail Survey :** Data may be collected by sending printed questionnaire to be respondents with a request to supply the written replies. It is presumed that while writing the answers sufficient thought will be given and therefore, it is more reliable than the oral answers provide to an interviewer. The answers can be collected in a standard form which will facilitate tabulation, computation and analysis. Questionnaire through mail can be sent to a large number of respondents scattered throughout the country. Thus, it is a cheaper method of collecting data. The bias on the part of the interviewers is also avoided. Questionnaire is prepared with great care. The written questions will be more precise and consistent than questions asked orally. A printed copy of the questionnaire with a covering letter and stamped reply paid envelope is posted to the respondent. A gift incentive may also be provided to ensure the quick return of duly completed questionnaire.

   Sometimes, the respondents are unwilling to provide certain information. Some people do not respond due to laziness while others do not send replies because they do not understand the questions.

3. **Focused Interview Method :** In this type of interview, the respondents are encouraged to talk freely, while the interviewer reports word for word. Sometimes guiding questions may be given to the interviewers to help them to keep the interview to the point. However, in the free story technique, even guiding questions are not put.

4. **Telephone Interview Method :** In this method, contact is established with the informants by telephone and the informants are asked a set list of questions relevant to the study. The questions may be modified or the informant may be asked to talk freely for some time. The method can be used only for telephone subscribers.

5. **Panel Method :** A consumer panel is a group of persons or families selected for getting information on the product and different aspects of the firm's marketing strategy. The panel selected after personal interviews may be given diaries in which the members enter all their purchases of the commodity being surveyed. The diaries may be examined periodically. Alternatively to this, the panel may be interviewed periodically regarding facts relevant to the survey. An adaptation of this method is the use of the panel for collecting reactions to a new product through post or personal interviews or by inviting the members at one place.

6. **Observational Method :** In this method, the observer does not rely on information given to him by a respondent which may be biased in some way. He records what he actually observes in the field. There can be many variations of this method. Some examples are :

   (a) **Stock audits :** checking up of the stock with samples of retailers to establish sales trends for certain commodities or brands.

   (b) **Pantry checks :** recording of the products in a housewife's kitchen or pantry to see what brands are bought.

   (c) **Dust-bin checks :** recording of the tins, wrappers and packages found in the subject's dust-bin.

   (d) Passenger or car counts for poster research.

   (e) **Behaviour research :** particular in self-service stores or department stores.

15

SALESMANSHIP

Salesmanship or personal selling is an important method of selling. It is the process of assisting and persuading a prospective buyer to buy a commodity in a face-to-face situation. It involves direct and personal contact between the seller or his representative with the prospective buyer. It is one of the most effective methods of selling the products. Personal selling is by far the major promotional method used to increase profitable sales by offering want-satisfying goods to the people over the long-run. Salesmanship is the process whereby the seller ascertains and activates the needs or wants of the buyer and satisfies the needs or wants to mutual continuous advantage of both the buyer and the sellers.

The purpose of personal selling is not the present sale alone but also winning a regular and permanent customer. It is persuasive in nature. It results not only in the benefit to the seller but also to the buyer. Aggressive sales-manship or selling is ethically not good. A good salesman should assist the prospect in satisfying his need by the purchase of products or services according to his capacity.

Significance of Personal Selling

Personal selling consists of individual and personal communication in contrast to the mass and impersonal communication of advertising and sales promotion. Because of this basic characteristic, personal selling has the advantage of being more flexible in operation. Salesmen can tailor their sales presentation to fit the needs, motives, and behaviour of individual customers. They can observe the customers' reaction to a particular sales approach and then make necessary adjustment on the spot. Thus, personal selling involves a minimum of wasted efforts. The seller can select the market and concentrate on the prospective customers. He need not communicate with the people who are in no way his real prospects. Personal selling is more effective as compared to advertising and sales promotion activities because it leads to actual sale in most case.

Personal selling is an important method of understanding the needs, nature and behaviour of the prospective customers and giving them full information about the product in question. It is easier to persuade a person to buy a product through personal explanation. In most situations, there is need of explaining the quality, uses and price of the product to the buyer to help him purchase the want satisfying products. Personal selling is also useful in knowing the tastes, reactions, habits and attitudes of the people and communicate the information to the manufacturers to help them to manufacture those products which are demanded by the customers.

Types of Salesmen : There are several methods of classifying a salesman's job. The most popular form of classification is by the type of employer the salesman represents. Accordingly, there are three types :

1. The manufacturer's salesman.
2. The wholesaler's salesman.
3. The retailer's salesman.

1. **Manufacturer's Salesman :** This type of salesman generally carries a very limited line of items in his portfolio. He has a highly specialised knowledge of those products. He deals directly with the middlemen and collects bulk orders to be supplied from headquarters. Such a salesman may again be :

   (a) **Promotional Salesman or Pioneer Products Salesman :** He is entrusted with the task of creating and cultivating outlets for a new product. He is a highly skilled salesman, out to sell to prospects the desirability of the product which never existed before. Such a salesman has to be aggressive and imaginative.

   (b) **Dealer Servicing Salesman :** He serves and supplies well-established regular dealers of his products. In addition, he keeps them well-informed about the products selling points and also trains the dealers' salesmen in effective selling methods.

   (c) **Speciality Salesman :** He is the representative of a manufacturer who calls upon consumers directly and makes door-to-door canvassing, selling household goods of office appliances, giving actual demonstration of their use (in the selling process) and removing doubts, if any, from the minds of the consumers about the products. This type of salesman must be alert, well-trained, fluent in speech, persistent, tactful and capable of working without direct supervision.

2. **Wholesaler's Salesman :** He is a representative of the wholesaler who generally deals with retailers or industrial consumers. He informs them about the various production stored and offered by the wholesalers, helps them in the selection of articles and counsels the retailer in evolving effective selling techniques. These salesmen may be outdoor

salesmen going out in the market and booking order, or indoor salesmen receiving the retailers and supplying their needs.

3. **Retailer's Salesman :** He is a salesman employed by a store, for receivng, attending on and serving the customers who visit the store. Some important requisites of success in retail salesmanship are given below :

To help customers buy wisely, the salesman must know his merchandise, i.e. stock, location of each item and facts about goods.

The salesman must understand and like people; i.e. get the customer's point of view, serve people as he would like to be served, be courteous, considerate and attentive, be friendly but no familiar, and treat customers as invited guests.

The salesman must have a wholesome attitude, i.e. be loyal to his store, be helpful to his customers, watch his health, keep his personal appearance neat and attractive, and keep enthusiastic about his job.

The salesman must use good selling methods; i.e. meet customers promptly and courteously, present his merchandise with respect and appreciation, give honest, convincing facts about his goods, answer questions and objection fully, help his customers to decide, suggest merchandise to satisfy additional needs, and show appreciation for his customer's patronage.

Sometimes salesmen may be classified on the basis of products and services which they may be called upon to sell. Thus there may be a category of salesmen who sell tangible goods. These salesmen sell products which can be seen, felt and handled physically. These may be producers' goods like machinery, tools, etc., or consumers' goods, say, a particular brand of soap, fan, or refrigerator. Another category of salesmen may be engaged in pushing up the sales of certain intangible things which relate to the mind. A salesman engaged to push up the sale of tickets for a movie or a theatrical performance will be selling entertainment, an intangible thing.

Yet another classification of the salesmen is into (i) creative, and (ii) service salesmen. A creative salesman is one who is charged with the important and difficult task of introducing a new brand or a new product in the market and pushing up its sales. Needless to say that such a salesman requires endless dynamism and appeal for establishing the new product. On the other hand, a service salesman may be described as one who has to sell such products as are already in demand or are at least known to the consumers. He performs the functions of maintaining the existing demand.

Methods of Remuneration for Salesmen : The compensation of salesmen is an important factor in their performance in so far as it will influence the quality and the amount of effort put in by them on their job. A good plan of remuneration of salesmen should combine the decent income and security, fairness, incentive to salesmen, flexibility, economy, salesmen's control over the basis of compensation and simplicity.

Types of Plans : Broadly speaking, there are two plans of remuneration for salesmen : (i) straight salary plan which provides fixed remuneration, and (ii) commission paln which makes remuneration variable with the sales volume achieved. However, certain combination plans have also been devised. Accordingly, the plans of remuneration for salesmen may be classified as under :

  (i) Fixed remuneration ...   Straight salary
 (ii) Fixed and variable remuneration
    (a) Salary and commission
    (b) Drawing account and commission
    (c) Salary and bonus
    (d) Salary, commission and bonus
(iii) Variable compensation
    (a) Commission
    (b) Commission and bonus
    (c) Bonus.

Straight Salary : This is the least complex plan of remuneration for salesmen. A salesman is paid a certain amount as salary like other employees. The salary is based on market rates of compensation and some measure of internal job evaluation. The amount of remuneration payable to a salesman remains the same whatever his contribution to the sales effort. Of course, if he performs miserably below the expectations of the management for some time, the management may well decide to get rid of him. This plan of salesman remuneration offers the following advantages :

  (a) It is simple to operate and reduces clerical work to the minimum.
  (b) It provides a sense of security and a measure of confidence to the sales people which will motivate them to effective selling.
  (c) Business risks arising out of factors beyond the control of salesman and affecting sales (say, a crop failure) do not affect the remuneration of a salesmen.
  (d) It keeps the morale of the sales force high and reduces the turnover among salesmen.
  (e) It minimises clash of interests between the management and the salesmen.
  (f) The salesmen do not have to adopt high-pressure selling tacties to increase sales under this plan.
  (g) Any readjustments in sales territories or management policies will be carried out without resistance from salesmen.

As against the above advantages, the straight salary plan suffers from the following drawbacks :

(a) It does not provide the incentive and the impetus to the salesmen to increase sales through additional effort.

(b) The plans tend to be inflexible in as much as these may lead to the over payment to shirkers and under-payment to sincere men.

(c) From the company's point of view, absence of variability in remuneration is a disadvantage as it makes salesmen's salaries a fixed burden on its earnings.

Commission Plans : Under such plans, an individual salesman is paid on the basis of a pre-determined ratio or ratios in accordance with the results which he can show in sales volume or some other measure of performance. The commission earned by an individual may be certain percentage (say, 5%) of all sales made or the rates of commission may vary according to the circumstances of sales made. There may be one rate (say, 5%) for sales up to Rs. 50,000 ; another (say, 5.5 %) for sales up to Rs. 75,000 ; and so on. Similarly, higher rates of commission may be paid for selling more profitable items. The rates of commission may, likewise, be higher for certain territories rated more difficult (say, sales in foreign countries). Sometimes salesmen may be offered higher rates of commission if they are able to sell at terms more favourable to the company than is done by others (say, 30 days' credit instead of 45 days extended by others).

The weaknesses of the straight salary plans are the strong points of the commission plans and vice versa. In short, these plans have direct incentive value and are flexible. They ensure economy and efficiency in the sales effort of an enterprise by placing premium on higher productivity and penalising inefficiency. On the other hand, these are relatively complex and may work out to be unfair where sales for due to factors beyond the control of salesmen. These plans encourage high pressure aggressive selling which may be harmful in the long run. Disputes may be frequent under these plans and the management control over salesmen is difficult.

Combination Plans : Considering the advantages and the drawbacks of both straight salary and commission plans, a combination of these may be tried through certain plans. Some important combination plans are :

(a) **Salary and Commission :** Under such plans, a salesman is entitled to a fixed salary or what may be called a drawing account and in addition, a commission based on sales volume or one or more of the various bases discussed in the foregoing section. The salary element gives the needed sense of security to the salesman while the commission element is meant to reward salesman for increased productive effort.

(b) **Salary and Bonus :** These plans provide for a higher salary than given with commission and give a certain percentage of the salesman's earnings (say, 20%) as bonus in addition. The incentive value of this plan is less than that of commission because it does establish a direct and immediate relationship between efforting reward.

(c) **Drawing account and commission :** A drawing account is in the nature of pre-paid commission. It is an advance paid to the salesman. The commission earned by the salesman is adjusted against the drawing account.

Points System : According to such a system, a salesman may be given a fixed monthly salary and a quota in points. Points may be awarded in differing amounts for sales of different products, roughly in proportion to the difficulties of selling. When the point quota is reached, the salesman may be given additional compensation either in a lump-sum or as a commission on the sales made.

Steps in the Personal Selling Process

The process of personal selling consists of the following steps :

(i) **Pre-sale preparation :** The first step in personal selling is the preparation of sales-persons. The sales-persons must be properly selected, trained and motivated for this job. They must be well acquainted with the product, the market and the techniques of selling. They should have the knowledge about the motivation and behaviour of the people to whom they are going to meet for the purpose of selling their products. They should also be well informed about the nature of competition and the nature of competitors' products.

(ii) **Prospecting or locating the potential buyers :** The sales-persons must locate the potential buyers and satisfactorily screen them to make sure that sales efforts will not be wasted. A sales-person can examine the records of past and present customers in his effort to determine the characteristics of his prospects. He may have to tap other sources of information also for this purpose.

(iii) **Approaching :** Before calling on the prospects, the sales-person should try to get information about their nature. He should try to ascertain what products or brands they are using. This information will help in approaching the prospective customers and making presentation in a better way. The sales-person must not be deceptive or he will lose the credibility that will be needed later in the sales presentation. The sales-person must introduce himself and his product to the prospective customer before he does anything else. He should not try to be over-clever and play with nerves of the prospective customers. He should be very polite while approaching the prospects so that he does not have much difficulty at the time of presentation.

A counter sales-person should also approach the customer properly to gain his attention. He should greet the customer and make him feel at home. He should make the customer feel that he is getting undivided attention from the sales-person. If the sales-person is busy with some other customers, he should assure the new customer that he would be attended very soon. Before making any presentation, the sale-person should try to understand the nature, need and spending capacity of the customer.

(iv) **Presentation :** The actual presentation of the sales-person starts with an attempt to attract the prospect's attention. The presentation should be such that the prospect takes continuous interest in the product during presentation. The sales-person should describe the features and price of the product briefly. He should also suggest the product's benefit and the need of the customer which will be fulfilled by the particular product. There is no specific approach which will be successful in all cases. The success of a sales-person will depend upon the degree to which he is able to match his approach with the attitude of the customer.

(v) **Demonstration :** Demonstration is one of the best methods of representation. Demonstration is frequently used to hold the prospect's interest and create desire for the product. Through demonstration and explanation, the prospect can be made to realise the suitability of the product for the satisfaction of his wants. Demonstration also achieves the involvement of the prospect and may create certain queries in his mind.

(vi) **Handling objections :** After demonstrating and explaining the products, its features, price and benefits, the salesman should entertain queries from the prospect. Handling queries or objections should not be considered to be an unpleasant task. A good salesman should realise that it is the golden opportunity to convince and persuade the prospect. This also gives him a chance to give additional information about the superiority of the product over the competitive products in the market. The salesman should not lose patience if the customer puts many queries and takes time in reaching any decision. A customer is a king. Even after handling all objections, if a customer does not buy, the salesman should part with him cheerfully without any design of temper.

(vii) **Closing the sale :** Closing the sale is not as easy as is considered by some people. A salesman has to act with patience with intelligence to close the sale. A salesman may periodically venture a trial close in order to sense the prospects' willingness to buy. He asks some 'either-or' questions from the prospect for his purpose. The trial close at various stages of the presentation will give the salesman an indication of how near the prospect is to a decision. Sometimes, prospects are convinced and are ready to buy even during the early stages of the presentation. They may change their mind afterwards by getting more information about the product. In such cases, sales are lost because of the failure of the salesman to ask for the order.

The trial close also brings out the buyer's queries and objections. This helps the salesman to change his sales approach quickly. He can bring out the additional benefits and features of the product or re-emphasize the previous stated points. After he is convinced that the customer has made up his mind to buy the product, he should close the sale by asking such questions as "What colour have you decided ?" "Do you want this gift-wrapped ?" or "What else would you like to buy ?" The sale would be closed in a cordial manner and the customer should be made to feel that he has made the right choice. The customer should also be reassured of better services in future.

Requisites of effective Salesmanship

A business enterprise can develop effective salesman to promote its sale. In order to achieve effective personal selling, the following requirements must be fulfilled :

1. **Personal qualities :** An effective salesman must possess certain physical, mental, social and vocational qualities.

2. **Training and Motivation :** In order to achieve effective personal selling, it is essential to train and motivate the sales-persons. The training programme for the sales-persons should be designed keeping in view the requirements of the business. The training programme should also aim at imparting knowledge of various selling techniques among the trainees.

3. **Wide Knowledge :** A salesman should have wide knowledge about the following :

   (a) **Self :** The salesman must know himself in order to make use of his personality in selling. He should try to know his strong and week points and remove his weak points through training and experience.

   (b) **Employer :** The salesman is a representative of his employer. He should have thorough knowledge of the origin and growth of the employer's business. He must know objects, policies and organisational structure of the employer's firm.

   (c) **Product :** The salesman must have full knowledge about the product he sells. He must know what the product is and what are its special features and uses. He should also know the whole process of production so that he may be able to answer the customer's queries and objections satisfactorily. Mostly, the customers are ignorant about the features and benefits of the product and they expect the salesman to give them sufficient information about it.

   (d) **Competitor's products :** The salesman must have complete knowledge about the competitive products because buyers often compare several before purchasing one of them. The salesman should know the positive and negative feature of the various sub-stitutes so that he is in a position to prove the superiority of his product.

(e) **Customers :** Before selling something, a salesman must have sufficient knowledge about the customers to whom he is going to sell. He must try to understand the nature of customers, their habits and their buying motives if he is to win permanent customers. The considerations which make the prospect to buy a particular product may be grouped under two categories of motives, namely (i) product motives, and (ii) patronage motives. Product motives explain why customers buy certain products and patronage motives determine why customers buy from specific dealers. A salesman can understand the motives of the customers by his intelligence and experience.

Qualities of a Successful Salesman : There are different types of salesmen in different lines of business because of which certain qualities may be relevant in some lines of business and irrelevent in others. The qualities required of a salesman also vary from situation to situation. Nevertheless, some of the common qualities which are often found among the effective salesmen are described below :

(i) **Personality :** A salesman should have good personality. The term 'personality' comprises several attributes like physical appearance, way of speaking, voice, posture, health, habits, etc. If any of these attributes is lacking substantially, a salesman may not be able to do his job effectively. A pleasing and charming personality always creates a good impression on the prospects. A salesman should possess good health because it is the key to his efficiency. His voice should be well-pitched. His tone of speaking should be natural so as to create receptivity among the listeners.

(ii) **Mental qualities :** An effective salesman must possess certain mental qualities like imagination, foresightedness, presence of mind, strong memory power and initiative. A salesman who is intelligent enough to understand to nature of the prospects and perceive their requirements is most likely to be successful. A good salesman must have the power of imagination so that he can enter into the shoes of the prospective customer to know what he wants and how he wants to be treated. These mental qualities will help a salesman in winning permanent and regular customers.

(iii) **Sociability :** A salesman should be social and have the ability to mix with people. He should not be shy and reserved. He should be able to have interaction with all types of people. He should be honest, sincere, dependable and co-operative. He should have the patience to listen to the customers and remove their objections. He should be polite and humble in talking to the customers. He should remain courteous with his customers throughout the presentation because his fate depends upon the attitudes of the customers. He should have the quality of adjusting with the customers of different natures.

(iv) **Vocational skills :** A salesman should have sound general education and have the specialised knowledge of selling techniques. Salesmanship is a highly skilled vocation. It requires certain training and a specific bent of mind. He should have ambition and enthusiasm to become a good salesman. A good salsman should know the features, benefits and other particular of the product he is going to sell.

(v) **Communication Ability :** Communication skill is an asset for the salesman. He should be able to speak freely, clearly and in a well-pitched voice. He must be a person who has a natural ability for conversation.

(vi) **Patience :** The salesman should not get provoked even under worst circumstances. He should have sufficient patience to listen to customers and clear their doubts.

(vii) **Determination :** The salesperson must have a sense of determination to secure the customer. He should not lose confidence and give up the customer so easily.

(viii) **Dependability :** The salesman can win permanent customers if he is honest, sincere and dependable. He should be able to win the confidence of the customers if he is to succeed in his vocation.

Employment of Salesforce : Utmost care should be taken in the selection of salesmen. Wrong choice of salesmen would cause higher employee turnover and prove injurious for the further development and growth of the concern. Before appointing the salesman, the management should clearly lay down the type of work which a salesman is expected to do. There should be proper description of the job of a salesman and the qualifications a person should possess to be appointed as a salesman.

The procedure for selection of salesmen involves the following steps :

1. **Advertisement :** In order to invite applications for the post of salesmen in the organisation, wide publicity is given to the number of vacancies and the qualifications required to fill them. Advertisement may be given in one or more newspapers to attract persons for the vacant posts.

2. **Receipt of Application :** The application form is provided to the candidates on request. It provides a written record of qualifications, experience and other qualities of the candidate. The blank application should be as simple as possible and incorporate questions having effect on the suitability of the applicant for the job. Application forms are received and processed by the office for further reference by the selection committee. The applications are screened to select the candi-

dates who are to be given the employment test and called for an interview.

3. **Employment Tests :** Employment tests are being widely used to select persons for various jobs. These tests helps in matching the characteristics of individuals with the vacant jobs so as to employ right types of personnel. Following are the types of tests given to the candidtes :

   (a) **Intelligence test :** It is used to judge the mental capacity of the applicant. It evaluates the ability of an individual to understand instruction and make decisions.

   (b) **Aptitude test :** It is used to measure an applicant's capacity and his potential for growth.

   (c) **Occupational or professional test :** It is designed to measure the proficiency of an individual in the skills required to perform a job.

   (d) **Personality test :** It tends to probe the qualities of the personality.

MEDICAL REPRESENTATIVE AS A SALESMAN

An industry contact the medical profession through a medical representative for promoting its products. The basic job of a medical representative is selling the products, concepts of health, and methods of treatment. A medical representative should be graduate in any subject like pharmacy, chemistry and biology. The educated medical representative can understand the products in a better way. He promotes the selling of the products to highly qualified persons such as doctors, chemists, hospital store incharges, etc. He can utilize the knowledge of qualities and uses of his products properly. He should learn the art of describing the information to motivate the doctors for buying or prescribing the products. He should be able to talk politely and precisely in a convincing manner. He is the vital link between the pharmaceutical industry and medical profession. He keeps the medical profession in touch with the latest development in medicine and thus perform a social duty by providing latest information to the medical profession. This helps in the elevation of standards of medical treatment.

A representative takes one type of sample. He has to express his facial impression according to the situation. In case of fatal diseases, he has to tell this with sad face. He should have good appearance as he deals with health products. A marketing executive appearance is achieved by wearing light coloured shirt, dark coloured pant, tie, polished shoes and neat bag. He should show manners while entering the doctors cabin. First of all he should give his visiting card. He should have fluent speech. He should stop at the end of every sentence and develop command over speech so that the doctor could understand his talk properly. He should be confident in discussing the technical matters.

The medical representative should possess knowledge about his products, customers, territory, industry policy and procedures, competition, ability for planning his activities and responding enquiries about the products. He should know about the ingredients, their concentration, rationale, dosage schedule, availability, bio-availability of products, etc. He should have the knowledge about physicians, their likes, dislikes, favourite brands, period for attending the call. The medical representative must have the detail knowledge about his area so that he can arrange his visit his visit for selling his visit for selling the products. For example, if he intends to visit a rural area, he should know the timings of transport, and clinic timings for doing his job in minimum period.

Industry's policy is important for selling its products. If the policy is to sell the products, e.g. cardiac drugs, to specialists, then the medical representative should not attend general practitioners. He should have a knowledge of the competitors products, their strategy and disadvantages. The activity of selling should be planned for a day, week, month or year. He may face objections from physicians, chemists, wholesalers. He should acquire a sound knowledge to handle the situation.

Attitudes of every person are controlled by emotions. For successful selling, the medical representative should develop correct attitudes. He should acquire the moral qualities such as sincerity for the job, determination for achieving goals, enthusiasm for new ideas and objects, patience to get result and dependability on customers, colleagues and superiors. He is responsible for his own time and prescribed number of persons to be visited. He represents an industry in his allocated area. His attitude and actions should project a good image on the visited persons.

16

ADVERTISING

Advertising is the dissemination of information concerning an idea, product or service to induce action in accordance with the intent of the advertiser. Advertising consists of all the activities involved in presenting to a group a non-personal oral or visual, openly sponsored message regarding a product, service or idea ; this message, called an advertisement, is disseminated through one or more media and is paid for by the identified sponsor. The message which is presented or disseminated is know as 'advertisement'. All activities necessary to prepare the message and get it to the intended people are part of 'advertisement '. The important features of advertising are discussed below:

(i) The purpose of advertising is to promote idea about the products and services of a business firm. It is directed towards increasing the sales of a business.

(ii) Advertising is a non-personal form of presentation and promotion of ideas, goods or services. There is no face-to-face direct contact with the customers.

(iii) Advertising is a paid form of communication. The advertisements are communicated through various advertising media and the advertiser has to pay for the space or time hired by him to communicate the message to the present and prospective customers.

(iv) Advertising is done by an identified sponsor. The identity of the advertiser is revealed in the advertisement itself.

Objective of Advertising

The fundamental purpose of advertising is to sell something - a product, a service or an idea. In addition to this general objective, advertising is also used by the modern business enterprises for certain specific objectives which are listed below :

1. To introduce a new product by creating interest for it among the prospective customers.
2. To support personal selling programme.
3. To reach people inaccessible to salesman.
4. To enter a new market or attract a new group of customers.
5. To fight competition in the market and to increase the sales.
6. To enhance the goodwill of the enterprise by promising better quality products and services.
7. To improve dealer relations. Advertising supports the dealers in selling the product. Dealers are attracted towards a product which is advertised effectively.
8. To warn the public against imitation of an enterprise's products.

Need and Significance of Advertising

Advertising helps in disseminating information about the advertising firm, its product, product qualities, place and availability of its products and so on. It helps to create a non-personal link between the advertiser and the receivers of the message. The significance of advertising has increased in the modern era of large scale production and tough competition in the market. Advertising is useful not only to the manufacturer and traders but also to the customers and the society. The benefits of advertising to different parties are discussed in the following paragraphs.

To Manufacturers and Traders : Advertising helps introducing a new product. A business enterprise can introduce itself and its products to the public through advertising. It can create new taste among the public and stimulate them to purchase the new product through effective advertisements. Advertising assists to increase the sale of existing products by entering new markets and attracting new customers. Advertising facilities creating steady demand of the products.

Advertising helps in meeting the forces of competition in the market. If a product is not advertised continuously, the competitors may snatch its market through increased advertisements. Therefore, in certain cases advertising is a necessity to remain in the market. Advertising is also used to increase the goodwill of a firm by promising improved quality to the customers. Advertisements also increase the morale of the employees because of the reputation of the firm. The salesmen feel happier because their task becomes easier if the product is advertised and made known to the public.

Advertising facilitates mass production of goods which enables the manufacturer to achieve lower cost per unit of product. Distribution costs are also lowered when the manufacturer sells the product directly to the customers. Advertising facilities direct distribution of the product through the retailers.

Retailers are encouraged to purchase and sell the well-advertised products.

To Customers : Advertising helps the customers to know about the existence of various products and their prices. They can choose among the various brands to satisfy their wants. Thus, they cannot be exploited by the sellers. Advertising educates the people about new products and diverse uses. Advertising also increases the utility of existing products for many people and increases the amount of satisfaction which they are already enjoying.

Customers get goods at lower prices because advertising helps to reduce cost by facilitating large scale production and eliminating whosesalers from the channels of distribution.

To Society : Advertising provides employment to persons engaged in writing, designing and issuing advertisement. Increased employment brings additional income with the people which stimulates more demand. More employment is generated to meet the increased demand. Advertising promotes the standard of living of the people by increasing the variety and quality in consumption, as a result of sustained research and development activities by the manufacturers. Advertising educates the people about the various uses of different products and this increases their knowledge.

Advertising sustains the press and other news media. Advertising provides an important source of income to the press, radio and television network. The customers are benefited because they get newspapers and magazines at cheaper rates. The publishers of newspapers and magazines are also benefited because of increased circulation of their publication. Lastly, advertising encourages commercial art.

Functions of Advertising

Advertising has become an essential marketing activity in the modern era of large scale production and severe competition in the market. It performs the following functions:

1. **Promotion of Sales :** It promotes the sale of goods and services by informing and persuading the people to buy them.

2. **Introduction of New Product :** It helps the introduction of new products in the market. A business enterprise can introduce itself and its product to the public through advertising. A new enterprise can't make an impact on the prospective customers without the help of advertising.

3. **Creation of Good Public Image :** It builds up the reputation of the advertiser. Advertising enables a business firm to communicate its achievements and its efforts to satisfy the customers' needs to the public. This increases the goodwill and reputation of the firm which is necessary to fight competition in the market.

4. **Mass Production :** Advertising facilitates large scale production. Mass production reduces the cost of production per unit by making possible the economical use of various factors of production.

5. **Research** : It stimulates research and development activities. Advertising has become a competitive marketing activity. Every firm tries to differentiate its product from the substitutes available in the market through advertising. This compels every business firm to do more and more research to find new products and their new uses.

6. **Education of People** : Advertising educates the people about new products and their uses. Advertising message about the utility of a product enables the people to widen their knowledge. It has helped people in adopting new ways of life and giving up old habits. It has contributed a lot towards the betterment of the standard of living of the society.

7. **Support to Press** : It sustains press. Advertising provides an important source of revenue to the publishers of newspapers and magazines. It enables to increase the circulation of their publications by selling them at lower rates. People are also benefited because they get publications at cheaper rates.

MEDIA OF ADVERTISING

Advertising media are the means to transmit the message from the advertiser to the particular class of people. A manufacturer can select any one or more of the following media of advertisement to promote his sales :

1. **Newspaper** : A newspaper is generally a daily publication containing news and opinions about current events and feature articles. Newspaper reading is a common habit of most educated people these days. Besides daily newspapers there are bi-weekly and weekly newspapers also. Newspapers reach almost every place and are read by all kinds of people. Therefore, newspaper can be used as a medium of advertisement with great advantage. While selecting a newspaper for this purpose, an advertiser has to take into consideration the strength of circulation, the class of readers it serves, the geographical region over which it is popular and the cost of space. Newspaper advertising has many advantages.

   (i) A newspaper has large circulation and a single advertisement in a newspaper can reach a large number of people.

   (ii) Continuous advertisement is possible because newspaper is published daily.

   (iii) Newspapers provide flexibility in advertising in the sense that advertisement campaign can be initiated and stopped quickly.

   (iv) Advertisements are the major source of income to the newspapers. This helps in selling the newspapers at reduced prices to the readers.

The limitations of newspaper advertising are as follows :

(i) The life of a newspaper advertisement is very short. Moreover, people devote only an insignificant part of their day's time in reading the newspaper.

(ii) Newspaper cannot be used for high class coloured advertisements. The advertisements are generally printed in black and white.

2. **Magazine :** Magazines or periodicals are an excellent medium of advertisement when a high quality of printing and colour is desired in an advertisement. Magazine advertisements can be directed towards a particular class of people and thus they avoid wasteful expenditure on advertising. Many specialised magazines or journals are published which can be used for transmitting the message to the specific class of customers.

Magazine advertising is considered to be superior to newspaper advertising because of the following merits:

(i) Magazines are read more carefully and at greater leisure. Advertising through magazines is more effective.

(ii) The life of the magazine advertisement is longer. Magazines are preserved for a long period of time and are read time and again.

(iii) Since advertisement copy is presented in a coloured form, it creates a better image of the product advertised.

Magazine advertising has the following limitations:

(i) Advertising through magazines is very costly.

(ii) The circulation of magazines is very small as compared to the newspapers.

(iii) Magazine advertisement are to be prepared and sent for publication well in advance. It is not possible to make the last minute change in the advertisement copy.

3. **Radio Advertising :** Radio advertisements have gained greater popularity these days. Advertisements are broadcast from the transmitting stations of the commercial service of All India Radio and picked up by the receiving sets owned by the public. Radio advertisements or commercials are normally broadcasted alongwith popular programmes of music. Even the sponsored programmes of interviews and plays can also be broadcast over the radio.

Radio advertising possesses the following merits:

(i) Radio advertisements carry an effective appeal and cover numerous listeners of different tastes.

(ii) Radio advertisements reach the illiterate people who cannot read the newspapers and magazines.

(iii) Radio provides selectivity to some extent because advertisements can be included in different programmes meant for different type of people.

(iv) Radio advertisement are highly suitable for the promotion of mass scale consumer goods.

The demerits of radio advertising are as under:

(i) Detailed message can't be broadcast over the radio. People may not remember the message.

(ii) It is non-visual. Thus, the usual impact of illustrating the product is not possible.

(iii) Sometimes, the message is not understood properly by the listeners. Many people switch off their radio or transistor sets when it is the time for commercial or advertisements.

4. **Television Advertising :** Television is the latest and fast growing medium of advertisement. It makes its appeals through both the eye and the ear. Products can be demonstrated as well as explained as in film advertisement. Advertising may take the form of short commercials and sponsored programmes. T.V. advertising has greater effectiveness as the message is conveyed at their homes to the people. Selectivity of message can also be achieved . Commercial may be given during that time period when the prospective buyers are supposed to watch television programmes.

T.V. advertising has got some demerits also. Television is a very costly medium of advertisement and can be made use of by the well established companies only. Another limitation of television advertisement is that once it is presented, its back reference is not possible as in the case of radio advertisement.

5. **Film Advertisement :** Films are an important medium of advertisement. Business concerns usually get a short motion picture prepared and distribute it to different cinema houses for displaying it before the commencement of the regular shows or during the period of interval. Such films are accompanied by running commentary to explain the features, uses and superiority of the product. But it involves high cost, small business firms can get cinema slide prepared for display in the cinema halls.

Film advertisement is very effective since it combines spoken words and visual presentation of pictures. It also helps in selective advertisement. A trader can advertise his product only in a particular locality if he wants to attract the local customers. The major drawback of film advertisement is that it is usually ignored by the people. Only a few persons are present in the hall before the start of the film and during the interval and they too are busy in talking.

6. **Direct Mail Advertising** : Direct mail is probably the most personal and selective of all the advertising media. Direct mail is used to send the message directly to the customer. For this purpose, the advertiser has to maintain a mailing list and the mailing list can be expanded or contracted by adding or removing names from the list. But a severe limitation is posed by the difficulty of getting and maintaining of good mailing list.

Advertisements that are sent by direct mail may be in the form of circular letters, leaflets, folders, calendars, booklets and catalogues. Circular letters are sent to the prospective customers to inform them about the merit of the product and to create their interest in the product. Booklets and catalogues contain the information about the products advertised. Information about the terms of sale and price of different varieties of the product are given to the prospective customers through catalogues.

The merits of direct mail advertising are as under :

(i) Mail advertising has a personal appeal since it is addressed to a particular person.

(ii) It maintains secrecy in advertising. The competitors do not get the information about the advertised material.

(iii) It gives flexibility in advertising. The message can be changed whenever the need arises

(iv) It gives an opportunity to the advertiser to provide detailed and illustrated information about the product to the prospects.

(v) It is the most selective medium of advertisement. The advertiser saves money also by directing his advertisement to the selected people.

The demerits of direct mail advertising are given below :

(i) The coverage of direct mail advertisement is limited. It is not suitable for all types of products.

(ii) It is very difficult to get the names and addresses of all the prospects whom the advertisement material should be sent by mail.

7. **Outdoor Advertising** : Outdoor advertising includes the use of poster displays, bill board displays and electrical displays. Posters are fixed or pasted on walls at important public place so that they may intercept the people on their way to work and home. Painted or bill board display involves the advertisement directly painted on the boards meant for that purpose. They are quite big in size and are fixed at outstanding locations like busy markets and crossing. Painted displays take the form of painted walls when the message is painted on the walls. Electrical display involves the use of electric lights or neon tubes to attract the attention of people particularly during night. Generally, a short mes-

sage is illuminated in tubes of different colours so that it is conspicuous and attractive. Electrical displays are fixed at heavy traffic centres.

Outdoor advertising is highly flexible and is a low cost medium. It is very useful for advertising consumer products because advertising can be displayed at various crowded centres. Outdoor advertisement attracts the attention quickly and requires much less time and effort on the part of the readers. Moreover, a complete picture of the product can be advertised through outdoor displays. Business concerns also use bill boards near the actual site of the business. The recent trend in outdoor advertisement is the use of public transport vehicles for advertising purpose.

Outdoor advertising is critical on the following ground :

(i) It can't carry long messages as posters, hoardigs, etc. are read by the people at a glance.

(ii) It has a low retention value because people don't devote special time to read the message.

(iii) It distracts the attention of the passers-by and may even cause accidents on busy roads.

8. **Vehicular Displays :** It has become a fashion these days to use modes of public transport for advertising. The space outside and inside the buses, railway carriages and other vans may be hired by the businessmen to spread their messages. Vehicles give mobility to the message.

Vehicular advertising has the following merits :

(i) Outdoor advertising is highly flexible and is a low cost medium.

(ii) It is very useful for advertising consumer products because posters, etc. can be displayed on the vehicles.

(iii) Vehicular advertisement attracts attention quickly and requires very less time and effort on the part of the readers.

9. **Speciality Advertising :** Many business firms offer speciality articles to the present and prospective customers. These articles may be diaries, pen holders, desk trays, key chains, purses, paper weights, cigarette cases and calendars. The name and address of the advertiser is printed in or inscribed on the speciality items. They also bear the brand name of the firm. Since these articles are of daily use, they have greater capacity to remind their users about the brand name of the firm offering such articles.

10. **Window Display :** Window display is an on sight method of advertising. Goods can be exhibited in artistically laid out windows at the shop fronts or at important busy centres like railway stations and bus stops. Large show rooms are organised by big manufacturers and wholesalers in the main markets to advertise their products and attend to the queries of the prospective customers. The retailers also organise attractive

display of goods in the windows of their shops. Window displays are very popular with the retailers since it helps in informing the customers about the types of goods available with them.

The main objective of window display is to draw the attention of the public and arouse their interest in the products displayed. Almost all the manufacturers insist that their products should be displayed at the retail shops. If a product is displayed properly at the point of purchase by the customers, it can make many customers buy it. Many people having no preference for a particular brand may discover a particular brand quite appealing and attractive and may purchase it. Thus, windows display creates the demand for the product. Window display acts as silent salesman. In order to achieve the purpose of window display, clealiness and a well-furnished appearance for the window are essential. Articles should be arranged in a systematic way and if possible price tags should also be attached with the articles. It is better if window displays are changed regularly to make the customers look at the displays everytime they visit the shop.

In preparing window display there are certain fixed units which must be arranged to produce a pleasing effect to increase selling power.

Window Decoration : The walls and floor behind the window, against which the merchandise and decorative materials are displayed, are known as backgrounds. They may add to or detract from the central figure of the display. The backgrounds should be exactly what the name implies. They serve only as a setting for the merchandise and should be un-obstructive rather intrusive. Backgrounds walls may be permanent or temporary. Permanent wood finished window panels are expensive. Dark backgrounds are not advisable for deep windows, unless the merchandise and display materials are all in the lighter shades. Mirror fittings at the back of the window should be avoided as they reflect distracting movements from the street. Temporary or movable background panels are more effective for drug store windows. Common wall board painted in flat solid shades can be used to attract customers. The colours of movable background panels can be changed easily. They can be decorated in different ways and used in different positions to change the size of the windows space. They can be used as mounts for small items , the panel being prepared prior to the installation of the display.

The floor of the display window may be decorated in different ways. Hard wood finish may be used or the floor may be permanently covered with monochrome carpet in neutral shade or with plain linoleum. Temporary effects may obtained by the use of fabrics, wall paper of suitable design or crepe paper. The floor should be un-obstructive, let it serve as a background only.

The ceiling, when it is visible should be lighter in colour. Fixtures are of great importance in the arrangement of drug store windows to display small items of merchandise. Fixtures may be obtained in wood, metal and /or glass. Simple arrangement is one of the desirable objectives in drug store window display. Fixtures consist of simpler units, which may be used separately or combined in many different patterns such as building blocks arranged by children. A series of cubical boxes may be arranged in graduated size , which may be placed in the window separately or in combination to make an interesting pattern for affording along position for the strategic placing of merchandise. Similarly, boxes of different length may be arranged . Another placement of fixtures includes wide, flat shapes, of different dimensions but all about 2 or 3 inches thick which may be rectangular, circular or oval in shape. They may be placed laid flat, tilted at an angle, or stood on sides or ends in the window in countless number of combinations. Another variation is the open shelf box in upto-date design.

Well-developed material is available in many attractive shades in larger rolls. Item may be used to prepare tube or column pedestals of various dimensions upon which small merchandise may be displayed. A piece of show cardboard cut to proper size and laid across to top of the later provides the floor for the merchandise. Painted boards or glass may be laid across several columns to form a shelf.

Artificial flowers and leaves of suitable colours enhance the appearance of show window or frontage and help in introducing personal atmosphere especially for products like cosmetics, lotions etc. The display of more merchandise does not attract more customers. All the other elements of window should be subordinate to the merchandise or in the institutional window. Modern type of stores may contain measurement of blood pressure, demonstration on diabetic regimen of diets and medicament.

Show cards playcards and other similar articles are intended to carry a brief selling message about the merchandise. Many customers would like to have the price-cards displayed in the window. The show cards and price levels should be printed in colour, size and style with the displays used.

Principles of Window Display : The fundamental purpose of the window display is to attract the passer-by, and develop interest in the merchandise displayed. The time required for the average person to walk past the average show window has been estimated to be 3 to 11 seconds.

The customers' attention must be arrested quickly or not at all. The window must be deliberately designed to attract the customer. People get impressions through the eye rapidly and then in any other way.

Some of the visual factors in getting attention for window displays are:

(1) Display is arranged within the normal range of vision of the passer by. The level of the show window should be about 1 foot above the floor of the usual window, which may be about 30 inches above the side walk. The central feature of the display should be placed somewhere within that area on the vertical dimension of the window. The other part of display should be used as the decorative portion and in such a way as to direct the attention down its natural point of focus.

(2) The window or the unit should be arranged to convey one dominant idea.

(3) The attracting devices, such as colour, motion, sound, novelty of arrangement, decorative features, spot lighting etc. should be used if the device itself will be so intense that the prime objective of the window will not be achieved, the attention device will thus defeat its own purpose.

(4) The display is kept pleasing and interesting. The quality or kind of attention must be taken into consideration.

(5) The arrangement of window background, colour, lines, etc. all attract the customers.

The display that brings all resources into play to make one distinct impression will most effectively attract attention . The display should have one major theme, such as the window display depicting the single themes of "Ever Supplies" "Baby Day". Every thing in the display should contribute to the development of such themes. The elements of display - the merchandise, cards, decoration, etc. can be arranged to receive successive periods of attention after the central theme has been impressed.

Some of the dominant ideas and methods adopted to drug store window displays are :

(a) The merchandise is made itself the central idea. The merchandise may be used as the primary focus of interest. The selling idea should be summarised or concentrated in a display card placed at the focal point of the display.

(b) The theme of display is developed around a timely event with season, holiday, national and local events, special store events such as industries.

(c) The dominant theme should be related to an associated idea such as an item in the news, a research achievement etc., which is currently engaging the interest of the public , or some timeless idea, such as the urge for romance, the desire for beauty, health, safety, parental love, etc.

(d) The window is built around an institutional theme such as professional integrity and service, quality, telephone and delivery service etc.

The pharmacist should know character, age, apparent income, status, sex etc. of the store customers and of the passers-by in order that the themes may be adapted to their principal interest. In certain locations of the city, there may be more women customers. In such a case the stores themes should be oriented towards women's interest.

The merchandise should be around the central object in a way that will balance. Balance (composition) means simply that the deposition of the unit must present a pleasing appearance.

Balance in window display must be considered in reference to the size of the objects, the shape of the objects and their colour.

Informal balance produces more interesting and dramatic effects. Symmetrical balance is easy to achieve and will suffer for most drug store window display.

In window display arrangement the units of display are placed in an interesting pattern. The flat, uniform, monotonous sheerily repetitive arrangements of units are to be avoided. An interesting rhythmic pattern is obtained by arranging the elements in groups of contrasting heights and width across the width of window. Smaller objects should be placed at the front of larger objects and taller display pedetral at the back.

In arranging drug store displays the related merchandise are grouped together. A whole window of shaving accessories, e.g., brushes, razor blades, creams, lotions, talcum power, shaving mirror, etc. is more logical and holds attention no better than a window where perfumes, pipes, toys and laxative remedies are mixed irregularly. If several lines of merchandise are displayed in the same window, the related lines should be grouped and separated from other groups. Many drugs stores prefer a separate large window into several sections. Colour is important in window to attract attention; and use harmoniously.

Some brightly coloured merchandise, show cards, plaques or other decorative accessory should be used in display. The order of arrangement of colour should be as :

(1) Red (2) Orange (3) Yellow (4) Green (5) Blue

It is better to use strong colours and contrasts in spots or splashes. In using colours in combination, one colour should predominate thus achieving unity in the display. Bright lightning is essential for window display. Lightning itself attracts people. Reflectors concealed at the top and front of the merchandise displayed and away from the eyes of the shoppers should be used. They should be not more than 35 cms apart, and the lamps of 150 to 500 watts should be used, depending upon the height and width of the window.

Coloured lightning of the entire window would not be effective for drug stores. However, a coloured spot may sometime be used to highlight effectively a particular item in the display.

The techniques of building and arranging the window display are important. But the success of the display depends on planning.

There are two purposes of planning ; (1) It assures the coordination of the window promotion with the other promotion activities of the store (2) It provides an outline of the details of the display.

Choice of Advertising Media

For the purpose of choosing the appropriate medium or media of advertisement, following factors should be taken into consideration :

(i) **Nature of Product :** Nature of the product to be advertised has an important bearing on the medium of advertisement. Products should be classified into two broad categories, namely, consumer goods and industrial goods. Consumer goods can be advertised in newspapers, magazines, radio and television and through outdoor displays. But industrial goods can be advertised profitably in the specialised trade, technical and professional journals.

(ii) **Nature of Market :** Nature and extent of market can be determined by various factors like geographical region, size of population and purchasing power of the population. The market may be either local or national. Film advertising and outdoor advertising are more suitable for local products. Newspapers are the most suitable for advertising products which can be sold throughout the country.

(iii) **Objectives of Advertising :** The objectives of the advertising programme are very important to determine the choice of advertising media. The objectives may be introduction of new product to increase demand of an existing product, or to avoid competition by the rivals. If advertising is not to be carried on a mass scale to have big impact in the short and long run, a combination of various advertising media may be chosen. Sometimes advertisements are inserted in the newspapers and magazines to complement the readers in order to enhance the goodwill of the advertiser.

(iv) **Circulation of Media :** If the media have greater circulation, the message of the advertiser will reach a larger number of people. It may be mentioned that newspapers have the widest circulation, but other media have limited and selective circulation.

(v) **Financial Consideration :** The cost of advertising media is an important consideration and it should be considered in relation (a) the amount of funds available, and (b) the circulation of the media. In the first instance, the amount of funds available may dictate the choice of a medium or a combination of media of advertisement and on the second account, the advertiser should try to develop some relationship between the cost of the medium and its circulation. The cost-benefit analysis will enable the advertiser to take right decision in regard to selection of the advertising media.

(vi) **Type of Audience :** If the message is to be conveyed to illiterate or less literate people, radio, television and cinema advertisement will serve the purpose in a better way. Newspapers, magazines, displays and direct mail may be used to convey the message to the educated people. Since different languages are popular in different regions, advertisements in different languages may be given to popularise the product.

(vii) **Life of Advertisement :** Outdoor display and magazines and direct mail have sufficiently longer life but the life of newspaper, radio and television advertisements is very short unless they are repeated regularly. Therefore, the advertiser should also take into consideration the duration for which he wants to create the impression in the minds of the prospective customers.

(viii) **Media used by Competitors :** The choice of advertising media also depends upon the media used by the competitors. If a product is being advertised in a newspapers, the producers of its substitutes will find it better to advertise them in the same newspaper. This practice has become more common these days in order to light competition in the market.

Themes of Advertisements

Different advertisers use different themes or central ideas to influence the instincts of different kinds of people. Some of the important themes are as follows :

1. **Prestige :** is used to popularise luxurious items like motor car, refrigerator and furniture.

2. **Comfort :** is used to advertise products like fans, air conditioners and refrigerators, etc.

3. **Health :** is the central idea used to advertise food stuffs and patented medicines.

4. **Beauty :** is very popular with the manufacturers and dealers of cosmetics, toilet soaps and perfumes.

5. **Parental affection :** is used for advertising products meant for children like toys, baby tricycles, baby foods, and baby dresses.

6. **Achievement :** is used to advertise products like number of units sold, foreign exchange earned, profit earned, etc.

7. **Fear :** is used by the insurance companies to stimulate people to go in

for insurance against death, accident, loss through fire, flood, burglary and so on.

8. **Patriotism :** influences the attitudes of the people who believe in purchasing goods made in India only.

9. **Economy :** is generally used for clearance sale or as a part of sale campaign on a mass scale.

Usually big times do not depend upon a single medium of advertisement. They choose a battery of advertising media in order to popularise their products and to sell on a massive scale. Subject to the availability of finance, they like to advertise their products through all the advertising media. It is because of the fact that advertisisng has become competitive these days and it is essential to advertise continuously in various media not only to increase the sales but also to remain in the market. Many people judge the superiority of a product from the point of view of the nature of its advertisement. However, advertisement expenses should be kept under control under the normal conditions. For this purpose a comparative evaluation of the effectiveness of various advertising media is necessary in order to choose the best combination of advertising media.

17

RECRUITMENT, TRAINING EVALUATION AND COMPENSATION

Definition of Recruitment

The process of identification of different sources of personnel is known as recruitment. Recruitment is the process of searching for prospective employees and stimulating them to apply for jobs in the organisation. It is a positive process as it attracts suitable candidates to apply for available jobs. The process of recruitment (i) identifies the different sources of labour supply, (ii) assesses their validity, (iii) chooses the most suitable source or sources, and (iv) invites applications from the prospective candidates for the advertised jobs.

SOURCES OF RECRUITMENT

The sources can be classified into the following two categories. :

(A) Internal Sources of Recruitment

There are two important internal sources of recruitment, namely, transfers and promotions which are discussed below.

1. **Transfer :** It involves the shifting of an employee from one job to another. At the time of transfer, it is ensured that the employee to be transferred to the new job is capable of performing it. In fact, transfer does not involve any major change in the responsibilities and status of the employee.

2. **Promotion :** It involves shifting an employee to a higher position carrying higher responsibilities, facilities, status and pay.

   Many companies follow the practice of filling higher jobs by promoting employees who are considered fit for such positions. Filling vacancies in higher jobs from within the organisation has the following merits :

(i) Employees are motivated to improve their performance.

(ii) Morale of the employees is increased.

(iii) Industrial peace prevails in the enterprise.

(iv) Filling of jobs internally is cheaper as compared to getting candidates from external sources.

Internal sources of recruitment have certain demerits also. These are listed below :

(i) When vacancies are filled through internal promotions, the scope for fresh talents is reduced.

(ii) The employees may become lethargic if they are sure of time bound promotions.

(iii) The spirit of competition among the employees may be hampered.

(iv) Frequent transfers may reduce the overall productivity of the organisation.

(B) External Sources of Recruitment

Every new enterprise has to tap external sources for various job positions. Running enterprises have also to recruit employees from outside for filling the positions whose specifications cannot be met by the present employees. The commonly used external sources of recruitment are discussed below :

1. **Direct Employment at Factory Gate :** An important source of recruitment is direct recruitment by placing a notice on the notice board of the enterprise specifying the details of the jobs available. It is known as recruitment at factory gate.

   Usually a large number of unemployed persons assemble everyday at the gate of every big factory. Whenever unskilled workers are required, the personnel manager will scrutinise in a general way the workers available and pick up the required number. This method of recruitment has the following advantages :

   (i) It is the direct method of recruitment. It does not involve any cost of advertising vacancies.

   (ii) It is the cheapest method to fill up casual vacancies.

   (iii) Whenever there is a rush of work or a large number of workers are absent, this source of labour may be easily used.

2. **Casual Callers or Unsolicited Applications :** Some organisations which are regarded as good employers draw a steady stream of unsolicited applications in their offices. This serves as a valuable source of manpower. The personnel department may find the unsolicited applications useful in filling some vacancies for which personnel are required immediately. The merit of this source of recruitment is that it avoids the costs of recruiting workforce from other sources.

3. **Advertisement :** Advertisement in newspapers or trade and professional journals is generally used when qualified or experienced personnel are not available from other sources. Most of the senior positions in industry as well as commerce are filled by this method. The advantage of advertising is that more information about the organisation, job designing and job specifications can be given in advertisement. It gives the management and wider range of candidates to choose from. Its disadvantage is that it brings in flood of response, and many times, from quite unsuitable candidates.

4. **Employment Agencies :** Employment exchanges run by the Government are regarded as a good source of recruitment for unskilled and skilled operative jobs. In some cases, compulsory notification of vacancies to employment exchange is required by law. Thus, the employment exchanges bring the job givers in contact with the job seekers. However, in the technical and professional area, private agencies and professional bodies appear to be doing most of the work. Employment exchanges and selected private agencies provide a nation- wide service in attempting to match personnel demand and supply.

5. **Educational Institutions :** Jobs in commerce and industry have become increasingly technical and complex to the point where school and college degrees are widely required. Consequently, many big organisations maintain a close liaison with the universities, vocational institutes and management institutes for recruitment to various jobs. Recruitment from educational institutions is a well-established practice of thousands of business and other organisations, organisations which require large number of clerks or which seek applicants for a continuing apprenticeship programme usually recruit from institutions offering vocational courses.

6. **Recommendations :** Applicants introduced by friends and relatives may prove to be a good source of recruitment. Many employers prefer to take such persons because something about their background is known. When a present employee or a business friend recommends a person, a type of preliminary screening takes place. Some organisations have agreements with their unions of employees to give preference to relatives of existing or retired employees if their qualifications and experience are suited to vacant jobs.

7. **Labour Contractors :** Labour contractors are an important source of recruitment in many industries in India. Workers are recruited through labour contractors who are themselves employees of the organisation. The disadvantage of this system is that if the contractor himself decides to leave the organisation, all the workers employed through him will follow suit. However, this system of recruitment is losing popularity these days.

SELECTION

The process of selection leads to employment of persons who possess the ability and qualifications to perform the jobs which have fallen vacant in the organisation. It divides the candidates for employment into two categories, namely, those who will be offered employment and those who will not be. This process could be called 'rejection' since more candidates may be turned away than hired. That is why, selection is frequently described as a negative process in contrast with the positive nature of recruitment.

The main purpose of the selection process is choosing right type of candidates to man various position in the organisation. A well organised selection procedure involves many steps and at each step more and more information is obtained about the candidates. A selection procedure is bound to prove ineffective if it does not derive the relevant information from the candidates which might be useful for offering them employment.

Importance of Selection

Hiring of employees is an important function of the personnel department. This function must be performed carefully because errors committed at the time of selection may prove to be very costly. If selection process is faulty, absenteeism will be too high and the rate of labour turnover will also be high. Whenever unsuitable candidates are appointed, the efficiency of the organisation will go down. Such persons will shirk work and will absent themselves from the work more often. In many cases, unsuitable employees have to leave their jobs. This will lead to wastage of time, energy and money in hiring such employees. The training cost incurred on them will also go waste.

SELECTION PROCEDURE

Selection has become a critical process these days because it requires a heavy investment of money to get right type of people. The major steps followed by modern organisations to get right type of persons are described below :

1. **Preliminary Interview :** In most of the organisations, the selection programme begins with preliminary interview which is generally brief and does the job of eliminating the total unsuitable candidates. The preliminary interview offers advantages not only to the organisation but also to the applicant.

2. **Application Blank :** An important step in hiring a person for the organisation is to get a written record of his qualifications, experience and any other speciality. Application blank is used to obtain information in the applicant's own handwriting sufficient to properly identify him and to make tentative inferences regarding his suitability for employment. Application blank should be as simple as possible and incorporate questions having bearing on the fitness of the applicant for the job.

3. **Employment Tests :** Individuals differ with respect to physical characteristics, capacity, level of mental ability, their likes and dislikes and also with respect to personality traits. The pattern of physical, mental and personal variables gives rise to thousand and one combinations and the particular pattern makes the individual suitable for several classes of activities, jobs or finds of work.

This will require the use of employment tests described below:

(a) **Intelligence Tests :** An intelligence test is used to judge the mental capacity of an applicant.

(b) **Aptitude Tests :** Aptitude means the potential which an individual has for learning the skill required to do a job efficiently.

(c) **Proficiency Tests :** Proficiency tests are those which are designed to measure the skill already acquired by the individuals.

(d) **Personality Tests :** Personality tests prone for the qualities of the personality as a whole, the combination of aptitude interest and usual mood and temperament.

4. **Employment Interview :** Interview may be used to secure more information about a candidate. The main purposes of an employment interview are : (a) to find out the suitability of the candidate,(b) to seek more information about the candidate,and (c) to give the candidate in accurate picture of the job with details of terms and conditions and some idea of organisation policies and employee relationship.

5. **Checking References :** A reference is potentially an important source of information about the candidate's ability and personality if he holds a responsible position in some organisation or has been the boss or employer of the candidate. Prior to final selection, the prospective employer normally makes an investigation on the references supplied by the applicant and undertakes more or less a thorough search into the candidate's past employment, education, personal reputation, financial condition, police record, etc. However, it is often difficult to persuade a referee to give his opinion frankly.

6. **Physical/Medical Examination :** The pre-employment physical examination or medical test of a candidate is an important step in the selection procedure. Medical test is located near the end, but this sequence need not be rigid. An organisation may place the medical examination relatively early in the process so as to avoid time and expenditure to be incurred on the selection of medically unfit persons.

7. **Final Selection :** After a candidate has cleared all the hurdles in the selection procedure, he is formally appointed by issuing him an appointment letter. The date by which the candidate must join the organisation is mentioned in the letter. The broad terms and conditions of employment, nature of job, pay scale, etc. may also be an integral part of the appointment letter.

PLACEMENT

The candidates selected for appointment are to be offered specific jobs. There must be a matching between the requirement of the job and the qualities of the employee concerned. Only then effective placement will take place. In practice, right placement is not easy task. It may take a long time before a candidate is placed on the right job. Generally, the candidate is appointed on a probation of one year or so. During this period, he is tried on different jobs. If his performance is satisfactory, he will be offered a permanent post.

Transfer or Job Rotation

Transfer means shifting of an employee from one job to another, one unit to another, or one shift to another. Transfers may be initiated by the organisation or by the employees with the approval of the organisation. Transfers have a number of objectives such as moving employees to positions with a higher priority in term of organisation goal, placing employees in position more appropriate to their interest or abilities, or filling department vacancies with employees from overstaffed departments.

Promotion

Promotion is a type of transfer involving placement of an employee to a position having higher pay, increased responsibilities, more privileges, increased benefits and greater opportunities. The purpose of a promotion is to staff a vacancy which, in general, is worth more to the organisation than the incumbent's present position. When the scale of salary of an employee is increased without corresponding change in job, it is called upgrading.

The promotion policy must consider the merit, potential for advancement and seniority of the employees. The merit factor requires a good procedure for evaluating the performance of employees. The quantity and quality of performance should be measured periodically and should form a part of the personnel records. The evaluation of performance should cover such factors as output, co-operation, initiative, willingness to accept responsibility and degree of reliability and dependability.

Seniority Vs. Ability

The management usually prefers to promote the person on the basis of ability while unions usually favour seniority or length of service as the basis for promotion. If seniority is adopted for promotion, the management will enjoy no discretion in this matter and everybody in the organisation will know for definite his place in order of importance. This will result in no, or at least fewer, disputes about promotion.

When workers are promoted to higher positions merely on the basis of the length of service, it is likely to have an adverse effect on the productivity of workers. Those who are about to be promoted on the basis of their seniority are apt to take work lightly because decline in efficiency cannot bar their chances for promotion. Thus it will not be advisable to adopt seniority of services as the sole basis for promotion. On the other hand, if ability is the sole consideration for promotion, standards of judgment may vary from individual to individual. A particular worker may be recommended for promotion by one superior while he may not be found suitable by another superior.

Trade unions are usually against the adoption of ability as the basis of promotion. They see in this basis a convenient opportunity for the management to abuse its powers and indulge in favoritism and nepotism on the pretext of being guided solely by consideration of ability. A sound promotion policy should therefore, consider both seniority and merit. "Seniority should be considered, but only when the qualifications of two candidates for better job are, for practical purposes, substantially equal."

TRAINING

Training is an organised activity for increasing the knowledge and skills of people for a definite purpose. The purpose of training is to achieve a change in the behaviour of those trained and to enable them to do their jobs in a better way. The trainees will acquire new manipulative skills, technical knowledge, problem-solving ability for attitudes, etc. Thus, training enables the employees to get acquainted with their jobs and also increase their skills and knowledge.

Need of Training

The responsibility for imparting training to the employees rests with the employer. If there is no formal training programme in the organisation, the workers will try to train themselves by trial and error, or by observing others. But this process will take a lot of time and will result in higher costs of training. Moreover, the workers may not be able to learn the best operating methods.

Training makes the new employees fully productive in the minimum of time. Even for the old workers, it is necessary to refresh them and to enable them to keep up with new methods and techniques as well a new machines and equipment. Training is valuable to the employees because it will give them greater job security and an opportunity for advancement. A skill acquired through training is an asset for the organisation and the employee. It can be taken away only by the complete elimination of the need for that skill because of rapid technological changes.

Advantages of Training to Employees

The major benefits of training are discussed below;

(i) **Less Learning Period :** A systematic training programme helps to reduce the learning time to reach the acceptable level of performance.

(ii) **Better Performance :** A well-trained employee usually shows a greater increase in and a higher quality of work output than an untrained employee. Training increases the skill of employee in the performance of a particular job. An increase in skill usually helps increase in both quantity and quality of output.

(iii) **Uniformity in Procedures :** With the help of training, the best available methods of performing the work can be standardised and made available to all employees. Standardisation will make high levels of performance rule rather than the exception.

(iv) **Economy in Operations :** Trained personnel will be able to make better and economical use of materials and equipments. Wastage will be low. In addition, the rate of accidents and damage to machinery and equipment will be kept to the minimum by the well-trained employees. These will lead to less cost of production per unit.

(v) **Fill Manpower Needs :** When totally new skill are required by an organisation, it has to face great difficulties in employment. Training can be used in spotting out promising men and in removing defects in the selection process. It is better to select and train from within the organisation rather than seek skilled employees from outside sources.

(vi) **Less Supervision :** If the employees are given proper training, the responsibility of supervision is lessened. Training does not eliminate the need for supervision, but it reduces the need for detailed and constant supervision.

(vii) **Good Human Relations :** The morale of the employees is increased if they are given proper training. A good training programme will mould employees' attitudes to achieve support for organisational activities and to obtain greater cooperation and loyalty. With the help of training, dissatisfaction, complaints, absenteeism, etc., can be reduced among the employees.

KINDS OF TRAINING

Depending upon the purpose of training, the following kinds of training programmes are used in industry:

1. **Induction or Orientation Training :** Induction is concerned with the problem of introducing or orienting a new employee to the organisation and its procedures, rules and regulations. When the new employee reports for work, he must be helped to get acquainted with the work environment and fellow employees. It is better to give him a friendly welcome when he joins the organisation, get him introduced to the organisation and help him to get a general idea about the rules and regulations, working conditions, etc. of the organisation.

2. **Apprenticeship Training :** Apprenticeship training involves imparting knowledge and skill in doing a craft or a series of related jobs. The Governments of various countries have passed laws which make it obligatory on certain employers to provide apprenticeship training to

the young people. The usual apprenticeship programmes combine on-the-job training and classroom instructions in particular subjects. Apprenticeship training is desirable in industry which requires a constant flow of new employees expected to become all-round craftsmen. It is very much prevalent in printing trade, building and construction, and crafts like machinists, electricians, welders, etc.

3. **Internship Training :** Under this method, the vocational institute enters into arrangement with a big business enterprise for providing practical knowledge to its students by gaining actual work experience. Internship training is usually meant for such vocations where advance theoretical knowledge is to be backed up by practical experience on the job. For instance, engineering students are sent to big industrial enterprises for gaining practical work experience and medical students are sent to big hospitals to get practical knowledge. The period of suckle training varies from six months to two years. The trainees do not belong to the business enterprises, but they come from the vocational or professional institutions. It is quite usual that enterprises giving them training absorb them by offering suitable jobs.

4. **Learner Training :** Learner training programmes are drawn up for those who do no have sufficient vocational background and knowledge about the jobs for which they have been selected. Such employees are sent to vocational schools for some time where they get some education and learn machine operations. Thus, learner training is a programme of education plus training. Such trainees are placed on regular work assignments after they complete the training programme.

5. **Refresher Training or Retraining :** The refresher training is meant for the existing employees of the enterprise. The basic purpose of refresher training is to acquaint the existing workforce with the latest method of performing their jobs and improve further their efficiency. The skills with the existing employees become obsolete because of technological changes and the tendency of human beings to forget.

6. **Training for Promotion :** The talented employees may be given adequate training to make them eligible for promotion to higher jobs in the organisation. Promotion of an employee needs a significant change in his responsibilities and duties. Therefore, it is essential that he is provided sufficient training to learn new skills to perform his new duties efficiently. The purpose of training for promotion is to develop the existing employees to make them fit for undertaking higher job responsibilities. This serves as a motivating force to the employees.

METHODS OF TRAINING

The important methods of imparting training to the operative employees are discussed below:

1. **On-the-job Training :** On-the-job training is considered to be the most effective method of training the operative personnel. Under this method, the worker is given training at the work-place by his immediate supervisor.

   On-the-job-training is suitable for teaching skills that can be learnt in a relatively short time. It has the chief advantage of strongly motivating the trainee to learn. It is not located in an artificial situation. It permits the trainee to learn at the actual equipment and in the environment of the job. On-the-job training methods are relatively cheaper and less time consuming. Another important factor about on-the-job training is that line supervisors play an important part in training their subordinates.

2. **Vestibule Training :** Vestibule schools are adapted to the same general type of training that is faced by on-the-job training. Vestibule training is suitable where a large number of persons are to be trained at the same time for the same kinds of work. A vestibule school is run when it is not possible to give training to the employees at the work-place. The training job is entrusted to the qualified instructors. The main emphasis is on learning rather than on production.

   A vestibule school is an attempt to duplicate as nearly as possible the actual conditions of the work-place. The learning conditions are carefully controlled. The trainees can concentrate on training only because they are not under any pressure of the work situation. Their activities do not interfere with the regular process of production. Thus, vestibule training is very much suitable where a large number of persons are to be trained and where more mistakes are likely to occur which will disturb the production schedules.

3. **Special Courses :** This is also known as 'class-room training'. It is more associated with knowledge than with skill. The special courses are designed to fit the needs of the organisation. These courses may be conducted by the line executives of the organisation or specialists from the vocational and management education institutes. Many firms also follow the practice of sending the selected employees to training and development programmes run by various educational institutions.

   Generally, the lecture method is employed under special courses. Lecturers are also supplemented by group discussions, films, demonstrations,etc. The main emphasis of the special courses is to enrich the workers with advanced knowledge in specific areas related to the effective performance of the job. Specific courses tend to prove more effective it. They ensure two-way traffic between the trainer and the trainee. Special courses may also be devised for the development of the executives at various levels in the enterprise.

JOB EVALUATION

Job evaluation is an orderly and systematic technique which aims at determining the worth of jobs. In other words, it is a formal system of determining the base compensation of jobs. Job evaluation may be defined as an attempt to determine and compare the demands which the normal performance of particular jobs make on normal workers, without taking account of the individual abilities or performance of the workers concerned. It is the task of determining the demands in terms of efforts and abilities which the normal performance of a job makes on normal workers. Job evaluation rates the job and not the man. It takes into account the demands of the job in terms of efforts and abilities, but it does not take into account the individual abilities and efforts which may, of course, be taken into consideration and reflected in the worker's earnings under a system of merit rating or performance appraisal.

Job evaluation involves the evaluation of various jobs in terms of certain factors. The important factors may be grouped as follows:

1. Skill : mental and manual,
2. Education,
3. Experience,
4. Efforts and initiative,
5. Responsibility to be undertaken,
6. Working environment, and
7. Supervision needed.

In general, the more difficult the job, the more it is worth. The more scarce the labour supply and higher the demand, the more a job is worth. The more skill, education and responsibility required in job, the more it is worth. These generalisations usually hold true for most jobs and serve as indicators of what the level of pay should be, but they are so general that they are of little use in translating specific jobs into rates of monetary compensation. That is why, several systems of job evaluation have been developed which take into account the above mentioned factors either directly or indirectly.

Significance of Job Evaluation

The benefits of job evaluation are as follows :

(a) Job evaluation is a valuable technique in the hands of management by which a more rational and consistent wage and salary structure can be evolved.

(b) Job evaluation helps in bringing or maintaining harmonious relations between labour and management since it tends to eliminate wage inequalities within the organisation and the industry.

(c) Because of increasing mechanisation and automation in industry, it has become unrealistic to pay workers primarily on the basis of their output. In many cases, it is the machine that determines the rate of production; so job evaluation will be of much use in fixing the wages.

(d) Job evaluation provides a rate for the job and not for the man. Because of division of labour and specialisation, any large enterprise may have hundreds or thousands of different jobs to be performed by a substantial number of workers. An attempt should be made to precisely define the jobs and fix wages accordingly. This is possible only by job evaluation.

(e) Job evaluation involves job analysis and appraisal which are of great use while recruiting new employees. Selection can be made objective by matching the qualifications of the candidate with job specifications.

Methods of Job Evaluation

Several methods of job evaluation are available which can be used either in their present form or in modified form to suit the particular needs of the individual organisation. There are four major methods from which choice can be made, viz : (i) Simple Ranking (2) Grading, (3) Point Rating, and (4) Factor Comparison. Simple ranking and grading represent non-quantitative methods. The point rating and factor comparison methods are, however, complex and are quantitative in nature.

(1) **Simple Ranking :** The simple ranking methods was first to be developed. In using this methods, jobs are compared with each other. The purpose is to determine whether a job involves the same level of duties, responsibilities and requirements as others in the series or a higher or lower level than they do. By comparing the jobs, the ranking of importance of each can be determined. In this methods, jobs are not split up into their component parts. Instead, comparison is made on the basis of whole jobs.

(2) **Grading :** The grading method of evaluation consists basically of establishing (1) job grades, (2) preparing of definition for each grade, and (3) classifying individual jobs according to how well their characteristics match those of the different grade definitions. These steps are explained below :

(1) **Job Grades :** Broad job groupings such as clerical, factory, sales and executive should first be decided upon. Then within each grouping an effort should be made to determine the significantly different levels of job difficulty, ranging from least demanding to most demanding. Quite frequently, the job ranking method is used in this preliminary stage.

(2) **Definitions of Grade Levels :** Definitions or descriptions of the grade levels are then carefully written. Usually these are made to cover the same basic elements, such as what types of duties are involved and what requirements or qualifications must be met. Benchmark or illustrative jobs are used liberally as examples to guide judgment.

(3) **Evaluation of Jobs** : Jobs are evaluated by carefully studying each job descriptions and placing each job in what seems to be the proper classification. Committees are usually used in order to provide representation to different departments and to attain the advantage of pooled judgment.

(3) **Point Method** : The method of job evaluation that enjoys widest acceptance is the point system. Fundamentally, this method consists of evaluating each job in respect of certain factors such as skill, efforts, responsibility and working conditions and combining the separate evaluations for each factor into a single point score for each job. The wage level appropriate for each job is fixed on the basis of total points scored by it.

The steps involved under the point method are listed below :

1. Determine type of jobs.
2. Decide upon job factors.
3. Construct scale of values for each factor.
4. Evaluate each job in terms of scales so constructed.
5. Conduct wage survey for selected key jobs.
6. Design the wage structure.
7. Adjust and operate the wage structure.

(4) **Factor Comparison Method** : This method takes a number of factors like mental requirements, physical requirements, responsibilities and working conditions as the basis of evaluation. These factors are listed on a sheet in columnar form. Then the salary for each key job is allocated to different factors as related to each job. Each key job is evaluated with regard to each of the given factors and entered in the factor column against the appropriate salary index. The salary components for each factor are added to get the appropriate salary level for each key job. Other jobs are ranked in relation to the ranking of key job.

Limitations of Job Evaluation

Job evaluation cannot really do what it looks as if it were doing and what some of its exponents have said it does. In practice, the technique of job evaluation suffers from the following limitations :

(a) It lacks scientific precision because there is no standard list of factors to be considered and, moreover, all factors cannot be measured accurately.

(b) It presumes that jobs of equal worth will be equally attractive to the employees, but it is not true in real life. If a job offers no prospects of a rise, while another of rated equal to its has bright prospects for employees, the latter will attract more people. The organisation may have to pay more for the former jobs so as to be able to attract the required number of persons even though both of them have been rated equal by job evaluation methods.

(c) Job evaluation tends to be inflexible in so far as it does not give right weightage to wage rates prevalent in the industry or region as a whole. It relies too much on internal standards and evaluation for fixing rates of wages.

(d) It suggests nothing about the absolute size of wage differentials appropriate to the evaluated job structure. Thus, it is not the complete answer to the wage problem.

COMPENSATION
Meaning of Wage and Salary

The term 'wage' is used to denote compensation to workers doing manual or physical work. Thus, wages are given to compensate the unskilled workers for their services rendered to the organisation. Wages may be based on hourly, daily, weekly or even monthly basis. But the term 'salary' is usually defined to mean compensation to office employee, foremen, managers and professional and technical staff. It is generally paid on weekly, monthly or yearly basis. Thus, the time period for which salaries are paid is generally greater than in case of wage payments.

Wages may be based on the number of units produced (i.e., piece wage system) or the time spent on the job. But salary is always based on time spent on the job. Where it is difficult to measure the production of the employee, the compensation is paid in the form of salary. Both wages and salaries constitute a significant portion of the cost of operation of business.

Factors Affecting Wages

In practice, the wages to be paid to the different categories of workers depend upon the following factors :

(i) **Demand for and Supply of Labour :** Wage is a price or compensation for the services rendered by a worker. The firm requires these services, and it must pay a price that will bring forth the supply which is controlled by the individual worker or by a group of workers acting together through their unions. The primary result of the operation of the law of supply and demand is the creation of the "going-wage rate".

(ii) **Ability to Pay :** Employer's ability to pay is an important factor affecting wages, not only for the individual firm, but also for the entire industry. This is a function of the financial position and profitability of the firm.

(iii) **Cost of Living :** Another important factor affecting the wage is the cost of living adjustment of wages. This tends to vary money wage depending upon the variations in the cost of living index following rise or fall in the general price level and consumer price index. It is an essential ingredient of long-term labour contracts unless provision is made to reopen the wage clause periodically.

(iv) **Productivity :** To achieve the best results from the worker and to motivate him to increase his efficiency, wages have to be productivity based.

(v) **Collective Bargaining :** Organised labour is able to claim better wages than the unorganized one. Higher wages may have to be paid by the firm to its workers under the pressure of unions of the workers. If the trade unions fail in their attempt to raise the wage and other allowances through collective bargaining, they resort to strike and other methods where by the supply of labour is restricted. This exerts a kind of influence on the employer to concede atleast partially the demands of the labour unions.

(vi) **Prevailing Wage Rates :** Wages in a firm are also influenced by the general wage level or the wages paid for similar occupations in the industry and the economy as a whole.

(vii) **State Regulation :** State regulation is an important factor having a bearing on employee remuneration. To protect the working class from the exploitation of powerful employers, the Government has enacted several laws. Laws on minimum wages, hours or work, equal pay for equal work, payment of dearness and other allowances, payment of bonus, etc. have been enacted and enforced to bring about a measure of fairness in compensating the working class.

Methods of Compensation

The various forms of wage payment fall into three classes :

  (a) those based on the time worked, or time wages;

  (b) those based on the quantity produced, or piece wages; and

  (c) those which combine the feature of both time and piece-rate, i.e., wage incentive plans.

A. TIME WAGE SYSTEM

Under this system, the worker is paid for the time spent on the job. This is the oldest and most common system and the wages are based on a certain period of time during the course of the work. The period of time may be an hour, a day, a week, a fortnight or a month, and the wage rate will depend upon the period of time. It must be remembered here that wages are paid after the time fixed for work is completed irrespective of output or completion of the work.

Wages can be determined by the following formula :

Wages = Number of Hours worked   × Rate per hour

Suppose that a worker is paid at the rate of Rs. 12/- per hour and he has spent 200 hours at work during a particular month. His wages for the month will be Rs. 2,400/-.

Situability : Time wage system is suitable in the following situations:

(a) When it is difficult to fix the standard time for doing a job.

(b) When quality of job is utmost importance.

(c) When the job relates to office or clerical work.

(d) When collective effort of a group of persons is necessary for the completion of a job.

(e) Where mental work is involved, such as policy-making and administration.

(f) Where machines, equipment and tools used for production are delicate and very costly.

(g) Where production process is complicated and demands higher degree skills.

Advantages : Time wage system offers the following advantages :

1. **Simplicity :** An important advantage of time wage system is its simplicity. It is very simple to calculate the amount earned and to measure the time spent on the job.

2. **Security to Workers :** It gives the worker a feeling of security as he knows in advance what will be his total remuneration at the end of the period. This will give him an assurance and he can plan his own expenditure accordingly. For the employer, it gives an adequate idea of his wage burden and he can make adequate provision for its payment. Thus, the absence of uncertainty benefits both.

3. **Equality of Wages :** All Workers doing similar jobs get the same rate of wages and a sense of equality prevails. There arises no cause for jealousy and malice as all the workers doing similar jobs are rated at the same level. Such sense of equality among the workers makes for the smooth working of the organisation.

4. **Better Quality :** Where the quality of products is more important than quantity or the materials worked upon are very costly, time wages prove cheaper than piece rates in their ultimate results.

5. **Less Wastage :** Under time wages, the workers need not speed up their operations to earn higher wages. There will be less wastage of materials and less wear and tear of tools and machinery.

6. **Adaptability :** This system can be adapted to all kinds of work. Even if a worker does a variety of jobs, he can be compensated on time wage basis.

7. **Acceptable to Trade Unions :** Labour unions always prefer time wages since this form of payment does not make any discrimination in wage matters between efficient and inefficient workers. This method ensures stable income to all the employees.

Disadvantages : The drawbacks of time wage system are as follows :

1. **Inefficiency :** This system does not check employees' inefficiency as there is no link between wages and productivity. The workers may deliberately slow down the pace of work.

2. **Lack of Motivation :** This system does not provide any incentive to greater effort or harder work. It makes no difference between an efficient and a lazy worker, and both are treated on the same footing.

3. **Increased Supervision :** Time wage system leads to lower productivity unless strict supervision is provided. Thus, there is a need of close supervision to ensure better productivity.

B. PIECE WAGE SYSTEM

Under this system, the output of work is the basis of payment. A worker under this system is paid according to the amount of work completed or the number of units of goods turned out irrespective of time taken to complete the work. The rate of wages is determined as so much per unit of output and is fixed in advance. Though the time is not of essence in this system, it is assumed that the worker will not take more than average time to complete a job. The earnings of a worker depend upon the speed of his work and his own skill and efficiency. As against time wage, under this system wages vary according to the number of units produced. An efficient worker would earn higher wages as compared to an inefficient worker. Wages may be calculated by following the simple formula.

Wages = Number of units produced   ×   Rate per unit.

Suitabiliy : Piece rate system is suitable in the following situations :

(a) When methods of production are standardised and the job is of repetitive nature.

(b) When productivity of the workers is to be increased.

(c) Where the degree of physical work is more than the mental work.

(d) Where output can be measured and quality control system exists to discourage low quality production.

(e) Where work does not require personal skills of higher order.

Advantages : The advantages of piece-wage system are as under :

1. **Incentive for Higher Production :** This system provides incentive to better workers to produce more and they are encouraged to realise their personal ambitions.

2. **Fairness :** This system ensures fairness by correlating wages and productivity. The inefficient workers are penalised as they get less wages.

3. **Costing :** Costing of production becomes easier as wages are a constant factor of the unit of output.

4. **Lesser Supervision :** Cost of supervision is less as the workers do not need constant supervision to lead them to work. They very attraction of greater reward for greater effort drives them to work harder.

5. **Personnel Decision :** Under this system, if a worker is constantly producing bad results, he may be shifted to another job. Thus, shifting of workers to jobs which suit them better takes place without creating difficulty for management.

6. **Economy :** The total unit cost of production comes down with larger output because the fixed overhead burden can be distributed over a greater number of units.

Drawbacks : The demerits of piece-wage system are as follows :

1. **Lower the Quality of Products :** To safeguard against his, a rigid inspection is required in those cases where piece rates operate.

2. **Insecurity of Workers :** The workers have a feeling of insecurity in their minds. They would get lower wages during a period when their efficiency may get reduced due to factors beyond their control. Thus, at times, the workers may be earning wages below the subsistence level.

3. **Strained Industrial Relations :** The relations between workers and employees becomes sour if their output is low due to some fault of management.

4. **Difficulty in Rate Fixation :** Fixation of piece rates poses a problem of the management. Lower rates may lead to resentment on the part of workers. Thus, industrial relations in the factory will be adversely affected.

5. **More Administrative Work :** Introduction of piece rate will involve increased administrative work as production records will have to be maintained for each worker. Daily record of production and rate of payment will have to be elaborately kept and preparation of pay-roll will entail a lot of calculations.

6. **Wastage :** The workers will increase the speed of work and this naturally leads to speeding up of machinery, waste of materials, fuel and power. This may result in greater loss to the industry. Excessive speed in running machines may cause break-down, accidents and frequent replacement resulting in loss to the concern.

7. **Health Hazard :** In their eagerness for increased earnings, workers may exert themselves to the point of exhaustion as to undermine their health and efficiency.

8. **Opposition by Trade Unions :** Differences in earnings cause dissatisfaction and resentment among workers. Trade unions are openly antagonistic to piece rates, as this form of wage payment encourage recovery between workers and endangers solidarity of labour unions.

C. INCENTIVE PLANS

The incentive plans have been designed to encouraged the workers to show higher productivity. Under these plans, workers are rewarded individually when their performance exceeds the pre-determined standared. The incentive plans may be either time based or production based.

Under time based incentive plans, a standard time is determined for doing a job. A standard time serves as the basis of giving bonus to the workers if they meet or exceed the standard. A worker is said to be efficient if he completes his job in less than the standard time. In order to reward him for his efficiency, he may be given bonus under an appropriate incentive plan. Followings are the important time based incentive plans:

(1) Halsey Plan
(2) Rowan Plan
(3) Emerson Plan
(4) Bedeaux Plan

Under the production based incentive plans, a standard of output is determined on scientific basis and payment of wages is made on the basis of number of units produced by a worker. A higher rate per unit is paid to the efficient worker. Production based incentive plans include the followings:

(5) Taylor's differential piece rate plan.
(6) Merrick's multiple piece rate plan.
(7) Gantt's task and bonus wage plan.

1. Halsey Premium Plan

Halsey premium plan is a simple combination of time and speed bases of payment. Under this plan, minimum time wage is guaranteed to every worker. A standard time is fixed for the completion of a job. If a worker performs his job in less than the standard time, he is given bonus. But there is no penalty for performing the job in more than the standard time fixed. The slow worker is paid the time wages and the efficient worker is paid some bonus in addition to the time wages. The bonus is in proportion to the wages earned during the time saved.

2. Rowan Plan

The Rowan plan is a modification of the Halsey plan. It also guarantees the minimum time wages and does not penalise a slow worker. A standard time is fixed for completion of job and bonus is paid to worker on the basis of time saved. Here, the bonus is that proportion of the wages for the time taken which the time saved bears to the standard time. It implies that as the time saved increases, time taken will be reduced and as such the bonus would increase at a diminishing rate. This will check over-speeding and overcome a major drawback of Halsey Plan.

3. Emerson Efficiency Plan

Under this plan, a minimum time wage is guaranteed to the workers. Conditions of work are standardised and a standard output is fixed which is to be completed within a specified period of time. This plan is similar to Gantt's Task and Bonus Plan and is an improvement over the Taylor's Differential Piece Rate Plan.

Under this plan, a worker is entitled for bonus if he is able to achieve 66.67 or more of the standard. If a worker's output is less than 66.67 of the standard output, he does not get any bonus, but he get the minimum time wages. The worker, whose output exceeds 66.67 per cent of the standard, gets incentives at a differential piece rate. A small bonus is paid for increases in efficiency from 66.67 per cent upwards, until at 80 per cent efficiency the bonus payable is 4 per cent, at 90 per cent efficiency, it is 10 per cent and at 100 per cent efficiency, it is as high as 20 per cent. After 100 per cent, 1 per cent bonus is given for every additional 1 per cent efficiency.

The important advantage of this plan to the workers is that their minimum wages for the day are secured. If a worker is unable to produce 66.67 of the standard output, he is not deprived of his daily wage. Secondly, there is enough scope for earning more and more for the efficient workers. The rate of bonus increases at an increasing rate. The plan is very beneficial to the extraordinary workers.

4. Bedeaux Point Plan

In this plan, the minute is the time unit described as the standard minute and accounted as Bedeaux point B. In determining the Bs, the time of operation and the time of rest are taken into account. Thus, B may be defined as a fraction of a minute of effort plus a fraction of a compensating rest always aggregating unity. The standard time for each job is fixed after undertaking time and motion study and expressed in terms of B. The standard time for a job is the number of Bs allowed to compete it. Thus, if the standard time required for a job is 5 hours, it will be expressed as 300 Bs.

The workers who are not able to or are just able to complete the work within standard time are paid at the normal rate. Those who are able to complete their work earlier are paid bonus equal to the wages for time saved as indicated by the excess of B point over the actual time taken.

Generally, the bonus paid to the worker is 75% of the wages for time saved. The remaining 25% goes to the foreman.

5. Taylor's Differential Piece Rate Plan

It is a system of wage payment under which earnings differ at different levels of a output. It does not guarantee minimum wages. It is modification of the simple piece wage system in order to provide greater incentive to efficient workers. Under this plan, standard output for the day is fixed after careful time and motion study. After this, two piece rates are set up for each job, a high piece rate and a low piece rate. High piece rate is given to those who produce equal to or more than the standard output, and low piece rate is offered to others. Suppose, the standard output per worker has been fixed at 8 units per day and the rate per unit for this standard output or above is Rs. 10 per unit and the rate for production below this standard is Rs. 9 per unit. The worker producing 7 units will get Rs. 63 and the worker producing 8 units will get Rs. 80.

6. Merrick's Multiple Piece-Rate Plan

This plan offers three grade piece rates than the two. The workers who produce less than 83% of standard output are paid at an ordinary piece rate. Those producing from 83% to 100% of the standard output are paid 110% of basic piece rate. Lastly, the workers producing more than 100% of standard output are paid 120% of basic piece rate. Thus, this system is an improvement over the Taylor's plan as it reduced the severity of the Taylor's plan.

Merrick's plan is liberal for the efficient workers. The workers producing more get their wages at increasing rates. This system also does not guarantee minimum wages for the workers. Another drawback of the system is the existence of a wide gap in slabs. As is obvious from the plan, all workers producing 1% to 82% of the standard output are considered as sub-standard workers and are paid at the same piece rate.

7. Gantt's Task and Bonus Wage Plan

Unlike Taylor's and Merrick's plans, minimum time wages is guaranteed to every worker under Gantt's task and bonus wage plan. A definite task representing first class performance is fixed as a standard after careful time and motion study. If a worker achieves or excels it, he gets extra wages varying between 25% to 50% of the hourly for the time allowed for the task. But if a worker fails to complete the task within the standard time, he receives only the wages for actual time spent at the specified rate. Suppose, the standard time for a job is 8 hours, time rate is Rs. 8 per hour, and bonus is 25% of the standard time. If a worker finishes his job within six hours, he will get Rs. 64 plus 25% of the day's wage, i.e., Rs. 16. Thus, he will get Rs. 80 in all for his work of six hours. The actual rate per hour paid to him comes out to be Rs. 13.33. The lesser the time he takes, the higher would be the actual rate per hour.

The benefits of Gantt's task and bonus wage plan are as follows :

(i)   The minimum wages to the workers are assured.

(ii) There is an incentive for the efficient workers. The more a worker produces in a given time, the higher is the remuneration he gets.

(iii) This plan motivates the employees to increase their efficiency because their remuneration is related to their efficiency.

Essentials of a Sound Wage System

A good wage system should aim at increasing productivity : reducing costs, improving efficiency and increasing employees' earnings while at the same time maintaining or enhancing employee morale and employer-employee relations. In order to achieve these, the following requirements must be fulfilled :

1. **Minimum Wage Guarantee :** The wage plan should guarantee minimum wage to protect the interest of the workers against conditions over which they have no control. As far as possible, the wages plan should take card of minimum wages and the essential needs of the workers in the given environment.

2. **Scope for Higher Earnings :** The wage incentive system should place no upper limit on the incentive earnings. This is so because the more the worker produces, the more the organisation will be benefited in general. Therefore, if a ceiling is put to the incentive earnings, it may also curtail the opportunity to achieve lower production costs per unit.

3. **Simplicity :** The successful operation of a wage incentive system is used upon the element of understandability and simplicity it embodies in itself. If the employee cannot understand how pay is to be calculated, the incentive is largely wasted. This problem is generally faced by the employees in cases when the plan involves a complex nature of mathematical exercise to arrive at figure of pay.

4. **Flexibility :** The wage plan should be flexible in order to meet changing conditions and should not involve excessive administrative cost.

5. **Wage Differentials :** Base wage for each job classification or skill should be related to others in terms of job requirements. Due consideration should be given to such factors as skill, length of time required in learning, versatility required and working conditions. Wage levels in different localities may vary, but the different skilled jobs should tend to bear the same general relationship to the common labour rate in each locality.

6. **Incentive for Higher Productivity :** The wage plan must include an incentive system for the efficient workers. The system should ensure higher pay to the workers who perform work at higher levels of efficiency.

7. **Based on Fair Standards :** Fair standard means the standard which an average workman can achieve in a given time under the prevailing conditions. A good wage payment policy must be based on fair standards. Such standards should be arrived at after careful study of an average worker, otherwise wages will not be fair.

8. **Fair to Employers and Employees :** A good wage system is one which is fair to both employers and employees. The system must secure a certain level of production at a certain cost and all the same time it must ensure reasonable wages to the workers.

18

BANKING SYSTEM

Banking system occupies an important place in a nation's economy. A banking institution is indispensable in a modern society. It plays a pivotal role in the economic development of a country and forms the core of the money market in an advanced country.

In India, though the money market is still characterised by the existence of both the organised and the unorganised segments, institutions in the organised money market have grown significantly and are playing an increasingly important role. The unorganised sector, comprising the money-lenders and indigenous bankers, caters to the credit needs of a large number of persons. Amongst the institutions in the organised sector of the money market, commercial banks and co-operative banks have been in existence for the past several decades. The Regional Rural Banks came into existence since the middle of seventies. A variety of specialised financial institutions have been set up in the country to cater to the specific needs of industry, agriculture and foreign trade.

In the field of industrial finance, the Industrial Development Bank of India (IDBI), set up in 1964, is the apex bank, which undertakes, refinancing of term loans granted by other financial institutions including the commercial banks. There are two prominent all-India institutions in this field, namely, the Industrial Finance Corporation of India (IFCI) and the Industrial Credit and Invested Corporation of India (ICICI). Besides, the State Financial Corporations (SFCs) and State Industrial Development Corporations (SIDCs) have been set up to meet the requirements of small and medium scale industries in the respective states. Industrial Reconstruction Bank of India (IRBI) has been set up to bring back to normalcy the industrial units which fall sick. Small Industries Development Bank of India was set as a subsidiary of Industrial Development Bank of India in 1990 to cater exclusively to the requirements of the Small Scale Sector in the country. All these institutions, engaged as they are in the task of development, are now designated as 'development banks' which are distinct from the traditional commercial banks. Development banking has had its genesis in the post-independence period in India and has contributed significantly to the industsrial growth of the country during this period.

For financing agriculture and allied activities in the rural areas, commercial banks began their active participation after the nationalisation of major banks in 1969. Long and medium-term credit to the agriculturists is being provided by another specialised institution, namely, the Land Development Banks which has a two-tier structure-Primary Land Development Banks at the district level and State Land Development Banks at the State level. National Bank for Agriculture and Rural Dvelopment (NBARD) is the full-fledged apex institution in the field of agriculture and rural development.

During 1988 two important financial institutions were established. National Housing Bank was set up in July 1988 as the apex banking institution in the field of housing finance. Discount and Finance House of India Ltd. was established to deal in money market instruments in order to provide liquidity in the money market.

There are a few other institutions, which are essentially engaged in the business of investing in the corporate and government and semi-government securities etc. They are the insurance institutions - Life Insurance Corporation of India (LIC), General Insurance Corporation of India (GIC) and the Unit Trust of India (UTI). These institutions mobilise the savings of the people and channelise them into desirable securities. Hence they are called the investing institutions or institutional investors.

To facilitate the banking business and to foster the growth of banking habit, two other institutions have been set up. The Deposit Insurance and Credit Guarantee Corporation of India undertakes the twin functions of extending the insurance over to the depositors in banks and protects the interest of banks by providing guarantees in respect of advances granted by them to small scale industries and the priority and neglected sectors of the economy. The Export Credit Guarantee Corporation (ECGC) provides protection to the banks in respect of risks inherent in financing the export trade. With the setting up and growth of all these institutions, Indian banking and financial system may be claimed to have the finest set-up comparable to any advanced country.

COMMERCIAL BANKS

Amongst the banking institutions in the organised sector, the commercial banks are the oldest institutions having a wide network of branches, commanding utmost public confidence and having the lion's share in the total banking operations. Initially, they are established as corporate bodies with share-holdings by private individuals, but subsequently there has been a drift towards State ownership and control. Today 28 banks constitute the strong public sector in Indian commercial banking.

Up to late sixties, they were mainly engaged in financing organised trade, commerce and industry, but since then, they are actively participating in financing agriculture, small business and small borrowers also.

The Commercial banks operating in India fall under a numbr of sub-categories on the basis of ownership and control of management.

Foreign commercial banks are the branches in India of the joint stock banks incorporated abroad. These banks, besides financing the foreign trade of the country, undertake banking business within the country as well.

Public sector in Indian banking reached its present position in three stages-first, the conversion of the then existing Imperial Bank of India into the State Bank of India in 1955 followed by the estalishment of its seven subsidiary banks; second, the nationalisation of 14 major commercial banks in July 1969 and last, the nationalisation of 6 more commercial banks on April 15, 1980.

Difference between State Bank and Nationalised Banks

(1) Though all the 28 public sector banks are corporate bodies, but the statutes under which they were established are different. The State Bank of India was established under the State Bank of India Act, 1955, the subsidiary banks under the State Bank of India (Subsidiary Banks) Act, 1959, and the nationalised banks under the Banking Companies (Acquisition and Transfer of Undertakings) Act, 1970. These banks are, therefore, governed by their respective statutes.

(2) The cent per cent ownership of the 20 nationalised banks vests in the Government of India, whereas the State Bank of India is owned, to a larger extent, by the Reserve Bank of India — there is still some private ownership in the share capital of the State Bank. The subsidiary banks are owned by the State Bank of India.

(3) The State Bank of India acts as an agent of the Reserve Bank of India. The Reserve Bank shall appoint the State Bank as its sole agent at all places in India where it does not have an office or branch of its Banking Department and there is a branch of the State Bank or branch of a subsidiary bank. The nationalised banks have not been conferred with this privilege of acting as agent of the Reserve Bank. The Reserve Bank has been empowered to appoint any nationalised bank to act as its agent at all places in India where it has a branch for the following purposes:

(i) paying, receiving, collecting and remitting money, bullion and securities on behalf of any government in India; and

(ii) undertaking and transacting any other business entrusted by the Reserve Bank from time to time.

THE CO-OPERATIVE BANKS

The co-operative banks also perform the basic functions of banking but differ from the commercial banks in many aspects as follows :

(1) The commercial banks have been organised either as joint stock companies under the companies Act, 1956, or as public corporations under separate Acts of Parliament. The co-operative banks have been established under the Co-operative Societies Acts of different States.

(2) The co-operative banks have a three-tier set-up. The State Co-operative Bank is the apex institution in a State, while Central/District co-operative banks function at the district level and Primary Credit Societies work at the village level. The commercial banks are organised on a unitary basis.

(3) Only the State Co-operative Banks have access to the Reserve Bank of India, whereas every commercial bank which is a scheduled bank is entitled to avail of the re-finance facilities from the Reserve Bank.

(4) Co-operative banks function within a given area. Their operations are restricted to a particular State in case of a State/Apex Bank, a particular district in case of a district co-operative bank and to a local area in case of a society. The commercial banks, on the other hand, function over a wide area which is not limited by the boundaries of a particular State or district. Most of them have branches over a number of States and many of them all over the country.

(5) Till 1969 the commercial banks were urban-oriented and financed organised trade and industry. The co-operative banks have been basically rural-oriented and have been financing agricultural and allied activities.

(6) The commercial banks are governed by all the sections of the Banking Regulation Act, 1949, but only some of the sections of this Act are applicable to co-operative banks. Thus the control of the Reserve Bank is partial over the co-operative banks.

(7) Co-operative banks proceed on the principles of co-operation, whereas commercial banks function on sound business principles. The former are, therefore, granted accommodation at concessional rates by the Reserve Bank.

THE REGIONAL RURAL BANKS

The Regional Rural Banks are relatively new banking institutions which were added to the Indian banking scene since October, 1976. There are 196 Regional Rural Banks with a network of branches in the states of the Indian Union. These banks have been established by the Government of India in terms of the provisions of the Regional Rural Banks Act, 1976. The distinctive feature of a rural bank is that though it is a separate body corporate with perpetual succession and common seal, it is very closely linked with the commercial bank which has sponsored the proposal to establish it. The Central Government while establishing a rural bank at the request of the commercial bank specifies the local limits within which it shall operate. The rural bank may establish its branches or agencies at any place within the notified area.

The necessity of rural banks was felt because the then existing credit agencies–the co-operative banks and the commercial banks–lacked in certain respects in meeting the needs of the rural areas. The weaknesses of these institutions in this regard may be summed up as follows :

(i) The co-operative credit structure is weak so far as the managerial talent and post-credit supervision and loan recovery are concerned. These institutions have not been able to mobilise adequate resources and, therefore, depend upon the Reserve Bank for re-finance to a large extent.

(ii) The commercial banks are basically urban-oriented. If they have to play a significant role in rural banking, their methods, procedures, training and orientation shall have to be adapted to the rural environment. This is not likely to be achieved easily and quickly. Moreover, the cost of their operations is quite high due to high salary structure, staffing pattern and high establishment cost. Thus the commercial banks are unable to provide credit at cheap rates to the weaker sections in the rural areas.

Rural Bank has been contemplated as an institutioln to combine the rural touch and local feel, a familiarity with rural problems and attitudinal identification with the rural economy which the co-operatives possess in large degree, with modern business organisation, commercial discipline, ability to mobilise resources and access to the central money markets which the commercial banks have. In other words the institution of rural banks is intended to be "locally bases,rural oriented and commercially organised:"

Capital : Initially the authorised share capital of each Rural Bank was Rs. 1 crore, divided into 1 lack shares of Rs. 100 each. Fifty per cent of the issued capital was subscribed to by the Central Govt., fifteen per cent by the concerned State Governments and thirty-five per cent by the sponsor bank.

Business of a Rural Bank : A Rural Bank carries on the normal banking business, and engages in one or more forms of business. A Rural Bank may, in particular, undertake the following types of business, namely :

(a) the granting of loans and advances, particularly to small and marginal farmers and agricultural labourers, whether individual or in groups and to co-operative societies (including agricultural marketing societies, agricultural processing societies, co-operative farming societies, primary agricultural credit societies or farmers' service societies) for agricultural purpose or agricultural operations or for other connected purposes; and

(b) the granting of loans and advances, particular to artisans, small entrepreneurs and persons of small means engaged in trade, commerce or industry or other productive activities within the notified area of a Rural Bank.

Regional Rural Bank are thus primarily meant to cater to the needs of the poor and small borrowers in the countryside. At the end of December 1987, their advances to the weaker sections accounted for 92% of their total direct advances. A sizable portion of indirect advances was also provided to the weaker sections.

Management : Each Rural Bank is managed by a Board of Directors. The general superintendence, direction and management of the affairs and business vest in the Board. In discharging its functions, the Board of Directors act on business principles and shall have due regard to public interest. A Regional Bank is guided by the directions issued by the Central Government in regard to matters of policy involving public interest.

The cost of operations of Rural Banks has been kept in strict control. The Central Government prescribes the salary scales of the employees after keeping in view the salary structure of the employees of the State Governments and the local authorities of comparable level and status in the notified area.

Responsibilities of Sponsor Banks : Apart from subscribing to the share capital, the sponsor banks shall assist the RRBs by imparting training to the personnel and providing managerial and financial assistance to the RRBs during the first 5 years of their functioning. The sponsor banks are empowered to monitor the progress of RRBs, to conduct inspections, internal audit and security and to suggest corrective measures, as and when necessary.

The Regional Rural Banks avail of the re-finance facilities from the National Bank for Agriculture and Rural Development in respect of the short-term, medium and long-term advances granted by them. The sponsor banks also provide them re-finance. The deposits with these banks are insured by the Deposit Insurance and Credit Guarantee Corporation.

LAND DEVELOPMENT BANKS

The long-term credit needs of the agricultural sector are met by another type of co-operative institutions known as Land Development Banks. The structure of these banks is a two-tier one at the State level, there are Central Land Development Banks and at the district or taluka level, there are Primary Land Development Banks. In a few States, e.g., Gujarat, Jammu & Kashmir and U.P., the structure is unitary, i.e., there are Apex Land Development Banks which operate directly through their own branches at the district level.

The Land Development Banks meet the requirements of the farmers for developmental purposes, viz., provision of equipment like pump-sets, tractors and machinery and land improvement in the form of levelling, bunding, reclamation of land, fencing, sinking of new well and repairs to old well. Loans are granted on the security of mortgage of immovable property of the farmers.

The Central Land Development Banks raise their resources by floating debentures in the market. These debentures carry the guarantee of the State Government and are subscribed by the Central and State Governments, Commercial Banks, Life Insurance Corporation and other Land Development Banks as a measure of mutual support. The Land Development Banks have availed of the re-financing facilities provided by the National Bank for Agriculture and Rural Development in respect of the term loans granted by them for the schemes of agricultural development. They also secure short-term accommodation from the State Governments, Commercial Banks and the State Co-operative Banks.

AGRICULTURAL FINANCE CORPORATION LIMITED

The Agricultural Finance Corporation Ltd. was promoted as a joint stock company in 1968 by the Indian Banks' Association. Today it was 37 banks-including of the State Bank and the nationalised banks-as its shareholders. The object of its establishment was to help the commercial banks in financial agricultural projects and to participate actively and extensively in the development of agriculture.

The AFC is now functioning as a Rural Development Consultancy Organisation. It has built up expertise in this field and is engaged in the formulation of projects and development plans at the instance of member-banks, State Governments and the Central Government. It locates and identifies potential areas or projects for investment by banks, also assists the banks in conducting surveys of the potential for investment, production and deposit mobilisation with a view to select operational areas. It has started consultancy work abroad as well.

INDUSTRIAL DEVELOPMENT BANK OF INDIA

IDBI is the apex banking institution in the field of long-term industrial finance. The assistance provided by IDBI falls in two broad categories, i.e., (i) direct assistance to large and medium industries, and (ii) indirect assistance. Major portion of the direct assistance is provided in the form of Project loans to industries. Besides, IDBI also provides assistance by way of under-writing and direct subscription to the shares/debentures of industrial undertakings. IDBI also provides soft loans for the modernisation of all industries.

Indirect assistance is provided by the Bank to tiny, small and medium enterprises, through other financial institutions in a number of way.

Besides the share capital of Rs. 703 crores as on March 31, 1991, wholly subscribed by the Central Government, the IDBI raises the bulk of its funds from (i) market borrowings by way of bonds, and (ii) the borrowings out of National Industrial Credit (Long-Term Operations) Fund of the Reserve

Bank. IDBI also takes short-term advances from the Reserve Bank against lodgement of usance bills. During recent years, IDBI has also raised resources in foreign currencies by way of loans and private placement of its bonds in foreign capital markets. Such resources are utilised for financing imports of capital goods and services required by the assisted projects.

INDUSTRIAL FINANCE CORPORATION OF INDIA

The Industrial Finance Corporation of India (IFCI) was the first development bank established in India in the year 1948. Its primary objective was to assist industry especially when accommodation from traditional sources of finance for the creation of fixed assets was felt inadequate or when recourse to capital market was difficult. IFCI provides assistance to the industrial concerns in various ways which are broadly classified into the following three categories:

(A) **Project Finance :** Under project finance assistance is provided in the following ways.

(1) Long-term loans - both in rupees and foreign currencies,

(2) underwriting of equity, preference and debenture issues,

(3) subscribing to equity, preference and debenture issues,

(4) guaranteeing the deferred payments in respect of machinery imported from abroad or purchased in India, and

(5) guaranteeing of loans raised in foreign currency from foreign financial institutions.

Financial assistance may be availed of by any limited company-in the public, private or joint sector-or by a co-operative society in-corporated in India, which is engaged or proposes to be engaged in the specified industrial activities. Such financial assistance is available for the setting up of new industrial projects and also for the expansion, diversification, renovation or modernisation of existing ones. The Corporation also provides financial assistance on concessional terms for setting up industrial projects in industrially less developed district in the States/ Union Territories notified by the Central Government.

(B) **Financial Services :** Under this category are included the merchant banking and allied services rendered by the IFCI. Besides, financial assistance, not tied to any project, provided by IFCI to industrial units is also included in this category. IFCI, thus, provides Equipment Financing, Equipment Leasing, Equipment Procurement, Equipment Credit, Instalment Credit, Suppliers' Credit and Buyers Credit.

(C) **Promotional Services :** They cover a wide range of services provided by IFCI. Important amongst them are funds support for technical consultancy, Risk Capital, Venture Capital, Technology Development, Tourism development and finance, entrepreneurship development, development of science and technology, etc.

Resources : The paid-up capital of IFCI (Rs. 143 crores as on 31st March 1991) has been subscribed by the Industrial Development Bank of India (50%) and by scheduled banks, co-operative banks, insurance concerns, investment trusts, etc.

The Corporaton raises its resources by way of (i) issue of bonds in the market, (ii) borrowing from Industrial Development Bank of India and the Central Government, and other financial institutions/organisations and (iii) foreign credits secured from foreign financial institutions and borrowings in the international capital markets.

INDUSTRIAL CREDIT AND INVESTMENT CORPORATION OF INDIA LIMITED

The ICICI was set up as a joint stock company in 1955 with the main objective to channelise the World Bank funds to industry in India and also to build up a capital market in India.

A significant feature of ICICI's operations is the predominance of foreign currency loans sanctioned by it. This has been made possible because of the facility it enjoys of raising funds in foreign currencies. The World Bank has been sanctioning to it lines of credit for lending to the private industrial sector. Recently, it has granted assistance for technology upgradation and modernisation of balancing equipment out of World Bank's lines of credit. New projects with export potentials have also been financed. ICICI has also raised foreign currency loans from other institutions abroad and has entered international capital markets also.

Besides lending to industries, ICICI is also playing a significant role in the development of the capital market. It undertakes underwriting activity and makes direct subscription to the shares and debentures of the companies. As merchant bankers, ICICI helps the corporate clients to raise resources in the capital market and otherwise also. ICICI also acts as Trustee for the holders of convertible and non-convertible debentures issued by companies.

Till recently, ICICI was having larger reliance upon the conventional source of rupee finance, namely government guaranteed bonds, borrowings from Industrial Development Bank of India and the Government of India. But during recent years emphasis has been shifted to public issue of equity, inter-corporate deposits, certificates of deposit and loans and depostis at commercial rates from other financial institutions. Thus while availability of funds from conventional sources has been reduced, non-conventional sources with low to medium maturities and close to market rate of interest have been tapped.

INDUSTRIAL RECONSTRUCTION BANK OF INDIA

The Industrial Reconstruction Corporation of India Ltd., which was set up in 1971 as a primary agency for rehabilitation of sick industrial units, has been reconstructed and renamed as the Industrial Reconstruction Bank of India

(IRBI). IRBI functions as the principal credit and reconstruction agency for industrial revival by undertaking modernisation, expansion, re-organisation, diversification or rationalisation of industry and also coordinates similar work of other institutions engaged therein and to assist and rehabilitate industrial concerns.

The IRBI is empowered :

(i) to grant loans and advances to industrial concerns,

(ii) to underwrite stocks, shares, bonds and debentures,

(iii) to guarantee loans/deferred payments and performance obligations of any contracts undertaken by industrial concerns, and

(iv) to act as an agent of Central and State Government, Reserve Bank, State Bank, Scheduled Commercial and State Co-operative banks, public financial institutions, SFC., etc.

Its functions also include development activities such as providing infrastructural facilities, raw materials, consultancy, managerial and merchant banking services for reconstruction and development of industrial concerns and providing machinery and other equipment on lease or hire-purchase basis.

The IRBI is empowered to take over management or possession or both and can transfer by way of lease and sale the property of defaulting industrial concerns. It can prepare schemes for reconstruction by scaling down the liabilities to submit the schemes of merger or amalgamation for approval of the Central Government. The Bank borrows funds from the Government and also by way of issuing bonds and debentures.

REGIONAL DEVELOPMENT BANKS

Besides the all-India industrial financing institutions, there are State level financial institutions also, which may be designated as Regional Development Banks. These institutions grant assistance to industrial units located within their own State/States.

STATE FINANCIAL CORPORATIONS

At present 18 State Financial Corporations are functioning. The SFCs are the State level agencies established for the development of small and medium industrial units within their respective States. Thus, they provide loans and underwriting assistance to industrial units having paid-up capital and reserves not exceeding Rs. 1 crore. The maximum amount that can be sanctioned to an industrial concern by SFC is Rs. 60 lakhs.

The Industrial Development Bank of India has made a significant contribution toward the share capital of the SFCs. Moreover, the SFCs depend upon the IDBI for re-finance in respect of the term loans granted by them. Apart from the above, SFC also resort to temporary borrowings from the Reserve Bank of India and borrowings from IDBI and by the sale of bonds.

STATE INDUSTRIAL DEVELOPMENT CORPORATIONS (SIDCs)

The State Industrial Development Corporation have been set up by the State Government as companies wholly owned by them. At present, 22 such SIDCs are functioning in India. SIDCs are not merely financing agencies, but are intended to act as instruments for accelerating the pace of industrialisation in the respective States. Besides providing financial assistance to industrial concerns by way of loans, guarantees and underwriting of or direct subscriptions to share and debentures, the SIDCs undertake various promotional activities such as conducting techno-economic surveys, project identification, preparaton of feasibility studies, selection and training of entrepreneurs. They also promote joint sector projects in association with private promoters. In such projects SIDCs take 26% of the equity, and the rest is offered to the investing public.

SIDCs also undertake the development of industrial areas, construction of sheds and provision of infrastructural facilities and also the development of new growth centres. They also administer various State Government incentive schemes.

The IDBI grants re-finance to SIDCs also against the term loans provided by them. SIDCs also borrow by way of bonds and from the Government and accept deposits to augment their resources.

THE INVESTING INSTITUTIONS

Life Insurance Corporation of India

The Life Insurance Corporation of India is the largest institutional investor in this country. The investments of LIC are regulated by Section 27-A of the Insurance Act, 1938. Consequently, a much larger portion of its investible resources is invested in Government and other approved securities and is given as loans to socially-oriented sector. However, the LIC provides assistance to the corporate sector in the following ways :

(i) By subscribing to the bonds and shares issued by the Development Banks like IDBI, IFCI, ICICI, SFCs.

(ii) By directly subscribing to, or underwriting the shares, bonds and debentures of the corporate sector. It also purchases corporate securities in the market.

(iii) By providing term loans to companies, singly or in participation with banks.

General Insurance Corporation of India

According to the guidelines issued by the Government, 70% of the accretions to the fund of GIC have to be invested in the socially-oriented sectors, which include Central and State Government's securities and loans to various public bodies engaged in housing. Out of the balance, the GIC invests in corporate sector by way of underwriting of new issues of companies and also by way of term loans/subscription to privately placed debentures.

UNIT TRUST OF INDIA

The Unit Trust of India (UTI) is a statutory public sector investment institution set up in 1964. It mobilises the savings of the community through the sale of its units under its various unit schemes. The resources thus mobilised are invested by the UTI mainly in the shares and debentures of the companies. Income received from these investments, after meeting the expenses of the Trust, is distributed to the unit holders annually as divided.

The UTI provides to investors, specially the small ones, opportunities for gainful employment of their savings. By buying units, they can share in the growing industrial prosperity of the country, diversify their risks, and at the same time, derive the benefit of professional management of their funds. The Unit Trust is always ready to buy back the units from the holders at prices determined by it. It has distributed dividends at constantly rising rates. The dividend declared by the UTI is exempted from income-tax subject to certain limits.

Mutual Fund Unit Scheme

In September 1986, the Unit Trust of India introduced a new Mutual Fund Unit Scheme wherein Master Shares of Rs. 10 each have been issued at par. The salient features of this scheme are :

(i) The master shares are listed on all the stock exchanges and thus provide liquidity to the investors.

(ii) The mutual fund will invest primarily in equity shares. It may also invest in money market instrument such as call deposits with, and bills discounted by banks, short-term borrowings by companies and variable rate debentures.

(iii) Master shares are freely transferable.

EXPORT IMPORT BANK OF INDIA (EXIM BANK)

Set up on January 1, 1982, the Export Import Bank of India is the apex banking institution in the field of financing foreign trade of India. The Exim Bank provides financial assistance to exporters and importers and functions as the principal financial institution for coordinating the working of other institutions engaged in financing of exports and imports of goods and sevices. It provides re-finance facilities also to the commercial institutions against their export-import financing activities. Broadly, the functions of Exim Bank include :

(i) financing of exports from and imports into not only India, but also third countries, of goods and services ;

(ii) financing of joint ventures in foreign countries ;

(iii) financing of export and import of machinery and equipment on lease basis ;

(iv) providing loans to an Indian party so as to enable it to contribute in the share capital of a joint venture in a foreign country.

The Bank also undertakes limited merchant banking functions such as underwriting of stocks, shares, bonds, or debentures of companies engaged in export or import and providing technical, administrative and financial assistance to parties in connection with export or import.

The Bank can raise resources form (i) the open market through the issue of bonds and debentures, (ii) from Reserve Bank of India, from its National Industrial Credit (Long Term Operations) Fund and (iii) can borrow foreign currency in or outside India.

Entire business of the Industrial Development Bank of India relating to export financing has been taken over by the Exim Bank.

Exim Bank operates three broad programmes of financing, viz., loans, rediscounting and guarantees. As present nine programmes are operated by the Bank as follows :

(a) Loans to Indian Companies are provided under its :

(i) Direct Financial assistance to exporters.

(ii) Technology and Consultancy Services.

(iii) Overseas investment financing for equity participation by an Indian company in joint venture abroad.

(iv) Pre-Shipment Credit in case of export contract for capital goods.

(b) Loans to foreign Governments, Companies and Financial Institutions are provided under its :

(i) Overseas Buyer's Credit Scheme.

(ii) Lines of Credit to foreign government.

(iii) Relending facility to banks overseas.

(c) Loans to Commercial Banks in India are available under :

(i) Export Bills Re-discounting Scheme (Short-term bills)

(ii) Re-finance of Export Credit.

Guarantee programme is available in case of construction and turnkey contracts.

NATIONAL BANK FOR AGRICULTURE AND RURAL DEVELOPMENT

The National Bank for Agriculture and Rural Development (NABARD) is the apex development bank for agriculture and rural development. It was set up on 12th July, 1982 by merging the Agricultural Credit Department and Rural

Planning and Credit Cell of the Reserve Bank of India and the entire undertaking of Agricultural Re-finance and Development Corporation.

NABARD has been entrusted with three types of functions, namely, (i) the credit functions, (ii) the developmental functions, and (iii) the regulatory functions :

(i) **Credit Functions :** It provides through the banking system all kinds of productive and investment credit to agriculture, small scale industries, cottage and village industries, handicrafts, and other allied economic activities. It provides different types of re-finance (i.e., short term, medium term and long term) to the eligible institutions, namely (a) State Co-operative Banks (b) Regional Rural Banks, (c) State Land Development Banks (excluding short term), (d) Commercial Banks (only long term) and other financial institutions approved by the Reserve Bank. NABARD has prescribed lower rates of interest on the re-finance provided by it and the rates payable by the ultimate borrowers.

(ii) **Development Functions :** NABARD coordinates the operations of rural credit agencies, develops expertise to deal with agricultural and rural problems, assists Government, Reserve Bank and other institutions in rural development efforts and acts as an agent to Government and Reserve Bank in relevant areas. It provides facilities for training and research and assists the State Governments to enable them to contribute to the share capital of eligible institutions.

(iii) **Regulatory Functions :** The Banking Regulations Act, 1949 empowers the NABARD to undertake inspection of Regional Rural Banks and Co-operative Bank (other than primary co-operative banks). If any such bank seeks permission of the Reserve Bank for opening branches, etc., it will have to obtain the recommendation of NABARD.

Resources : The paid-up capital of NABARD is Rs. 100 crores at present contributed equally by the Government of India and the Reserve Bank. Besides the National Rural Credit (Long Term Operations) fund and the National Rural Credit (Stabilisation) Fund, the NABARD is authorised to raise resources by issue of bonds and debentures guaranteed by the Central Government, and also to borrow from the Reserve Bank, Central Government or any other organisation approved by the Central Government. It can also raise funds externally through the Government of India.

NATIONAL HOUSING BANK

National Housing Bank is the latest apex bank set up in India. The Bank has started functioning on 9th July, 1988 with its head office in New Delhi.

Functions : The Bank is the apex housing finance institution in the country and has been entrusted with the following functions :

(i) The Bank's primary responsibility is to promote and develop specialised housing finance institutions for mobilising resources and extending credit for housing.

(ii) The Bank is empowered to extend re-financing facilities to housing finance institutions and to Scheduled Banks. The Bank has also been given the power to inspect the books and accounts of any housing finance institution to which it has given financial assistance.

(iii) Its other functions will include :

   (a) to provide guarantee and underwriting facilities to housing finance institutions.

   (b) to formulate schemes for mobilisation of resources and extension of credit for houses (including that for the economically weaker sections of society which may be supported by subsidies).

   (c) to provide guidelines to housing finance institutions to ensure their growth on sound lines.

   (d) to provide technical and administrative assistance to the housing finance institutions and to coordinate with various agencies connected with housing.

(iv) The Bank will also provide advisory services to the Central and State Governments, local authorities and other concerned agencies on all matters concerning housing.

Resources : The Bank is empowered to raise resources through issue of bonds and debentures. It can borrow from the Central Government, and other approved institutions and accept deposits of long-term duration. In addition, the Bank can also borrow in foreign currency from banks and financial institutions in India and abroad. It can also avail of short-term loans for fixed periods upto 18 months from Reserve Bank of India also long-term loans from the recently established National Housing Credit (Long Term Operations) Fund by Reserve Bank.

Collection of Credit Information : The Bank is also authorised to collect credit and other information from housing finance institutions, the Central and State Governments, local authorities etc., to publish the same.

Power to Regulate Corporate Housing Finance Institutions : The Housing Bank is also empowered to exercise control over the Corporate Housing Financing Institutions, which was hitherto exercised by the Reserve Bank. The Housing Bank can now regulate or prohibit the issue by any housing finance institution, which is a corporate body, of any prospectus or advertisement soliciting deposit of money from the public. The Bank can collect information from such institutions regarding deposits and give them directions regarding acceptance of deposits and can also inspect them.

Home Loan Account Scheme : The Housing Bank has launched a Home Loan Account Scheme with effect from July 1, 1989 which is operated through the commercial and co-operative banks. The Housing Bank will be a re-financing institution. Under the Scheme any individual can open a home loan account. After 5 years, he will be entitled to a housing loan within specified limits.

DISCOUNT AND FINANCE HOUSE OF INDIA LTD.

Discount and Finance House of India Ltd. (DFHI), a unique institution of its kind, was set up in April 1988. The Discount House has been established to deal in money market instruments in order to provide liquidity in the money market. Thus the task assigned to DFHI is to develop a secondary market in the existing money market instruments.

The establishment of a Discount House was recommended by a Working Group on Money Market. The main objective of DFHI is to facilitate the smoothening of the short term liquidity imbalances by developing an active money market and integrating the various segments of the money market.

At present DFHI's activities are restricted to :

(i) dealing in 182 Days Treasury Bills,

(ii) re-discounting short term commercial bills,

(iii) participating in the inter-bank call money market and term deposits, and

(iv) dealing in Commercial paper and Certificates of deposits.

The DFHI is authorised to augment its resources with lines of credit from public sector banks and re-finance lines from the Reserve Bank. The amount and the rate of interest charged by Reserve Bank on re-finance would be flexible, so that Reserve Bank can have its impact on the money market by varying the quantum of re-finance and the rate of interest thereon.

SMALL INDUSTRIES DEVELOPMENT BANK OF INDIA

In the field of financing of small scale industries in India, a separate Apex Development Bank has started its operations from April 2, 1990. The Small Industries Development Bank of India (SIDBI) has been set up for promotion, financing and development of industry in the tiny and small scale sector. It coordinates the functions of other institutions engaged in similar activities.

The SIDBI has been established as a wholly-owned subsidiary of the Industrial Development Bank of India. It has taken over IDBI's financing activities relating to the small scale sector.

The major activities undertaken by this Bank are as follows :

(i) re-financing of term loans granted by banks and other eligible financial institutions, namely the State Financial Corporations and State Industrial Development Corporations.

(ii) direct discounting as well as re-discounting of bills arising out of sale of machinery or capital equipment by manufacturers in small scale sector on deferred credit.

(iii) equity type assistance under National Equity Fund and by way of seed capital to entrepreneurs.

(iv) re-discounting of short term trade bills arising out of sale of products of small scale sector.

(v) resources support to National Small Industries Corporation and other institutions concerned with small industries.

(vi) Share capital and resources support to factoring organisations.

DEPOSIT INSURANCE AND CREDIT GUARANTEE CORPORATION (DICGC)

The Deposit Insurance Corporation was established by an Act of Parliament on January 1, 1962. The Corporation performs the following two functions :

(a) **Deposit Insurance :** With a view to provide protection to small depositors in commercial banks, regional rural banks and co-operative banks, the corporation provides insurance cover up to a certain amount. Under the scheme in the event of liquidation, reconstitution or amalgamation of an insured bank, every depositor of that bank is entitled to re-payment of his deposits held by him in the same right and capacity in all branches of that bank up to Rs. 30,000. The Corporation charges premium from the insured banks for this purpose and credits the same to Deposit Insurance Fund, maintained by it.

(b) **Credit Guarantee :** The Corporation provides guarantee cover to credit facilities extended to certain categories of small borrowers belonging to the weaker sections of the society and also to the small scale industries. Such guarantees are extended to the participating institutions, viz., Commercial banks, Regional Banks, Co-operative Banks, State Financial Corporation and other term lending institutions.

EXPORT CREDIT GUARANTEE CORPORATION OF INDIA LTD. (ECGC)

Export Credit Guarantee Corporation of India Ltd. is a Government of India undertaking which plays a very important role in the field of export promotion and export finance. As the Indian exporters offer competitive credit terms to foreign buyers in the world markets, ECGC offers them protection from the risk inherent in selling goods on credit to foreign buyers. The standard policies issued by the ECGC cover the following commercial and political risks inherent in an export transaction :

(i) **Commercial risks :** include isolvency of the importer, default on his part to pay for the goods or failure of the importers to accept the goods.

(ii) **Political risks :** include restrictions placed on transfer of payments in rupees by the importer's government, war between the two countries, war, revolution or civil commotion in the importer's country, imposition of new import licensing restrictions in the buyer's country or cancellation of a valid import licence, additional handling, transport or insurance charges arising from interruption or diversion of voyage which cannot be recovered from the importer.

The Corporation re-imburses the exporter a specified percentage of loss incurred. These policies insure the risks of the exporters and thus enables them to get finance from the bankers on the collateral security of the policies.

The ECGC also issues a number of financial guarantees to the banks to protect their interest in financing exports. The guarantees have been designed to encourage banks to give liberal credit-pre-shipment and post-shipment for producing, packing and exporting goods. The ECGC re-imburses the banks specified percentage of their loss and charges guarantee fees in lieu thereof.

RESERVE BANK OF INDIA

As the central bank of the country, the Reserve Bank of India performs both the traditional functions of a central bank and a variety of developmental and promotional functions. The Reserve Bank of India Act, 1934, confers upon it the powers to act as note-issuing authority, banker's bank and banker to the Government.

Reserve Bank as Note-Issuing Authority

The currency of our country consists of one-rupee notes and coins (including subsidiary coins) issued by the Government of India and Bank notes issued by the Reserve Bank. As required by Section 38 of the Reserve Bank of India Act, Government puts into circulation one-rupee coins and notes through Reserve Bank only. The Reserve Bank has the sole right to issue bank notes in India. The notes issued by the Reserve Bank and the one-rupee notes and coins issued by the Government are unlimited legal tender. Reserve Bank also bears the responsibility of exchanging notes and coins into those of other denominations as required by the public.

As required by the Reserve Bank of India Act, the issue of notes and the general banking business of the Bank are undertaken by two separate departments of the Bank. The Issue Department is responsible for the issue of new notes. It keeps its assets, which form the backing for the note issue, quite separate from the assets of the Banking Department.

The business of banking is undertaken by the Banking Department which holds stock of currency with itself. Whenever necessary, the Banking Department replenishes the stock of currency from the Issue Department against equivalent transfer of eligible assets. Similarly, if the stock of currency with the Banking Department becomes surplus to its normal requirements, the excess is returned to the Issue Department in exchange of equivalent assets.

The assets of the Issue Department against which bank notes are issued consists of the following, namely :

(i)   gold coins and bullion,
(ii) foreign securities,
(iii) rupee coins,
(iv) Government of India rupee securities, and
(v)   the bills of exchange and promissory notes payable in India which are eligible for purchase by the Bank.

The aggregate value of gold coins and bullion shall not at any time be less than Rs. 115 crores and together with foreign securities (i.e., the total of (i) and (ii) above) not less than Rs. 200 crores. The Reserve Bank is also empowered to reduce its holding of foreign securities in the Issue Department to any lesser amount, with the previous sanction of the Central Government.

Currency Chests : The Reserve Bank has made adequate administrative arrangements for undertaking the function of distribution of currency notes and coins. The Issue Department has opened its offices in 10 leading cities for this purpose. Moreover, currency chests have been maintained all over the country to facilitate the expansion and contraction of currency in the country. Currency chests are receptacles (i.e., boxes or containers) in which stocks of new or re-issuable notes are stored along with rupee coins. The total number of currency chests and repositories as at the end of June 1981 was 3,841 which were run by the Reserve Bank, State bank, and its subsidiaries, public sector banks and Government Treasuries and Sub-Treasuries. The stock of new notes is thus held in currency chests scattered over the entire country and maintained by the public sector banks in most of the cases. There are several advantages to the bank or the Treasury maintaining a currency chest :

(1) If its payments on a particular day exceeds its own balance, it can immediately withdraw funds from the chest. Likewise, if the funds are in surplus it can deposit into it any such surplus funds. Thus the necessity for the physical transfer of cash at frequent intervals from one place to another is avoided. The Treasuries and bank branches work with relatively small balances.

(2) The currency chests facilitate the exchange of rupees coins for notes and supply of notes of lower denomination for those of higher denominations and vice versa and also the issue of new notes for old and soiled notes.

(3) The currency chests also serve as the basis for providing remittance facilities to banks and the public.

Reserve Bank as Banker to Government

The Reserve Bank of India acts as banker to the Central and State Governments. It is obligatory for the Bank to transact government business including the management of the public debt of the Union. Central Government entrusts the Bank all its money, remittance, exchange and banking transactions in India and in particular deposit free of interest all its cash balances with the Bank.

The Bank is also required to maintain currency chests of its Issue Department at places prescribed by the Government and to maintain sufficient notes and coins therein.

The Reserve Bank is also authorised to make to the Central and State Governments ways and means advances which are repayable within 3 months from the date of making the advance. The Bank also acts as adviser to the government on important economic and financial matters.

Reserve Bank as Bankers' Bank

Reserve Bank is the banker to the banks - commercial, co-operative and Regional Rural Banks.

Functions Rendered by Banks

The range of functions offered differs from bank to bank depending mainly on the size and type of banks, but the acceptance of deposits from the public and provision of credit form the mainstay of the banking business. The services offered by commercial banks may be classified into (i) services to depositors and borrowers for providing credit to them, and (ii) ancillary services.

Services Rendered to Depositors and Borrowers

Banks open various types of deposit account and render the following services to the depositors and borrowers :

1. Collection of cheques, demand drafts, bills of exchange, promissory notes, hundis, inland and foreign documentary and clean bills.
2. Purchase of local and foreign currency documentary/clean bills, negotiation of bills under inland and foreign letters of credit, advising of inland and foreign letters of credit established by branches and correspondents.
3. Carrying out the standing instructions for the payment of insurance premia, subscriptions, certain taxes and gift remittances.

Ancillary Services

1. Performance Guarantees and Financial Guarantees,
2. Safe Custody of Deeds, Securities,
3. Safe Deposit Vault,
4. Purchase and Sale of Securities,
5. Collection of Interest on Securities/Debentures and Dividend on Shares, Collection of Pension Bills,
6. Remittance of Funds - Bank Drafts, Mail Transfers, Telegraphic Transfers,
7. Executor and Trustees,
8. Personal Tax Assistance, Preparing Income Tax, Sales Tax, Wealth Tax Returns,

9. Investment Facilities - Underwriting, Banker to new issues, Guidance to investment, Stock Exchange assistance,

10. Credit Transfers,

11. Credit Cards,

12. Travellers Cheques and Gift Cheques,

13. Emergency Vouchers,

14. Sale of Units of Unit Trust of India.

19

FINANCIAL PLANNING

Need for Finance : Finance may be defined as the provision of money at the time it is wanted. It is undoubtedly the lifeblood of business. The ambitious plans of businessman would remain mere dreams unless adequate money is available to convert them into reality.

The financial function of management will have particular responsibility for the following :

(a) ensuring a fair return on investment to the shareholders.

(b) generating and building up surplus and reserves for growth and expansion,

(c) planning, directing, and controlling the utilisation of finances so as to ensure maximum efficiency of operations and proper relations with suppliers, financiers, workers and members, and

(d) coordinating the operations of the various wings or departments through appropriate measures to ensure discipline in the use of financial resources.

Meaning of Financial Planning : Once the promoters of a company are convinced of the commerce worthwhileness of a business proposition, they will take steps to chalk out the finance plan of the proposed company.

(1) they will try to determine the amount of capital which will be needed for implementing the business plans. This will naturally involve estimation of the amount of promotion expenses, expenses on organisation, cost of fixed assets, operating costs, and the cost of getting the business established.

(2) they will relate to the form and proportion of the securities which can be issued to raise the required amount to be collected by the issue of shares and debentures and also what should be the proportion of shares and debentures.

(3) the promoters will also make up their mind about the policies which they will pursue with regard to the administration of capital.

Capitalisation refers to the process of determining the plan or patterns of financing. It includes not merely the determination of the quantity (amount) of finance required for a company but also the decision about the quality of financing. Capitalisation is the sum-total of all long-term securities issued by a company and the surpluses not meant for distribution. Capitalisation may be said to be composed of (1) the value of shares of different kinds, (2) the value of surpluses, whether capital surpluses or earned surpluses, and (3) the value of bonds and debentures issued by a company still not redeemed. The term capitalisation is used only in relation to companies and not in respect of firms or sole-proprietorships. Thus capital includes all the loans and reserves of the concern, but 'capitalisation' includes only long-term loans and retained profits besides the capital.

Theories of Capitalisation : There are two recognised bases for capitalising new companies :

(i) **Cost Theory :** According to the cost theory of capitalisation, the value of a company is arrived at by adding up the cost of fixed assets like plants, machinery, patents, etc., the capital regularly required for the continuous operation of the company (working capital), the cost of establishing business and expenses of promotion. The true value of an enterprise is judged from its earning capacity rather than from the capital invested in it.

(ii) **Earning Theory :** The true value (capitalisation) of an enterprise depends upon its earnings and earning capacity. The value or capitalisation of a company is equal to the capitalised value of its estimated earnings. For this purpose a new company has to prepare an estimated profit and loss account. For the first few years of its life, the sales are forecasted and the manager has to depend upon his experience for determining the probable costs.

In case of new companies, therefore, the cost theory provides a better basis for capitalisation than the earnings theory.

Over-Capitalisation : If a company raises more capital (by the issue of shares and debentures and through long-term loans) than is warranted by the figure of capitalisation of its earning power, the company will be said to be over-capitalised. In other words, a company is over-capitalised when its actual profits are not sufficient to pay interest and dividends at proper rates. It follows that an over-capitalised company is unable to pay a fair return on its capital investment.

Overcapitalisation results in the following ways :

(i) The enterprise may raise more money by issue of shares and debentures than it can profitably use. In other words, there may be large amounts of idle funds with the company. This may be done intentionally or unintentionally.

(2) If a company borrows a large sum of money and has to pay a rate of interest higher than its rate of earning, the result will be over-capitalisation.

(3) Over-capitalisation may often result when an excessive amount is paid for goodwill and for fixed assets acquired from the vendor company or from promoters or other people associated with the company, or when unduly high amounts are spent on establishment.

(4) Sometimes a company acquires assets like plant, machinery and buildings during a boom period. The price paid is naturally high. If the boom disappears and a slump sets in, the real value of such assets will decline greatly and a large part of the company's capital would be lost. Such a company is over-capitalised because its real earning capacity will suffer a setback due to a fall in the value of assets, whereas the capital will stand at its original figure.

(5) If a company does not make sufficient provision for depreciation and replacements and distributes higher rates of profit amongst the shareholders, the company will find after some time that, while the book value of assets is high, the real or market value is extremely low.

(6) High rates of taxation may leave little in the hands of the company to provide for replacements and dividend to shareholders. This may adversely affect its earning capacity and lead to over-capitalisation.

(7) when the promoters underestimate the capitalisation rate, the capitalisation may not support the expected rate of earnings and over-capitalisation may result.

Watered Capital : 'Water' is said to be present in the capital when a part of the capital is not represented by assets. It is considered to be as worthless as water. Sometimes the services of the promoters are valued at an unduly high price. Similarly the concern may pay too high a price for an asset acquired from a going concern. The capital becomes watered to the extent of the excess price paid for an asset.

Evils of Over-capitalisation : Over-capitalisation has evil consequences from the point of view of the company, the society and the shareholders.

From the Point of View of the Company

(a) Over-capitalisation will result in considerable reduction of the rate of dividend of the equity shares issued.

(b) with the disappearance of reduction of dividends, the market value of the shares falls, and the investors lose confidence in the company.

(c) Sometimes the compnay resorts to questionable practices including 'window dressing' in order to show a respectable figure of profits. Some people are downright dishonest and merely cook up an increase. Others avoid necessary expenditure so that the debit in the profit and loss account is reduced.

(d) Over-capitalised company has to go into liquidation, unless drastic steps are taken to re-organise the share capital.

From the Point of View of Society

(a) Over-capitalisation is an indication of reduced efficiency. An over-capitalised concern is compelled to raise the prices of its products. With diminished efficiency, it is usually not able to maintain the quality of its products.

(b). An over-capitalised company may try to raise its profits by effecting cuts in wages of workers. This may affect industrial relations.

(c) Since an over-capitalised concern is unable to compete with other concern, it may have to close down.

(d) Over-capitalisation results in misapplication of society's resources. The capital lying idle or being under-utilised by an over-capitalised concern can be better utilised by other concern which are in need of funds.

The shares of an over-capitalised conceren provide scope for gambling on the stock exchange. It is undesirable from the social point of view.

From the Shareholder's Point of View

(a) Over-capitalisation means depreciation of investment. The shares of an over-capitalised company sell below par in the market.

(b) The shareholders have also to suffer due to a low return on their investment which, too, is not always certain and regular.

(c) The shares of an over-capitalised company have relatively small value as security for loans which a shareholder may like to raise.

(d) The low-priced shares of an over-capitalised concern are subject to speculative gambling. This harms the interests of the real investors.

(e) When an over-capitalised concern tries to set its house in order through re-organisation, the shareholders are the worst sufferes. Re-organisation would usually take the form of reduction of capital for writing off past losses.

Remedies

The following remedial steps may be adopted to this end :

    (i) Redemption of bonds through outright re-organisation.

    (ii) Reduction of interest on bonds.

    (iii) Reduction of preferred stock.

    (iv) Reduction of par value on stock.

    (v) Reduction in the number of equity shares.

Under-Capitalisation : Under-capitalisation is just the reverse of over-capitalisation. Sometimes a company, on the face of it, may have an insufficient capital but it may have large secret reserves. Thus, in case of well-established companies, there is a very large appreciation in the value of assets specially of building, plant and goodwill. Such appreciation is generally not brought into the books. Nevertheless these assets do bring and, therefore, the profits in such a company would appear to be much larger than are warranted by the book figure of the capital. In such a case, the dividends will be high and the market quotations of the shares of such companies will be higher than the par value of the shares of other similar companies. A company is under-capitalised when its actual capitalisation (i.e., total long-term resources) is lower than its proper capitalisation as warranted by its earning capacity. Such a company will earn considerably more than the prevailing rate on its outstanding securities. Under-capitalisation, too, has its own disadvantages : (i) competition is encouraged and made acute by the higher earnings of such companies; (ii) the high dividend rates give an opportunity to workers to ask for increase in wages ; (iii) it may give the consumers a feeling that they are being exploited by the company ; (iv) it may tempt the management to manipulate share values ; (v) it may limit the marketability of shares due to which the shares may not enjoy so high a market value as is justified by the earnings ; and (vi) it may attract government control and higher taxation.

Remedies

    (i) Splitting-up of shares

    (ii) Increase in par value of shares

    (iii) Issue of bonus shares

Comparison : Having examined the various disadvantages of over-capitalisation and under-capitalisation, it is clear that there is little to choose between them. At the most, one may like to know which of the two is the lesser evil. As has been pointed out above, over-capitalisation can prove more dangerous to the company, the shareholders and the society than under-capitalisation. The only solution in over-capitalisation is a thorough reorganisation which would mean considerable loss for the shareholders and the creditors. Under-capitalisation characterised by high share values and high rates of dividend may be avoided by capitalisation of reserves. This would distribute the earnings over a large number of shares. Thus, under-capitalisation may be called the lesser evil, though both are bad. The goal of every company should be 'proper' or 'fair' capitalisation, i.e., capitalisation related to the normal earning capacity in an industry for firms of a certain size.

Estimation of Capital Requirements

A company should be properly capitalised and that the actual capital should be neither more nor less than the amount which is needed and which can be gainfully employed. It is, therefore, necessary for a new concern to estimate its requirements of funds properly. The financial requirements of a new company may be outlined under the following heads :

1. Cost of fixed assets including land and building, plant and machinery, furniture, etc. The amount invested in these items is called fixed capital.

2. Cost of current assets including cash, stock of goods, book debts, bills, etc.

3. Cost of promotion including the expenses on preliminary investigation, accounting, marketing and legal advice, etc.

4. Cost of setting up the organisation.

5. Cost of establishing the business, i.e., the operating losses which have generally to be sustained in the initial periods of a company.

6. Cost of financing including brokerage on securities, commission on underwriting, etc.

7. Cost of intangible assets like goodwill, patents, etc.

8. Margin money required for raising working capital loans.

Fixed Capital : The fixed capital of an industrial concern is invested in fixed assets like plant and machinery, land, building, furniture, patents, etc. These assets are not fixed in value ; in fact, their value may record an increase or decrease in course of time. They are fixed in the sense that without them, the business of the concern cannot be carried on. This means that the fixed capital is used for meeting the permanent or long-term needs of the concern. While making an assessment of fixed capital requirements, a list of the fixed assets needed by the concern will have to be prepared. Having compiled a list of the fixed assets which will be required, it is not difficult to estimate the amount of funds required for the purpose. The prices of land are generally known, or can be ascertained easily. A contractor can be relied upon to give a proper estimate of the cost of the building to be erected. Those who supply machinery and plant will certainly give quotations for the plant and equipment to be installed. Similarly, the amount to be paid for patents, trade marks, goodwill, etc., will not be difficult to ascertain.

The total of all these items will give the amount to be invested in fixed assets. The amount of fixed capital requirements of a concern depends on : (a) nature of the business, and (b) size of the business unit. For instance, a public utility concern (say, an electricity supply company, water supply undertaking or, for that matter, a railway company) would require heavy investment in fixed assets and equipment. On the other hand, a trading concern represents the other extreme. It requires comparatively much less equipment of fixed nature. Its fixed capital requirements would, therefore, be relatively much less. The fixed capital needs of a manufacturing concern would vary with the scale of production. Usually, the larger the scale, the heavier would be the investment in fixed assets.

Fixed capital may be needed not only for financing the acquisition of fixed assets, but also for the initial periods of its working when it is trying to establish itself, even for providing margin money for working capital loans and for improvements in, and expansion of its existing set-up. These requirements may be met with long-term and medium-term capital.

Working Capital : The working capital is required for the purchase of raw materials, and for meeting the day-to-day expenditure on salaries, wages, rents, advertising, etc. Modern industrial concerns produce in anticipation of demand. Payment has, therefore, to be made for the purchase of raw materials, the storage of finished and semi-finished goods, the work done by the staff and the worker. But, this sum cannot be got back immediately. Some time will pass before the goods are sold out and the amount spent on all these items is recovered. The working capital is needed for this purpose. It may be defined as the capital invested in the working or current assets like stock of raw materials, semi-finished and finished products, debtors, bills receivable, etc. The working capital is invested, recovered and re-invested repeatedly during the life-time of the concern. In other words, it keeps on revolving or circulating from cash to current assets and back. The working capital requirements can be met with short-term funds. At least a part of the working capital can be called 'regular' or 'fixed' working capital. This is needed to meet the requirements of a rise in the volume of production during the peak periods of the year.

The requirements of working capital will depend upon a number of factors which differ from industry to industry and even from company to company. For example, in a business like banking almost the whole of the capital required is for working capital requirements. But in case of a transport company or an electricity undertaking the requirements of working capital are small, while a huge sum has to be invested in fixed assets. The working capital differs from company to company because management might decide upon diferent degrees of mechanisation in plants of their respective companies. It should also be noted that funds required for working capital purposes will also differ from time to time. If, for example, prices of raw materials and wage rates rise, there will be an immediate increase in the requirements. If sales are slack, then also the working capital requirements will increase. If it is a seasonal industry, the reverse is also true during the slack season.

Factors of Working Capital : The following are the factors which determine a concern's requirements of working capital :

(i) The proportion of the cost of raw materials to total cost.

(ii) **Importance of Labour :** In industries where there is a great degree of mechanisation, the working capital requirements are correspondingly small.

(iii) **Length of Period of Manufacture :** The time which elapses between the commencement and the end of the manufacturing process has an important bearing upon the requirements of working capital.

(iv) Stocks of raw materials and other stores

(v) Rapidity of turnover.

(vi) Terms of credit.

(vii) Seasonal variations

(viii) **Requirements of Cash :** Cash may be needed for the payment of salaries, rents, taxes, etc., or for meeting the obligations of trade and other creditors, etc. The greater the requirements on these counts, the higher will be the working capital needs of the company.

CAPITAL STRUCTURE

Capital structure of a company (or financial structure) "refers to the make-up of its capitalisation". In a broader sense, capital structure includes all the long-term capital including loans, debentures, bonds, share issues, reserves, etc., and the components of the total capital. A company engaged in making a financial plan will be faced with problems regarding the proportion of funds to be raised by issue of its shares and the amount to be raised through borrowing. There is an important difference between these two methods. Funds raised from shareholders require the payment of dividends only out of profits earned by the company and the amount will be given back to the shareholders only if the company is wound up. In case of borrowings, however, interest has to be paid, no matter whether there is profit or loss, and the amount of loan must be repaid on the stipulated date. In case of capital raised from shareholder, too, there is one class of shares, namely, preference shares on which dividends have to be paid at the fixed rate before the equity shareholders get any share of profits. The proportion of that part of the funds on which a fixed rate of interest or dividend is to be paid to the total funds required shows the gearing. In other words, capital gearing means the decision about the ratio which different types of securities will bear to total capitalisation. A company is said to be high geared when it has agreed to pay a fixed rate of interest or dividend on a very large proportion of its funds. On the contrary, it may be described as being low geared, if it is not bound to pay a fixed return on a large proportion of its capitalisation. In other words, a company which raises a major proportion of its long-term funds by the issue of bonds, debentures and preference shares is high geared, while a company, which has raised funds largely by the issue of equity shares is low geared.

Considerations in Proper Capital Gearing : The following factors generally govern the capital gearing of a company :

1. **Trading on Equity :** A company earns profits at a certain rate on capital employed by it whether the capital is borrowed or raised from shareholders. On the borrowed capital, only a fixed rate of interest or dividend is to be paid. If this fixed rate is lower than the general rate of the company's earnings, the other sharesholders, known as equity shareholders or ordinary shareholders, will have an advantage in the form of additional profit being distributable to them in the shape of dividend. This is referred to as 'trading on equity'.

   Limitations :

   (a) If the rate of earnings is less than the rate of interest, even reliance upon borrowing at fixed rates of interest will depress the rate of dividend below the rate of earning.

   (b) Fixed interest and dividends impose a recurring burden on the company. Payment of a fixed rate of interest must be made even if there are no profits. Since a company may not always earn profit, the payment of interest would be a big burden in those years in which it incurs losses or makes little profits. If there is a prolonged slump or depression, the company may find it very difficult to make these fixed payments.

   (c) The fact that every increase in borrowings raises the rate of interest places yet another limitation on the principle of trading on equity. As a company borrows more, the risk for the subsequent lenders gets enhanced. As a result, borrowings become costlier and their profitability in the interests of equity shareholders may decline.

2. **Retaining Control of the Company :** Quite often the promoters want to raise capital from the general public while retaining effective control of the affairs of the company. For this purpose, they raise a large part of funds by the issue of debentures and preference shares. The debentureholders and the preference shareholders are usually not given the voting rights enjoyed by the equity shareholders. Thus the company is able to collect its requirements of funds from the public, though the control rests with the promoters. The profits of the company may also be utilised in part for meeting the financial requirements without the surrender of control to outsiders.

3. **Nature of Enterprise :** The financial plan is the nature of enterprise, i.e., whether it is the manufacturing, merchandising, financing, extraction or public utility type. All these enterprises differ in regard to the amount of investment, subject to risks of failures and trade cycles and freedom from competition. These differences enable one type of enterprise to issue securities which may be not be available for the other enterprise to issue. Public utilities are well suited to financing through fixed interest securities (like bonds) because of freedom from competition and stability of income. Manufacturing enterprises do not always

enjoy these advantages and, therefore, they have to rely, to a greater extent, on equity share capital.

4. **Legal Requirements :** One must comply with the legal provisions regarding the issue of different securities. Not all business may be subject to these legal provisions but for some these do apply. In India, banking companies are not allowed by the Banking Companies Act to issue any type of securities except the equity shares.

5. **The Purpose of Financing :** An important consideration is the purpose of which the funds are raised. The funds may be required either for betterment expenditure or for some productive purposes. The betterment expenditure does not, directly add to the earning capacity of the business. Such expenditure may be incurred out of funds raised by share issue or still better out of retained earnings. Borrowing should be used only for purposes of financing definite productive projects. Usually, borrowed funds are of little help in avoiding losses. If such funds are used only for buying new plant and machinery, so that more goods can be produced, or the productive efficiency is otherwise increased the interest can generally be paid out of the profits thus earned. In such a case, borrowed funds will not become a burden.

6. **Period of Finance :** Normally, funds which are required for a comparatively short period are raised through borrowings, because then the loan can be repaid as soon as the company comes into possession of its own funds. To raise funds through issue of preference shares for, say, 5 or 10 years, will present certain difficulties because legal sanction must be obtained for repayment. There is a class of shares which can be redeemed even during the life-time of the company, viz., redeemable preference shares, but in such a case too, there are certain legal restrictions.

7. **Market Sentiment :** The above-noted considerations govern 'capital gearing' from the point of view of the company. It is, however, the investors who have to decide whether they will buy shares or debentures, and their decisions will often depend upon the general mood or sentiment in the investment markets. There are periods when people want to play for absolute safety. At such a time, funds can be raised only through issue of debentures or bonds, even if the company wants it otherwise. There are other periods when the investors do not care about safety and want to earn high speculative incomes. At such times, equity shares will be in great demand.

8. **Requirement of Investors :** Different types of securities must also be issued to meet the requirements of the different classes of investors. Investors who want the security of the principal and stability of income usually go in for debentures and preference shares. Equity shares appeal most to those who can, and would like to, take risks for higher incomes. The nominal value of the shares should also be adjusted so as to secure subscription from the middle-class sections of the society.

TIME FOR FLOATATION

An important factor in financial planning is the selection of a suitable time for the floatation of a company. If enough care is not exercised in this matter, the company may find itself in financial straits long before it can consolidate its position. It will do well to take advantage of the changes in the business activity which occur more or less regularly at intervals of three to five years. These changes are in the nature of 'ups' and 'downs' in the economy and are referred to as 'trade cycles'. A trade cycle consists of alternating periods of prosperity and depression. In fact, it usually has four marked phases, viz. :

(i) **Boom :** It is the period of peak prosperity when the factories are fully employed and economy shows signs of inflation.

(ii) **Recession :** Production runs ahead of demand during a boom period. This leads to a downward trend in the business activity. Recession, as it is called, is the period of falling prices, reduced incomes and lower levels of employment. Due to a fall in the volume of business activity, loans are in great demand. The interest rates, therefore, rise for some time.

(iii) **Depression :** The downward trend started by a recession is completed by the depression. This is the direct opposite of a boom. During a period of depression, economic activity is at its lowest. The levels of prices, incomes, and employment are all low. It is a period of crisis for business.

(iv) **Recovery :** The depression has the germs of improvement which come to life after the worst has happened to business. The low prices of securities begin to attract investors. There is a revival of business activity and an upward trend is set in motion. The levels of prices, incomes and employment show an improvement and the stage is gradually set for another boom period.

A company has the best opportunity for the sale of securities when the period of improvement is on, and the economy is experiencing a boom. The best time to raise funds is when business is booming and people are optimistic. The funds so raised can be used for the purchase of equipment and other fixed assets during the recession and depression. This would mean considerable economy, because, during such periods, prices are low. Production may be started towards the end of depression so that the products are put in the market with the beginning of the 'recovery'. In this way, products can be sold at a profit. Thus, the most appropriate time for the floatation of company and raising funds is a boom. An existing concern interested in a fresh issue of securities should also follow this principle.

20

SOURCES OF FINANCE

Every company requires for investment in the form of fixed capital and working capital. Funds may be required for long-term, for medium-term and for short-term period. It is the period of fiannce which determines the source or sources of finance to be tapped and the method of financing to be use. The term 'source' implies the agencies from which funds are procured and the method of raising finance is linked with the period for which funds are required and it deals with the mode of raising finance.

Sources : According to the length of the period for which funds are required, sources of raising finance may be classified as follows :

(i) **Long-term Finance :** It is required for investment in fixed assets like land, building, plant and machinery, and for financing extension programmes. Long-term funds are raised for a minimum period for 10 years. The following are the sources of long-term financing : (a) shareholders ; (b) debentureholders ; (c) financial institutions ; and (d) retained earnings.

(ii) **Medium-term Finance :** It is required for investment in working capital and for repayment of assets. It is raised for a period ranging from more than one year and less than ten years. The following are the sources of medium-term financing: (a) debentureholders; (b) financial institutions ; (c) public deposits ; (d) commercial banks ; and (e) Industrial finance institutions.

(iii) **Short-term Finance :** It is required for meeting the short-term needs of working capital. Its period is less than 12 months and it can be raised from the following sources : (a) public deposits ; (b) trade credits ; (c) commercial banks etc.

Methods : It has already been observed that the management of company can use different methods of raising finance for different periods and purposes.

On the basis of the term for which the funds are required, the methods of financing can be classified into the following categories :

(i) For long-term requirements :
- (a) Issue of shares ;
- (b) Issue of debentures ;
- (c) Assistance from special Industrial Finance Institutions ; and
- (d) Ploughing back or reinvesting of retained earnings.

(ii) For medium-term requirements :
- (a) Issue of preference shares ;
- (b) Issue of debentures ;
- (c) Assistance from Special Industrial Finance Institutions ;
- (d) Receiving public deposits ; and
- (e) Borrowing from commercial banks.

(iii) For short-term requirements :
- (a) Borrowing from commercial banks ;
- (b) Trade credit ;
- (c) Instalment credit ;
- (d) Accounts receivable financing ;
- (e) Customer advance ;
- (f) Leasing ; and
- (g) Commercial papers.

ISSUE OF SHARES

Issue of ownership securities of shares is the most important method of raising long-term finance for permanent investment in the companies. Funds raised from issue of shares provide a financial floor to the capital structure of a company. A share may be defined as a unit of measure of a shareholder's interest in the company. The share capital of a company is divided into a large number of equal parts and each part is individually known as a share. According to Section 86 of the Companies Act, 1956, a public company limited by shares can issue two types of ownership securities, viz., equity shares and preference shares. An independent private company can issue deferred shares as well.

Preference Shares

Preference shares are those which carry preferential rights as to the payment of dividend at a fixed rate either free of or subject to income tax, and as to the repayment of capital. Thus, preference shareholders enjoy two preferential rights over the other category of shares. Firstly, they are entitled to receive a fixed rate of dividend out of the net profits of the company prior to declaration of dividend on equity shares. Secondly, the assets remaining after the payment of debts of the company under liquidation are first appropriated for returning the capital contributed by the preference shareholders.

Preference shares may be classified into following categories :

(i) **Cumulative and Non-cumulative Preference Shares :** The holders of cumulative preference shares are entitled to arrears of dividend on their shares to be paid out of the profits of subsequent years, if in any year the dividend on them cannot be paid. Thus, they are sure to receive dividend on the preference shares held by them for all the years out of the earnings of the company. If in a particular year they are not paid the dividend, they will be paid such arrear in the next year before any dividend can be distributed among equity shareholders. But the dividend on non-cumulative shares does not accumulate if dividend is not paid in any year.

(ii) **Participating and Non-participating Preference Shares :** The holders of participating preference shares are entitled to a share in the surplus profits if they remain after paying dividend to preference shares and equity shares. Thus, participating shareholders obtain return on their investment in two forms : (i) fixed dividend ; and (ii) share in surplus profits. The preference shares which do not carry the right to share in the surplus profits are known as non-participating preference shares.

(iii) **Redeemable and Irredeemable Preference Shares :** Redeemable preference shares are those which in accordance with the terms of their issue, will be repaid on or after a certain date. The preference shares which cannot be redeemed during the life time of the company are known as irredeemable preference shares.

(iv) **Convertible and Non-convertible Preference Shares :** If the preference shareholders are given a right to convert their shares into equity shares within a fixed period of time, such shares will be known as convertible preference shares. The preference shares which cannot be converted into equity shares are known as non-convertible preference shares. A Company can also issue partially convertible preference shares. Under this scheme, only a part of preference shares will be converted into equity shares.

Evaluation

The issue of preference shares has the following benefits :

(i) The preference shares attract funds from those investors who prefer safety of their investments and a fixed rate of return on their investment.

(ii) The management can retain control over the company by issuing preference shares to outsiders because the preference share-holders have only restricted voting rights.

(iii) Preference shareholders are entitled to a fixed rate of dividend which enables the equity shareholders to get higher dividend.

(iv) Preference shares do not impose heavy burden on the company because they carry a fixed rate of dividend.

(v) Redeemable preference shares may be issued to bring flexibility in the financial structure of the company as they can be redeemed whenever it is necessary.

(vi) A company can raise finance for a long-term without creating any charge over its assets.

There are certain limitations of raising funds by issuing preference shares. The investors may not like these shares because preference shareholders have restricted voting rights only. The issue of preference shares is costlier than the issue of debentures because these shares have to be given a rate of dividend which is higher than the prevailing rate of interest on debentures. The existence of preference shares in the capital structure of a company may also affect credit-worthiness of the company.

During 1977-78, the public limited companies offered preference shares worth Rs. 278 lakhs for public subscription. But public subscribed for preference shares worth Rs. 7 lakhs only. The underwriters subscribed for the remaining amount Rs. 175 lakhs as investors and Rs. 96 lakhs as underwriting obligations. This clearly reveals that the preference shares are not popular with the general public. On the other hand, the general public subscribed for equity shares worth Rs. 3,071 lakhs out of the public offer of equity shares worth Rs. 5,436 lakhs. This also shows that companies prefer equity capital as compared to preference share capital.

EQUITY SHARES

Equity Shares are also called 'ordinary shares'. Equity shares provide capital on permanent basis to the company. Equity shareholders are the real owners of the company and they bear the risk of business. They get dividend only after the dividend on preference share is paid out of the profits of the company. At the time of winding up, equity capital can be paid back only after every claim including that of preference shareholders has been settled. Since equity shareholders bear higher risk, they also stand a chance of getting higher dividend if the company's earnings are higher.

Equity shareholders control the affairs of the company as they have the voting right in the general body meetings of the company. They elect the board of directors of the company and frame the policies of the company in the general meetings.

Evaluation

Equity shares are regarded as the cornerstone of financial structure of a company as they offer the following advantages :

(i) Equity share capital constitutes the permanent resources of the company. The company is not bothered by the problem of refunding the capital raised by issuing equity shares.

(ii) Equity shares do not impose any obligation on the company to pay fixed dividend to their holders.

(iii) A company with sufficient paid-up equity capital is viewed with considerable favour by the lenders.

(iv) Equity shares do not create any charge over the assets of the company. The assets may be utilised as security for further financing.

Equity share capital has certain drawbacks also. If the equity shares are issued excessively, it may result in over-capitalisation which may be difficult to cure. In such a case, the company will also lose the benefit of trading on equity. Since control of the company rests with the equity shareholders, the affairs of the company may be manipulated by a powerful group of equity shareholders.

No-par Shares : In the U.S.A. and Canada, many companies issue shares which have no-par or face value. The total owned capital of the company is divided into a certain number of shares. The share certificate merely states the number of shares held by a particular holder and does not mention the face value of the shares. The dividends on such shares are paid at the rate of a given amount per share instead of as a certain percentage of the par value of each share. Such shares cannot be issued in India, because the law requires every share to have fixed nominal value. The advantages usually claimed for such shares are :

(i) The balance sheet presents a realistic picture with such shares because the capital is equal to the net worth (assets minus liabilities), and is not an imaginary amount as with shares of nominal value.

(ii) Since the value of such shares is related to the earnings, the shareholders always know the real value of their holdings.

(iii) The shareholders are not liable to pay further calls because the total value of a no-par share is collected in the beginning.

(iv) The shares need not be marketed at a discount because there is no minimum par value of these shares. This avoids a lot of legal formality.

(v) Since the value of the shares is automatically adjusted with the earning capacity, no reduction of capital is necessary.

On the contrary, the no-par value shares suffer from the following drawbacks :

(i) The no-par value shares may easily be used to deceive ignorant investors. In case of such shares there is no standard by which fluctuations in share values can be ascertained.

(ii) Such shares make the balance sheet unduly complex and difficult to understand. This makes the task of investors, creditors and tax authorities difficult.

(iii) Unscrupulous management gets an opportunity to manipulate the sale proceeds of shares and pay dividend out of capital.

(iv) The creditors lost the additional security of uncalled capital which they get in case of party paid shares with par value.

(v) Since the capital account remains fluctuating from time to time, the promoters may snatch unduly high amounts of remuneration for themselves.

ISSUE OF DEBENTURES

Debentures are creditorship securities which provide funds to the company on loan basis rather than on capital basis. A debenture may be defined as an acknowledgement of a debt by a company. The debentureholders are entitled to periodical payment of interest at a fixed rate and are also entitled to redemption of their debentures as per terms of debenture issue. The debentureholders are the creditors of the company. Their rights depend upon the type of debentures issued by the company. A company may issue the following types of debentures :

(i) **Secured and Unsecured Debentures :** Secured debentures represent the fixed or floating charge on the assets of the company.

When the particular assets are charged by way of security, it is known as fixed charge. Such debentures are also known, as 'mortgage debentures'. When the charge is created on assets which are of general nature like stock, it is called a floating charge. Under floating charge, the company is free to deal with the property forming the subject-matter of the charge until the said charge becomes fixed by default of company in paying the interest or some other event stipulated in the deed of charge. Unsecured debentures, also known as simple or naked debentures, do not carry any charge or security on the assets of the company.

(ii) **Registered and Bearer Debentures :** In case of registered debentures, the name of the debenture holder is entered in the debenture certificates and books of the company. They can be transferred by filling in the transfer deed. But bearer debentures can be transferred by filling in the transfer deed. But bearer debentures can be transferred by mere delivery without any notice to the company. Debenture coupons are annexed with such debenture certificates. The bearers of the debentures can fill in the coupons and claim interest after sending them to the company. But in case of registered debentures, the company pays interest to the registered debenture holders.

(iii) **Redeemable and Irredeemable Debentures :** In case of redeemable debenture, the companies reserve the right of paying off the principal on or before particular date. In case of irredeemable or perpetual debentures, the company does not fix any date by which they should be redeemed and the holders of such debentures cannot demand payment from the company so long as it is a going concern.

(iv) **Convertible and Non-convertible Debentures :** The convertible debentures can be converted into equity shares of the company after the expiry of a specified period. But non-convertible debentures cannot be converted into equity shares. The practice of issuing partially convertible debentures has also gained popularity. Under this scheme, only a part of the debenture amount is convertible into equity shares on a specified date.

Evaluation

Debentures offer the following advantages :

(i) Debentures are liked by the investors who give weightage to safety of principal and a continuous fixed rate of income on the principal.

(ii) Debenture-holders do not possess voting right. They do not weaken the control of existing shareholders.

(iii) Debentures offer an opportunity to the company to trade on equity and thereby increase the return of equity shareholders.

(iv) Debentures provide financial flexibility as they can be redeemed when the company has surplus funds.

(v) Interest paid on debentures is deductible from the profits of the company for income tax purpose. Thus, the company enjoys tax benefit by issuing debentures.

Debentures are also not free from drawbacks. Debentures require a company to bear a fixed burden of interest every year irrespective of profits earned. If a company does not have stable earnings, this liability will create problems. Debenture-holders prefer safety of their investments and so they like secured debentures. A company which is not willing to offer its assets as security may not be able to raise finance by issuing debentures. If the capital structure of a company is loaded heavily with debentures, banks and other institutions do not show a favourable attitued towards the company.

Popularity of Debentures

Despite their limitations, the issue of debentures as a method of raising long-term finance is gaining popularity these days. The response of the investors, both individual and institutional, has been encouraging because of following factors :

(i) Debentures with more attractive terms particularly having a convertible clause have been issued. The conversible of debentures into equity shares encourages the institutional investors to invest in debentures. Leading companies in the country like TELCO and Reliance Textiles have issued convertible debentures succesfully.

(ii) Statutory restrictions on the institutional investors like Life Insurance Corporation and Industrial Finance Corporation have been relaxed. They can have more debentures in their investment portfolio. Debentures are issued by the flourishing companies also to have the benefit of trading on equity. This has changed the attitude of banks and others towards the companies having issued the debentures. Formerly, the companies having issued debentures were considered to be less creditworthy concerns.

(iii) Companies prefer to issue debentures because of low cost of financing through debentures. Less formalities have to be observed while issuing debentures. Moreover, the interest paid on debentures is allowed as deductible expenditure against the profits of the company.

(iv) Debentures bring about flexibility in the capital structure as they can be redeemed after a stipulated period.

(v) Underwriting of debenture issues by the leading brokers and financial institution has also increased their popularity.

RETAINED EARNINGS

The use of retained earnings as a method of itself financing is commonly used by the established companies. It is also known as 'ploughing back of profits'. Under this method, the undistributed or retained profits of the company are used to finance the requirements of the company. The main feature of this method is that it is an internal source of finance. Every good company does not distribute its entire earnings in the form of dividend but rather retains a part of it every year. Such a policy helps the company to build up reserves which can be used for financing expansion programmes.

The practice of ploughing back of profits is influenced by many factors. Firstly, it depends upon the net profits of the company. If a company has earned huge profits in a particular year, its capacity to retain profits will be higher. Secondly, dividend policy of the company determines the extent to which profits can be retained for ploughing back. For instance, if a company follows a policy of declaring a consistent rate of dividend every year, it will not be able to retain much if in a particular year it earns less profits. Lastly, the age of the company affects the policy of ploughing back of profits. New companies generally do not retain much profits because of their desire to satisfy their shareholders. But an older company can declare less profits for distribution to shareholders and retain the major portion of its profit for reinvestment in the business.

Evaluation

The advantages of ploughing back of profits are as follows :

(i) It is a very economical method of financial because no return is to be paid on retained earnings and no fixed obligations are created.

(ii) It makes the company financially strong, increases credit-worthiness and enables it to float new securities in the market and borrow from the public and financial institutions without any difficulty.

(iii) The reserves, created by ploughing back of profits, can also be used for redeeming debts and for replacing obsolete assets.

(iv) Retained earnings can be a good source of stabilising the rate of dividend on equity shares.

(v) Reinvestment of earnings increases capital formation which is necessary for the economic development of the country.

(vi) Retained earnings enable the company to absorb the shocks due to depression and uncertainty of the capital market.

Excessive ploughing back of profits may be associated with certain drawbacks and limitations which are as follows :

(i) The management of a company may misuse the retained earnings by investing them in unprofitable areas or by spending them unnecessarily.

(ii) The management may also utilise the retained earnings for issuing bonus shares to the equity shareholders which may lead to over-capitalisation.

(iii) The practice of retained earnings may be used to manipulate the price of shares in the stock exchange with a view to purchase the shares. This will lead to deceiving of genuine investors and concentration of economic wealth in a few hands.

(iv) The existing shareholders may be dissatisfied with the company because low dividend is available to them.

PUBLIC DEPOSITS

Besides the issue of securities, the companies have been counting public deposits for a long time in order to meet their medium term and long-term requirements. The practice of receiving public deposits was very popular mainly with the cotton textile mills of Bombay, Ahmedabad and Sholapur and tea gardens of Assam and Bengal during the first quarter of the 20th century. The reason for this was the lack of banking facilities in the country. There was no financial institution to provide term loans to the industrial enterprises. People preferred to deposit their savings with the reputed industrialists because of their lack of faith in the banks and the low rate of interest offered by the banks.

In the recent years the method of raising finance through public deposits has again become popular for varying periods at rates of interest which are higher than those offered by the commercial banks. The rate of interest on deposits varies from 11 percent to 15 percent per annum depending upon the period of deposit and reputation of the company. Companies generally receive public deposits for different periods ranging from 1 year to 3 years and allow for renewal of deposits. They also take the help of stock brokers to receive public deposits. Any person who is interested to deposit the money with a company can fill up a specified form and deposit the money with the company. The company in return issues a deposit receipt which is an acknowledgement of debt by the company. The terms and conditions of the deposit are mentioned on the back side of the deposit receipt.

A company has to follow the directions issued by the Reserve Bank of India and the provisions of the Companies Act in order to accept deposits from the public. A company can receive secured and unsecured deposits up to the extent of 10 and 25 percent respectively of the paid up share capital plus free reserves. The Central Government may prescribe the conditions, limitations and the manner of accepting deposits by the company from the public. The Central Government has laid down that no company shall invite a deposit unless an advertisement, including a statement showing the financial position of the company, has been issued in the prescribed form. Companies accepting public deposits must regularly file returns giving detailed information regarding such deposits. Under the rules framed by the Government, the deposits can not be invited initially for a period of more than 3 years. However, they can be renewed later on.

Evaluation

Companies raise finance for medium-term requirements through deposits because of the following advantages :

(i) It is beneficial to the company since it receives funds at lower rates of interest as compared to the rates charged by banks and special financial institutions.

(ii) Cost of administering public deposits is lower as compared to issue of shares and debentures. The company has to fulfil less formalities and follow a simple procedure. It receives money and issues a deposit receipt to every depositor.

(iii) Public deposits helps in trading on equity if the company is earning more than the rate of interest paid on public deposits. A company can pay a higher dividend to its shareholders and thus raise its reputation.

(iv) The depositors do not have any right to interfere with the internal management of the company. Thus, there is no dilution of control of shareholders.

(v) The public deposits are usually not backed by any security or assets of the company. The company can use its assets as security for raising loans from other sources like commercial banks and financial institutions. Public deposits introduce flexibility in the financial planning. Public deposits can be re-paid when they are not required.

The method of raising funds through public deposits has the following demerits :

(i) This method is not dependable because it is difficult to predict whether public deposits would be forthcoming to the desired extent. Such deposits are termed as 'fair weather friends'. The depositors may not respond when the conditions in the economy are uncertain. They may think it better to deposit their savings with the commercial banks. They may think it better to deposit their savings with the commercial banks. They may withdraw their money when they visualise, even on false grounds, the shaking position of the company. This may put the survival of the company into danger.

(ii) Depositors do not get any security for their deposits. Money deposited by them may be used by the management in any way it likes.

(iii) Public deposits are generally available for a short period though they can be renewed, but it is not a wise thing to depend on them for long-term financing.

(iv) New companies and companies with uncertain earnings cannot raise finance through public deposits.

(v) Receiving public deposits create unhealthy trends in the capital market. There are numerous rates of interest offered by different companies. This is detrimental to the development of the capital market.

Popularity of Public Deposits

Companies resort to public deposits as a method of short-term and medium-term financing because it is cheaper to raise funds through public deposits than from the commercial banks. Public also prefer to deposit their saving with the sound companies as they get higher rate of interest (varying from 11% to 15%) as compared to the bank deposits (varying from 5% to 10%). It is estimated that the amount of public deposits with the companies has exceeded Rs. 6000 crores (uptodate data is not available with the Reserve Bank). Deposits held by Joint Stock Companies on March 31,1982 were Rs. 5,491.80 crores as compared to Rs. 4,188 crores a year earlier.

The Government companies have also started receive deposits from the public in the recent years. BHEL, ITI and SAIL are the examples in this regard. Some investors prefer Government companies to private companies even though the Government companies offer a slightly lower rate of interest as compared to the companies in the private sector.

ASSISTANCE FROM THE INDUSTRIAL FINANCE INSTITUTIONS

A notable feature of the present-day capital market is the existence of special finance corporations set up by the Government with the object of stimulating industrial development in the country by cheapening and widening the channels of industrial finance. These include the Industrial Development Bank of India, the Industrial Finance Corporation of India, Industrial Credit and Investment Corporation. Unit Trust of India, Life Insurance Corporation of India and the State Finance Corporation of India. Here, it will be useful to note that assistance from these institutions has become an important method of financing the requirements of new companies as well the going concerns. The assistance of these institutions may take the form of direct subscription to company securities, underwriting of new security issues, grant of loans, guaranteeing of loans and debentures, and guaranteeing of deferred payment against imports of capital goods, etc. Some of them, particularly the ICICI, provide technical know-how and all of them make available to the eligible companies expert advice on the planning and execution of projects. In fact, a company receiving assistance from these institutions receives a boost in the market because it is widely known that these will assist only solid companies and the priority projects. Not merely this, these institutions ensure that the assistance granted is effectively utilised for the declared purpose by the recipient companies. Assistant from the Industrial Development Bank of India can be secured either directly (if the project is very expensive and is beyond the reach of the other institutions) or through banks or other institutions under the refinancing scheme or the participation scheme.

The procurement of assistance from the special industrial finance institutions offers the following advantages :

(i) Availability of finance for modernisation, expansion, etc. at reasonable interest rates making it possible for the company to develop a sound and balanced capital structure without depressing dividends on equity shares.

(ii) Facility of underwriting and equity participation for new companies.

(iii) Deferred payment facilities for import of capital equipments.

(iv) Facility of repayment of loan in easy instalments.

(v) Availability of expert advice in planning and executing projects and financial plans.

(vi) Reasonable security requirement for loan assistance.

(vii) Availability of finance during periods of depression when the other methods of financing fail.

In short, assistance from these institutions is suitable (a) for the floatation of new companies, (b) for financing schemes of expansion and modernisation, which generate additional income and make it possible for the borrowing company to repay in instalments, and (c) for meeting financial requirements during recessions and depressions. These institutions are important sources of long-term and medium-term finance now and many companies get even their finance from these.

BORROWING FROM BANKS

The Commercial Banks provide for financial assistance to industries for short term, medium term purposes, recently also for long-term loans.

Most of the joint-stock banks in India are modelled on the lines of the British banks which are purely commercial banks. Their funds are mainly the accumulated deposits a large number of individual members of the public, and are withdrawable at short notice or after the agreed period. If all depositors wanted their money at the same time, there would not be sufficient cash to pay them all because these funds are used in lending activity. For this reason, a bank is generally cautious in granting loans to its clients. These loans are made on the full backing of tangible and readily marketable securities. These are meant for financing particular pieces of business and are avowedly for short periods.

Provision of Short-term Funds : The commercial banks have played important part as suppliers of short-term or working capital requirements. The short-term requirements of companies are met by the commercial banks in the following ways :

   (i) by granting advances, loans, cash credits, etc.,

  (ii) by discounting bills and other commercial papers, and

 (iii) factoring.

The most popular of these has been the assistance through cash credits. For obtaining a cash credit, the company has generally to pledge its stock of finished or semi-finished products, or even or raw materials. The borrowing company can borrow up to an agreed limit. Interest has to be paid on the amount actually withdrawn and also the commitment charges for not utilising the sanctioned limits fully. In some cases where the banks are favourably inclined and are assured of the borrower's financial soundness, the goods pledged may remain in the physical possession of the borrower though the banks have legal line on them. This is called 'hypothecation of goods'.

Term Loans : The short-term assistance provided by a bank can be converted into medium-term finance through renewal and extension from time to time. In other words, a cash credit or an overdraft may be "turned over" or rolled over and converted into a medium-term loan. But these are called for meeting short-term or working capital requirements. The assistance is generally renewed if the enterprise is a growing one with improved profitability.

The other method of securing medium-term assistance from a bank is through a 'term loan' for a duration of, say, 3 to 7 years. Banks were hesitant in extending such loans for a long time, but with the extension of re-financing facilities since 1958, banks found it possible to engage in term lending to industrial enterprises. Under the refinancing scheme, the bank can grant loans for periods ranging between 3 and 7 years and get them re-financed at a relatively lower interest rate. This avoids pressure on the short-term deposits of the banks. The refinancing facility is now extended by the Industrial Development Bank of India. The generally accepted banking criteria for the grant of term loans may be listed as under :

  (i) **Type and Size of Business :** Businesses engaged in relatively stable line or showing growth characteristics and large scale or medium-size firms are usually preferred for term assistance.

 (ii) **Management :** The record of performance of management is looked into for determining the suitability of a firm for such assistance.

(iii) **General Record of the Borrower :** The borrower's markets, the competition faced by him, and the general outlook of the industry are carefully analysed and considered.

(iv) **Operating Efficiency :** The financial accounts of the borrowing concern are analysed to determine their efficiency of operations. Profit-expenses relationships are also considered for this purpose.

 (v) **Financial Condition :** The balance sheet of the company is scrutinised to determine the financial soundness of the company. A proforma balance sheet may also be prepared to assess the position after the loan is given.

(vi) **Ability to Repay :** The earnings record of the concern is looked into to determine whether it will generate enough cash to be able to meet the repayment requirements according to schedule of repayment.

With the encouragement provided by the re-financing facility, banks are gradually taking to term-lending though it has yet to become a normal routine function of commercial banks in India. However, some banks have also started participating with the financial institutions in term loan assistance. The availability of cheaper finance from the Reserve Bank of India for loans in the priority industries has also encouraged such lendings by banks.

Financing of Long-term Requirements : The banks have done little to finance the long-term capital requirements of the industry. In fact, after World War I, and even before, when the Swadesh Movement started, attempts were made to introduce industrial banking on the lines of the German example so that long-term finance could be provided for industries by the banks. But the experiment was a failure. The Tata Industrial Bank has to merge with the Central Bank, and other banks have to close down. Ever since then, the banks have confined themselves to purely commercial banking functions. The idea of mixed banking, i.e., combining long-term financing of industry with commercial banking, seems to have been given up for good. At present, a small percentage of banks investments is put into the purchase of shares and debentures of industrial companies.

Critical Evaluation : Bank accommodation by way of term loans offer the following advantages to the borrowing companies :

   (i) **Timely Assistance :** This applies to short-term as well as medium term accommodation. A company can usually rely upon the bank for amounts to the credit limit sanctioned for it.

   (ii) **Flexibility :** The accommodation can generally be got extended. Also, if the amount or a part of it is no longer needed, interest on it can be saved by repaying it.

   (iii) **Non-interference with Management :** Generally banks do not interfere with the management of the borrowing companies. A company is able to get finance without strings attached to it.

   (iv) **Secrecy :** This is by far the greatest advantage of bank finance. The information supplied to the bank is treated in utmost confindence and is not to be made public in any circumstances.

   (v) **Economy :** Bank assistance entails the payments of only interest and does not involve the kind of costs which are to be incurred in the issue of securities.

As against the above-noted advantages, bank accommodation and loans suffer from the following drawbacks :

   (i) **Burden of Mortgage / Hypothecation :** This applies particularly to the stock of finished or semi-finished goods that may have to do kept in bank-sealed godowns in case of pledge limits, otherwise it is hypothecated to the bank.

   (ii) **Short Duration of Assistance :** The bank accommodation was generally available for periods less than a year and extension or renewal was uncertain. There is some liberalisation of this policy in the wake of nationalisation of major banks.

   (iii) **Cumbersome Terms :** Generally, the banks grant assistance only to the extent of 75% of the industrial assets. The stock has usually to be taken to bank's godowns in case of pledge limits.

In conclusion, it may be said that bank accommodation is available, by and large, for short-term and marginally for medium-term requirements, but not for long-term financing except in case of participation with the financial institutions.

SOURCES OF SHORT-TERM FINANCE

Short-term financing deals with raising money required for a short period, i.e., less than one year. It is raised to meet the short-term working capital requirements of the business. Various sources of short-term financing include trade credit, instalment credit, accounts receivable financing, customer advance, and bank credit. It is important to point out that requirements of regular or permanent working capital for the business are financed through sources of medium-term and long-term finance. The main feature of short-term financing is that it is raised and paid back within a short period of time.

1. Trade Credit

Just as a firm grants credit to its customers, so it often gets credit from its suppliers. It is known as trade or mercantile credit. Trade credit may be defined as the credit extended by the sellers to buyers at all levels of production and distribution processes down to the retailer. It does include consumer credit on instalment. It arises due to difficult transfer of goods and is unsecured. Usually, business enterprises buy supplies on a 30 to 90 days account basis. This means that the supplies are delivered but not paid for until the period of credit. No security is required for getting trade credit from the supplier. The supplier makes supplies on credit to those customers who have sufficient financial reputation and goodwill.

Trade credit does not make available the funds in cash, but it facilitates the purchase of supplies without immediate payment. It is a very simple method of raising finance for short period. No interest is payable on trade credits. The actual cost is the loss of cash discounts. Moreover, no charge is created against the assets of the buyer of goods. The suppliers readily agree to grant trade credits to the reputed customers. The period of trade credit depends upon the nature of product, location of the customer, customs of trade, degree of competition in the market, financial resources of the supplier and the eagerness of suppplier to sell his stocks.

2. Instalments Credit

Business firms may get credit from equipment suppliers. The supplier may allow the purchase of equipment with payments extended over a period of 12 months or more. Some portion of the cost price of the asset is paid at the time of delivery and the balance is paid in a number of instalments. The supplier charges interest on the instalment credit which is included in the amount of instalment. Sometimes, instalment credit is granted by financial companies or commercial banks which have special arrangements with the suppliers. Equipment may also be supplied on hire purchase basis. Under this system the ownership of the equipment remains with the supplier until all the instalments have been paid by the buyer.

3. Accounts Receivable Financing

Under this arrangement, the accounts receivable of a business concern are purchased by a financing company or money is advanced on security of accounts receivable. The finance company usually make advances up to 60 per cent of the value of the accounts receivable pledged. The debtors of the business concerns make payment to it which in turn forwards to the finance company. If there is any bad debt, it is to be borne by the business concern itself.

4. Customer Advance

Many times, the manufactures of goods insist on advance by the customers, particularly in cases of special orders or big order. The customer advance represents a part of the price of the products that have been ordered by the customer and which will be delivered at a later date. Customers are prepared to make part payment in advance when they are placing big orders and insist that the goods are supplied in time, and when goods are not easily available in the market.

5. Bank Credit

Commercial banks play an important role in financing the short-term requirements of business concerns. They provide finance by way of the following methods :

(a) **Loans :** When a bank makes an advance in lump sum, the whole of which is withdrawn in cash immediately by the borrower who undertakes to repay it in one single instalment, it is called a loan. Here advance is kept in separate loan account to which the whole amount of loan is immediately credited. The borrower is required to pay the interest on the whole amount from the date of sanction, whether he draws the full account from the loan account or not.

(b) **Cash Credits :** Cash credit is the most popular method of financing by commercial banks. It is an arrangement under which a borrower is allowed to borrow up to a certain limit against the security of tangible assets or guarantees. It is also known as secured credit. But if the cash credit is not backed by any security, it is known as clean cash credit. In case of clean cash credit the borrower gives a promissory note which is signed by two or more sureties. Unlike loan account, cash credit account is a running account from and to which withdrawals and deposits can be made frequently. The customer has to pay interest only on the amount actually utilised.

(c) **Overdrafts :** Under this arrangement, the commercial bank allows its customer to overdraw his current account so that it shows the debit balance. Any business concern can enter into this arrangement to tide over a temporary shortage of funds. The customer is charged interest on the account actually overdrawn and not on the limit 'sanctioned'.

(d) **Discounting of Bills :** Commercial banks finance the business concern by discounting their credit instruments like bills of exchange, promissory notes and hundies. These documents are discounted by the bank at the price lower than their face value.

Generally, banks insist on security when they grant credit facilities to their customers. The security is provided in the form to pledge, hypothecation or mortgage. The important types of securities which may be lodged with a bank are (i) goods, (ii) documents of title to goods, (iii) stock exchange securities, (iv) real-estate, (v) Life Insurance policies, (vi) fixed deposit receipts, and (vii) book debts.

Recently, commercial banks have also started 'term lending'. The encouragement for 'term lending' is provided by the refinancing facilities by the Industrial Development Bank of India. Banks have also started underwriting of new issues of shares and debenturers of industrial enterprises. They invest in the securities of industrial enterprises. But the commercial banks mainly provide short-term financing facilities. However, the short term facility granted by the banks is converted into medium-term finance by renewal from time to time. While granting credit facility to a business concern, a commercial bank considers the following points :

(i) nature and size of the business unit, (ii) type of management, (iii) financial soundness and profitability of the business unit, and (iv) ability to repay its loans.

It is better to get short-term accommodation from the banks because they maintain utmost secrecy of the information supplied to them. The banks do not interfere in the management of the borrowing concerns. Bank credit can be repaid whenever the business concern has surplus money. Thus, it brings flexibility in financial planning for short-term period. But sometimes, it creates certain problems also. The duration of bank credit is very short and there is no certainty of its renewal. Sometimes, banks insist on security of tangible assets whose value should not be less than one and a half times the amount of credit facilities granted. But despite these problems business concerns usually find it convenient to approach commercial banks for short-term credit facilities.

6. Hire-Purchase

It means a transaction where goods are sold and purchased with the condition that (a) its payment will be made in instalments (b) each instalment will be treated as hire charges in case any default is made. The seller will be entitled to take away the goods without compensating the purchaser if default is made in paying all the agreed instalment. (c) The ownership of goods shall pass on to the purchaser only when all the instalments are paid. Till then he shall not be the owner of goods. Before entering into hire-purchase agreement, the purchaser has to make cash down payment (initial payment) and the balance is payable in instalments with agreed interest thereon. This is sometimes called instalment credit also.

7. Lease Finance

This is a new concept acquiring fixed assets for a business. The lessor purchases the asset and hires to the lessee for use against payment of monthly lease rentals comprising cost of asset and interest thereon. At the end of lease period after payment of all dues and agreed lease rentals, the lessor may sell the asset to the lessee on the agreed amount or may take it back for leasing to other lessee considering the residual life of that particular asset. It may be a Finance Lease or Operating Lease. In financial lease the lessor is not responsible for any financial risk or operational maintenance, viz., insurance etc. whereas it is there in case of operating lease.

Hire-purchase business is very old in India whereas the lease business is relatively new, but is coming only as a boon for the rapid industrialisation of the country.

In industry both the systems of financing have been used, generally by the transporters for financing of vehicles for business. It has rarely been in practice or preferred for acquisition of other fixed assets on account of higher rate of interest as compared to commercial banks and as well as the financial institutions. This has also been used to boost the sales of consumer products.

8. Commercial Paper

With a view to enabling high rated companies to reversify as well as to raise their short term borrowings and to provide an additional instrument to investors, the commercial paper was introduced in 1990. It was also to meet the short term requirements of funds by the corporate sector. The companies with a net worth (paid-up capital plus free reserves) of at least Rs. 5 crores are permitted ot issue commercial paper maturing between 91 days and 6 months and the rate of interest will be freely determined. Their shares should have been listed on one or more stock exchanges and have obtained credit rating from Credit Rating Information Services of India Ltd. (CRISIL) and from Investment Information Rating Agency of India Ltd. (ICRA) and it should not be older than 2 months and are availing the working capital limits (fund based) not less than Rs. 5 crores from the commercial banks. The minimum current ration should be 1.33 : 1 ; as per the latest audited Balance Sheet and their credit account should have been classified under Health Code No. 1 by the financing bank(s). The aggregate amount of commercial paper shall not exceed 70% of company's working capital (fund based) limit. It shall be issued in the form of usance promissory notes negotiable by endorsement and delivery and to be issued at such discount to face value as determined by the issuing company.

9. Factoring

Suppliers of goods and services, particularly the smaller ones face working capital problems because purchasers often delay payments. Factoring services started in 1989, generally being provided by the banks and investment companies, is a tool for assisting the suppliers in the matter of financing and collection of their commercial receivables. Under this, financing companies or institutions assume the credit and collection functions for their clients, purchase their receivables as they arise. The priority of factoring depends upon the creditworthiness of the customer, his track record, quality of portfolio, turnover, average size of invoice etc. The most important the cost and the amount of funds involved, generally the factors cost of funds is 13.5 per cent per annum and try to charge less than the rate being charged by commercial banks on account of competition. But this service can be performed well by the banks as they have considerable experience in financing, they have a network of branches to collect credit information on both sellers and buyers. Accordingly this service is performed by the subsidiaries of the banks. For the time being there in no such agency in India which would supply credit information on clients to the factors. They have to rely upon for this on the banks or other available sources.

This being newly started and on account of less experience, the factors have initially started helping known or big concerns and where the amount involved is less. Making it an efficiency service, a conductive environment is yet to be created by government by promoting various legislations and making amendments in the existing laws. But this is a fact that this service is really beneficial for industrial concerns in meeting their short term or working capital requirements which was thought as a hinderance to their growth in business and meeting short term funds requirement.

21

INTRODUCTION TO ACCOUNTING

ACCOUNTING

Accounting in the art of recording, classifying and summarising in a signifi-cant manner and in terms of money transactions and events which in part, at least of a financial character, and interpreting the results thereof. It may be defined as "the process of identifying, measuring, and communicating economic information."

From the above the following attributes of accounting emerge :

(i) It is the art of recording and classifying business transactions and events. Business transactions are analysed in such a way that it may be possible to determine profit or loss made by the business and its financial condition on a specified date. Business transactions may relate to the receipt and payment of cash, purchase or sale of goods on credit, incurring an expense or receiving an income or relating to mis-cellaneous items.

(ii) The transactions or events of a business must be recorded in monetary terms. If there are certain events which cannot be measured in terms of money, they will not be recorded in financial accounting. For example, a quarrel between production manager and financial manager may be affecting the business but it cannot be measured in terms of mc. ey and thus will not be recorded in the books of accounts.

(iii) It is an art of making summaries, analysis and interpretation of these transactions. The accounting information must be summarised, analy-sed and interpreted by calculating various ratios and percentages or other relationship in order to evaluate the past performance of the business and to make sound plans for the future.

(iv) The results of such analysis must be communicated to the persons who are to make decisions or form judgments. All information must be provided in time and presented to the different categories of the persons so that appropriate decisions may be taken at the right time.

The main purpose of accounting is to ascertain profit or loss during a specified period, to show financial condition of the business on a particular date and to have control over the firm's property. Such accounting records are required to be maintained to measure the income of the business and communicate the information so that it may be used by the management.

FUNCTIONS OF ACCOUNTING

The main functions of accounting can be given as follows:

1. It keeps a record of income and expenses in such a manner so that net results of the business can be quickly known for any period.
2. It keeps a record of assets and liabilities in such a way that financial position of the business can be readily had at any point of time.
3. It keeps a systematic and permanent record of all financial transactions of the business.
4. It protects the property of the business by designing such a system of accounting which may be helpful to achieve this purpose.
5. It keeps a track of all changes in the value of assets and liabilities.
6. It keeps a control on expenses in order to minimise the same.
7. It communicates the results of the business to the various categories of persons as owners, investors, creditors, employees, management, government, etc.
8. It provides information for meeting various legal requirements as income tax returns, return for sales tax, etc.
9. It helps in making decisions concerning the acquisition, use and preservation of scarce resources.
10. It helps in devising remedial measures for the deviation of the actual performance from the planned performance.

Accounting is useful in all types of organisations. Business executives, public accountants, hospital administrators, school and college administrators and politicians are better equipped to perform their duties when they have an understanding of accounting data. An effective accounting system provides information to managers, for use in strategic planning and to stockholders, government and other outside parties.

CLASSIFICATION OF ACCOUNTING

Accounting can be classified into the following categories :

1. **Financial Accounting :** The main purpose of this type of accounting is to record business transactions in the books of accounts in such a way that operating results for a particular period and financial condition on

a particular date can be known for the information of the various groups of persons.

2. **Cost Accounting :** It relates to the collection, classification. ascertainment of cost and its accounting and cost control relating the various elements of cost, i.e. materials, labour and overheads.

3. **Management Accounting :** It relates to the use of accounting data collected with the help of financial accounting and cost accounting for the purpose of policy formulation, planning, control and decision-making by the management.

USERS OF ACCOUNTING SYSTEM :

A. **External Users of Accounting Information :** External users are those groups or persons who are outside the organisation for whom accounting function is performed. Following can be the various external users of accounting information :

1. **Investors :** Those who are interested in investing money in an organisation are interested in knowing the financial health of the organisation to know how safe the investment already made is and how safe their proposed investment will be. To know the financial health, they need accounting information which will help them in evaluating the past performance and future prospects of the organisation.

2. **Creditors :** Creditors (i.e. supplier of goods and services on credit, bankers and other lenders of money) want to know the financial position of a concern before giving loans or granting credit. They want to be sure that the concern will not experience difficulty in making their payment in time i.e. liquid position of the concern is satisfactory. To know the liquid position, they need accounting information relating to current assets, quick assets and current liabilities which is available in the financial statements.

3. **Members of Non-Profit Organisations :** Members of non-profit organisations such as schools, colleges, hospitals, clubs, charitable institutions etc. need accounting information to know how their contributed funds are being utilised and to ascertain if the organisation deserves continued support or support should be withdrawn keeping in view the bad performance depicted by the accounting information and diverted to another organisation. In knowing the performance of such organisations, criterion will not be the profit made but the chief criterion will be the service provided to the society.

4. **Government :** Central and state governments are interested in the accounting information because they want to know earnings or sales for a particular period for purposes of taxation. Income tax

returns are examples of financial reports which are prepared with information taken directly from accounting records. Government also needs accounting information for compiling statistics concerning business which, in turn helps in compiling national accounts.

5. **Consumers :** Consumers need accounting information for establishing good accounting control so that cost of production may be reduced with the resultant reduction of the prices of goods they buy. Sometimes, prices for some goods are fixed by the government, so it needs accounting information to fix reasonable prices so that consumers and manufacturers are not exploited. Prices are fixed keeping in view fair return to manufacturers on their investments shown in the accounting records.

6. **Research Scholars :** Accounting information, being a mirror of the financial performance of a business organisation, is of immense value to the research scholar who wants to make a study into the financial operations of a particular firm. To make a study into the financial operations of a particular firm, the research scholar needs detailed accounting information relating to purchases, sales, expenses, cost of materials used, current assets, current liabilities, fixed assets, long term liabilities and shareholders' funds which are available in the accounting records maintained by the firm.

B. **Internal Users of Accounting Information :** Internal users of accounting information are those persons or groups which are within the organisation. Following are such internal users :

1. **Owners :** The owners provide funds for the operations of a business and they want to know whether their funds are being properly used or not. They need accounting information to know the profitability and the financial position of the concern in which they have invested their funds. The financial statements prepared from time to time from accounting records tell them the profitability and the financial position.

2. **Management :** Management is the art of getting done through others, the management should ensure that the subordinates are doing work properly. Accounting information is an aid in this respect because it helps a manager in appraising the performance of the subordinates. Actual performance of the employees can be compared with the budgeted performance they are expected to achieve and remedial action can be taken if the actual performance is not upto the mark. Thus, accounting information provides "the eyes and ears to the management."

Two of the most important functions of management are planning and controlling. Preparation of various budgets, such as sales budget, production budget, cash budget, capital expenditure budget etc., is an important part of planning function and the starting point for the preparation of the budget is the accounting information for the previous year. Controlling is the function of seeing that programmes laid down in various budgets are being actually achieved, i.e. actual performance ascertained from accounting is compared with the budgeted performance, enabling the manager to exercise control in case of weak performance. Accounting information is also helpful to the management in fixing reasonable selling prices. In a competitive economy, a price should be based on cost plus a reasonable rate of return. If a firm quotes a price which exceeds cost plus a reasonable rate of return, it probably will not get the order. On the other hand, if the firm quotes a price which is less than its cost, it will be given the order but will incur a loss on account of price being lower than the cost. So selling prices should always be fixed on the basis of accounting data to get the reasonable margin of profit on sales.

3. **Employees :** Employees are interested in the financial position of a concern they serve particularly when payment of bonus depends upon the size of the profit earned. They seek accounting information to know that the bonus being paid to them is correct.

LIMITATIONS OF ACCOUNTING

The following are the main limitations of accounting :

1. **Records Transactions Measurable in Monetary Terms :** Accounting records only those transaction which cannot be measured into monetary terms. Non-monetary transactions such as conflict between production and marketing manager, efficient management etc. may be very important for a concern but not recorded in the business books.

2. **Effect of Price Level Changes not Considered :** Accounting transactions are recorded at cost in the books. The effect of price level changes is not brought into the books with the result that comparison of the various years becomes difficult. For example, the sale to total assets in 1990 would be much higher than in 1980 due to rising prices, fixed assets being shown at cost and not at market price.

3. **No Realistic Information Due to Different Concepts and Conventions:** Accounting information may not be realistic as accounting statements are prepared by following basic concepts and conventions. For example, going concern concept gives us an idea that the business will continue and assets are to be recorded at cost but the book value which the asset is showing may not be actually releasable. Similarly, by following the principle of conservatism the financial statements will not reflect the true position of the business.

4. **Personal Bias of Accountant Affect the Accounting Statement :** Accounting statements are influenced by the personal judgment of the accountant. He may select any method of depreciation, valuation of stock, amortisation of fixed assets and treatment of deferred revenue expen-

diture. Such judgment if based on integrity and competency of the accountant will definitely affect the preparation of accounting statements.

SYSTEMS OF ACCOUNTING

The following are the main systems of recording business transactions:

1. **Cash System :** Under this system, actual cash receipts and actual cash payments are recorded. Credit transactions are not recorded at all until the cash is actually received or paid. The Receipt and Payments Account prepared in cash of non-trading concerns such as a charitable institution, a club, a school, a college, etc. and professional men like a lawyer, a doctor, a chartered accountant, etc. can be cited as the best example of cash system. This system does not make a compete record of financial transactions of a trading period as it does not record outstanding transactions like outstanding expenses and outstanding incomes. The system being based on a record of actual cash receipts and actual cash payments will not be able to disclose correct profit or loss for a particular period and will not exhibit true financial position of the business on a particular day.

2. **Merchantile (Accrual) System :** Under this system all transactions relating to a period are recorded in the books of account i.e., in addition to actual receipts and payments of cash income receivable and expenses payable are also recorded. This system gives a complete picture of the financial transactions of the business as it makes a complete record of the financial transactions. It discloses correct profit or loss for a particular period and also exhibits true financial position of the business on a particular day.

3. **Mixed System :** Under this system both cash system and merchantile systems are followed. Some records are kept under cash system whereas others are kept under merchantile system.

22

ACCOUNTING PRINCIPLES, CONCEPTS, CONVENTIONS AND POLICIES

Accounting is the language of business. To make the language convey the same meaning to all people, accountings all over the world have developed certain rules, procedures and conventions, which represent a consensus view by the profession of good accounting practices and procedures and are generally referred to as Generally Accepted Accounting Principles (GAAP). Accounting statements are prepared in confirmity with these principles in order to place more reliance on them. The need for the common accounting principles becomes more apparent when we contemplate the chaotic conditions that would prevail if every accountant could follow his own principles about the measurement of revenue and expenses.

CHARACTERISTICS OF ACCOUNTING PRINCIPLES

The following are the main characteristics of accounting principles :

1. Accounting principles are man made so they do not have the authoritativeness as universal principles like the principles of physics, chemistry and other natural sciences have. They represent the best possible guidelines based on reasons and observations and have been developed by accounting to enhance the usefulness of accounting data in an ever changing society.

2. The science of accounting is not in a finished form ; it is the process of evolution. Consequently, accounting principles are fast developing. These are influenced by business practices and customs, government agencies and other business groups.

3. The general acceptance of an accounting principle usually depends on how well it meets three criteria: relevance, objective and feasibility. A

principle is relevant to the extent that it results in information that is useful to those who want to know something about a certain business. A principle is objective to the extent that the accounting information is not influenced by the personal bias of those who furnish the information. The accounting information given in the financial statements should be free from the personal bias of the persons have taken part in the preparation of such statements. A principle is feasible to the extent that it can be applied under complexity or cost.

Accounting principles can be classified into two categories :

1. ACCOUNTING CONCEPTS

According concepts may be considered as postulates, i.e. basic assumptions or conditions upon which the science of accounting is based. There is no authoritative list of these concepts but most of the concepts have fairly general support.

2. ACCOUNTING CONVENTIONS

The term 'conventions' denotes customs or traditions which guide the accountant while preparing the accounting statements.

Accounting concepts and conventions are significant to the development of accounting theory in two ways. First, they are themselves part of an empirical process for developing principles of accounting. In this respect, they may be taken as belonging to the corpus of accounting theory. Second, they reflect the influence of the social, economic, historical and legal forces which shape the philosophy of accounting in a given environment. Their origin lies in a historical process of development of viable theories of accounting.

The above concepts and conventions are explained below:

ACCOUNTING CONCEPTS

1. **Business Entity Concept :** This concept implies that a business unit is separate and distinct from the persons who supply capital to it. Irrespective of the form of organisation, a business unit has got its own individuality as distinguished from the persons who own or control it. The accounting equation (i.e. Assets = Liabilities + Capital) is an expression of the entity concept because it shows that the business itself owns the assets and interm owes the various claimants. Business is kept separate from the proprietor so that transactions of the business may also be recorded with him. In case this concept is not followed affairs of the business will be mixed up with the private affairs of the proprietor and the true picture of the business will not be available.

ACCOUNTING PRINCIPLES

ACCOUNTING CONCEPTS

1. Business Entity
2. Money Measurement
3. Going concern
4. Cost
5. Dual Aspect
6. Accounting period
7. Matching
8. Realisation
9. Objective Evidence.

ACCOUNTING CONVENTIONS

1. Consistency
2. Full Disclose
3. Conservation
4. Materiality

Thus, in the books of a sole trader, a firm or a limited company, only business transactions are recorded and no note is taken of the personal transactions of a sole proprietor, the partners of the firms and the shareholders of the company. But their transactions with the business (e.g., capital provided to the business, goods and amount withdrawn from the business for the personal use of the sole trader and the partners of the firm, income tax or life insurance, etc.) are recorded so that true financial position and profitability of the business may be disclosed.

The business entity concept employed in accounting for a sole proprietorship is distinct from the legal concept of a sole proprietorship. The non-business expenses, incomes, assets and liabilities of a sole proprietor are excluded from the business accounts. Legally, however, a sole proprietor is personally liable for his business debts and may be required to use non-business assets (i.e. his private assets) to make the payment to his business creditors. Conversely, business assets are not immune from claims of the sole proprietor's personal creditors. In the eyes of law business and non-business assets and liabilities are treated alike in case of a sole proprietor. Similarly, in case of a partnership firm, business assets of the firm are used first for paying business liabilities of the firm and if a surplus remains after paying the firm's liabilities, a partner can use his share of the surplus for the payment of his private liabilities. In the same way, private assets of the individual partners are first utilised for the payment of their individual private liabilities.

In case of joint stock companies, there is a legal distinction between the owners (i.e. shareholders) and the business. Shareholders are not liable for the debts of their company beyond the amount of capital they have agreed to subscribe. The accounting treatment of capital contributed by shareholders is the same as it is in case of sole trader and partnership, except of course that the capital of a joint stock company is divided into a number of shares.

2. **Money Measurement Concept :** Money is the only practical unit of measurement that can be employed to achieve homogeneity of financial data, so accounting records only those transactions which can be expressed in terms of money though quantitative records are also kept. The advantage of expressing business transactions in terms of money is that money serves a common denominator by means of which heterogeneous facts about a business can be expressed in terms of numbers (i.e. money) which are capable of additions and subtractions. It can better, be illustrated by taking the following example.

The items given in different units of measurement cannot be added together to get an idea of the total value of the assets owned by the business; to get an idea of the total value of the assets, all items should be expressed in terms of money.

The money measurement concept restricts the scope of accounting as it does not record the fact that there is a strike in the factory or the sales manager is not on speaking terms with the production manager. Accounting, therefore, does not give a complete account of the happenings in a business unit. Money provides a common denominator for measuring, but it does not take care of inflation which takes place with the passage of time. Money is expressed in terms of value at the time a financial transaction is recorded in the books. Subsequent charges in the purchasing power of money due to inflation do not affect this amount.

3. **Going Concern Concept :** It is assumed that a business unit has a reasonable expectation of continuing business at a profit for an indefinite period of time. A business unit is deemed to be a going concern and not a gone concern. It will continue to operate in the future. Transactions are recorded in the books keeping in view the going concern aspect of the business unit. It is because of this concept that suppliers supply goods and services and other business firms enter into business transactions with the business unit. Suppliers will not supply goods and services and other persons will not have business dealings with the business entity if they have the feelings that the concern will be liquidated. This assumption provides much of the justification for recording fixed assets at original cost (i.e. acquisition cost) and depreciating them in a systematic manner without reference to their current releasable value. It is useless to show fixed assets in the Balance Sheet at their estimated realisable values if there is no immediate expectation of selling them. Fixed assets are acquired for use in the business for learning revenues and are not meant for resale, so they are shown at their book values and not at their current realisable values. But when the concern is not a going concern and is to be liquidated, current realisable values of fixed assets become relevant.

Similarly, the going concern concept supports the treatment of prepaid expenses as assets even though they may be virtually unsaleable. Prepaid expenses are made assets on the assumption that the business entity will continue in future and the benefit of prepaid expenses will be utilised in future. A less direct effect of the going concern concept is that it lays emphasis on the determination of net income rather than on the valuation of assets. The earning capacity of the business entity is more significant than the market value of its individual assets in judging the overall worth of a business. Because of this emphasis on the earnings, the accountant directs his attention to the proper allocation of incomes and expenses to the current period and does not bother about the market value of fixed assets which will not be sold.

4. **Cost Concept :** A fundamental concept of accounting, closely related to the going concern concept, is that an asset is recorded in the books at the price paid to acquire it and that this cost is the basis for all subsequent accounting for the asset. This concept does not mean that the asset will always be shown at cost but it means that cost becomes basis for all future accounting for the asset. Asset is recorded at cost at the time of its purchase but is systematically reduced in its value by charging depreciation. The market value of an asset may change with the passage of time, but for accounting purpose it continues to be shown in the books at its book value i.e., the cost at which it was purchased minus depreciation provided up to date.

The cost concept has the advantage of bringing objectivity in the accounts. Information given in the financial statements is not influenced by the personal bias or judgment of those who furnish such statements. In the absence of cost concept, assets will be shown at their market values which will depend on the subjective views of persons who furnish financial statements. However, on account of high degree of inflation in the economy in the recent past, the preparation of financial statements on the basis of cost concept has become irrelevant for judging the financial position and ascertaining the profitability of the business entity. To overcome the drawbacks of cost concept, inflation accounting is advocated which makes a provision for recording all items regularly in the financial statements at their current values. But keeping in view the practical difficulties and absence of legal provisions for inflation accounting, historical cost accounting based on cost concept still serves as a fair and adequate basis for reporting business performance.

According to this concept, it is possible to remove the cost of fixed assets from the accounts altogether by writing off their cost as depreciation against income even though assets are still in good condition and are being used in the business. As a result of this drawback, secret reserves are created and the auditor may overlook the verification of assets showing zero book value because their accounts will no longer appear in the books.

5. **Dual Aspect Concept :** This is the basic concept of accounting. According to this concept, every financial transaction involves a two-fold aspect, (a) yielding of a benefit and (b) the giving of that benefit. For example, if a business has acquired an asset, it must have given up some other asset such as cash or the obligation to pay for it in future. Thus a giver necessarily implies a receiver and a receiver necessarily implies a giver. There must be a double entry to have a complete record of each business transaction, an entry being made in the receiving account and an entry of the same amount in the giving account. The receiving account is termed as debtor and the giving account is called creditor. Thus every debit must have a corresponding credit and vice versa and upon this dual aspect has been raised the whole superstructure of Double Entry System of Accounting. The accounting Equation [i.e. Assets = Equities (or Liabilities + Capital) is based on dual-aspect concept. The term 'Assets denotes the resources owned by the business while the term 'Equities' denotes the claims of various claimants including the proprietors of the business against the assets.

6. **Accounting Period Concept :** The measurement of income or loss of a business entity is relatively simple on a whole-life basis. A complete and accurate picture of the degree of success achieved by a business unit cannot be obtained until it is liquidated, converts its assets into cash and pays off its debts. On liquidation, it is possible to determine with finality its net income. But the owners, the investors and overall the Government, all are impatient and do not want to wait, until the dissolution of the concern, to know what has been the results of the business activities. All these persons are interested in regular reports and accounts at proper intervals to know "how things are going"? This means that the final accounts must be prepared on a periodic basis rather than waiting till the business is terminated.

Under the going concern concept it is assumed that a business entity has a reasonable expectation of continuing business for an indefinite period of time. This assumption provides much of the justification that the business will not be terminated, so it is reasonable to divide the life of the business into accounting periods so as to be able to know the profit or loss of each such period and the financial position at the end of such a period. Normally accounting period adopted is one year as it helps to take any corrective action, to pay income-tax, to absorb the seasons fluctuations and for reporting to the outsiders. A period of more than one year reduces the utility of accounting data.

The principle of segregating capital expenditure from revenue expenditure is based on the accounting period concept. The revenue expenditure for a particular period is transferred to the Profit and Loss Account of that period whereas capital expenditure is carried forward to the extent its benefit will be utilised in future accounting periods. Thus, the accounting period concept plays a very important role in determining the income of a particular accounting period. It is also helpful in ascertaining the true and fair view of the financial position of a business entity on a particular date at a particular point of time.

7. **Matching Concept :** This concept is based on the accounting period concept. The most important objective of running a business is to ascertain profit periodically. The determination of profit of a particular accounting period is essentially a process of matching the revenue recognised during the period and the costs to be allocated to the period to obtain the revenue. It is,thus, a problem of matching revenues and expired costs, the residual amount being the net profit or net loss for the period. Revenue is considered to be earned on the date at which it is realised, i.e. on the date when the goods are delivered or services rendered to the customer even though payment may be received at some future date. Revenue may also be considered to be earned at the time the cash is collected, regardless when the sale is made or service is rendered as is the practice with physicians, attorney and other enterprises in which professional services are source of revenue. It has the practical advantages of simplicity of operation and avoidance of the problem of estimating losses on account of bad debts. It is also advantageous from income tax point of view because income tax is paid only on cash income.

Like revenue, all costs incurred during the period are not taken,but only costs related to the accounting period are taken. The purchase price of fixed assets is not taken but only depreciation on fixed assets related to the accounting period is taken. Expenses paid in advance are excluded from the total costs and expenses outstanding are added to the total costs to arrive at the costs attached to the period.

Application of matching concept, however, is beset with certain difficulties. There are some expenses like preliminary expenses, share issue expenses, advertisement expenses, etc. which are not readily identified against the revenue of a particular period. Similarly, how much of the capital expenditure should be written off by way of depreciation during the particular period poses the question of finding out the expected life of the asset. Likewise, in case of long term contracts when amount is not received in proportion to the work executed may present some difficulties.

8. **Realisation Concept :** According to this concept, revenue is considered as being earned on the date at which it is realised, i.e. on the date when the property in goods passes to the buyer and he becomes legally liable to pay. This can be made clear by taking the following example:

A customer at Kanpur places an order with a manufacturer at Delhi on 1st January. On receipt of order, the manufacturer manufactures goods and delivers them to the customer at Kanpur on 1st February who makes payment of goods on March 1 after enjoying the credit period of one month. In this case, revenue was realised not on January 1, when order was received nor on March 1, when cash was realised but on February 1, when goods were delivered to the customer.

However, in case of hire-purchase sales, the ownership of goods sold on hire-purchase does not pass to the purchaser when the goods are delivered but it passes when the last installment is paid. But sales are presumed to have been made to the extent of down payment, installments received and installments due, but not received.

The realisation concept is criticised by economists on the ground that if an asset has increased in value then it is irrelevant because it has not yet been sold. In other words, unrealised gains are not considered in accounting. As a result of this concept, distinction is made between holding gains and operating gains. Holding gains arise as a result of increases in value from holding an asset and operating gains are realised as a result of selling assets. Holding gains are not recorded because property in goods has not yet transferred but operating gains are reported because they have resulted as a result of sale.

9. **Objective Evidence Concept :** Objectivity connotes reliability, trustworthiness and verifiability, which means that there is some evidence in ascertaining the correctness of the information reported. Entries in accounting records and date reported in financial statements must be based on objectively determined evidence. Without close adherence to this principle, the confidence of many users of the financial statements could not be maintained. Invoices and vouchers for purchases and sales, bank statements for amount of cash at bank, physical checking of stock in hand, etc. are examples of objective evidence which are capable of verification. As far as possible, every entry in accounting records should be supported by some objective evidence. Evidence should be such which will minimise the possibility of error and intentional bias or fraud. Evidence is not always conclusively objective for there are numerous occasions in accounting where judgments and other subjective factors play part. In such situations, it should be seen that most objective evidence available should be used. For example, the Provision for Doubtful Debts Accounts is an estimate of the losses expected from failure to collect sales made on credit.

Estimation of this account should be made on such objective factors as past experience in collecting debtors and reliable forecasts of future business activities.

ACCOUNTING CONVENTIONS

1. **Convention of Consistency** : Accounting rules, practices and conventions should be continuously observed and supplied i.e. these should not change from one year to another. The results of different years will be comparable only when accounting rules are continuously adhered to from year to year. For example, the principle of "valuing stock at cost or market price whichever is lower" should be followed year after year to get comparable results. Similarly, if depreciation on fixed assets is provided on straight line method, it should be done year after year. Consistency serves to eliminate personal bias because the accountant will have to follow consistent rules, practices and conventions year after year. The rationale behind this concept is that frequent changes in accounting treatment, would make the financial statements unreliable to the persons who use them.

   Consistency also implies external consistency, i.e., the financial statements of one enterprise should be comparable with another. It means that every enterprise should follow the same accounting methods and procedures of recording and reporting business transactions. The development of international and national accounting standards is due to the convention of consistency.

2. **Convention of Full Disclosure** : According to this convention, all accounting statements should be honestly prepared and to that end full disclosure of all significant information should be made. All information which is of material interest to proprietors, creditors and investors should be disclosed in accounting statements. An obligation is placed on the accounting profession to see that the books of accounts prepared on behalf of others are as reliable and informative as circumstances permit. The convention is becoming popular these days because most of big business units are in the form of joint stock companies where ownership is divorced from management. The Companies Act, 1956 has prescribed the forms in which financial statements are to be prepared. The Act makes ample provisions for the disclosure of essential information that there is no chance of any material information being left out. For example, the basis of valuation of fixed assets, investments and stock should be clearly stated in the Balance Sheet because it is of material interest to the proprietors, creditors and prospective investors. If there is no detailed disclosure in the profit and loss account, undisclosed reserves accumulated in the past periods may be used to swell the profits in years when the company is failing badly and the shareholders may be misled into thinking that company is making profits.

3. **Convention of Conservatism on Prudence :** Literally speaking, conservatism means taking the gloomy view of the situation. It is a policy of caution or playing safe and had its origin as a safeguard against possible losses in a world of uncertainty. It compels the businessman to wear a "risk-proof" jacket, for the working rule is; anticipate no-profits but provide for all possible losses. For example, closing stock is valued at cost or market price whichever is lower. If market price is higher than the cost, the higher amount is ignored in the accounts and closing stock will be valued at cost which is lower than the market price. But if the market price is lower than the cost, the higher amount of cost will be ignored and stock will be valued at market price which is lower than the cost. Thus, the principle of conservatism is inherent in the valuation of stock.

Overoptimism in reporting results is more undesirable results than overoptimism results because it shows position better than what actual financial position is. But the excessive application of the convention of conservatism could result in the creation of secret reserves, a practice which is contrary to the convention of full disclosure. Conservatism carried beyond what is warranted by reasonable doubts distorts earnings in as much as net profit in one period may be understated than what actual profit is. Keeping in view this, current accounting thought has shifted somewhat from the principle of conservatism. The concepts of consistency, full disclosure, materiality and objectivity take precedence over conservatism and the letter should be a factor only when the others do not play a significant part.

4. **Convention of Materiality :** Whether something should be disclosed or not in the financial statements will depend on whether it is material or not. Materiality depends on the amount involved in the transaction. For example, minor expenditure of Rs. 10 for the purchase of a waste basket may be treated as an expense of the period rather than an asset. Customers also influence materiality. For example, any round figures (to the nearest rupee) may be shown in the financial statements to make the figures manageable without affecting the accounting data. Similarly, for income tax purposes the income has to be rounded to nearest ten rupees.

The term "materiality" is a subjective term. The accountant should record an item as material even though it is of small amount of its knowledge seems to influence the decision of the proprietors or auditors or investors. For example, commission paid to sole selling agents should be disclosed separately in the Profit and Loss Account. Similarly, amount due to directors or other officers of the bank should be disclosed separately in the Balance Sheet of a bank to know the amount of advances due from the directors or officers who are managing the affairs of the bank.

23

DOUBLE ENTRY SYSTEM

Every business transaction has two astpects, i.e., when we receive something, we give something else in return. For example, when we purchase goods for cash, we receive goods and give cash in return ; similarly in a credit sale of goods, goods are given to the customer and the customer becomes debtor for the amount of goods sold to him. This method of writing every transaction in two accounts is known as Double Entry System of Accounting. Of the two accounts, one account is given debit while the other amount is given credit with an equal amount. Thus, on any date, the total of all debits must be equal to the total of all credits because every debit has a corresponding credit.

RULES OF THE DOUBLE ENTRY SYSTEM

There are separate rules of the double entry system in respect of personal, real and nominal accounts which are discussed below :

1. **Personal Accounts :** These accounts record a business's dealing with persons or firms. The person receiving something is given debit and the person giving something is given credit. For example, if Anand sells goods to Sanjay on credit, Sanjay's Account will be given debit (in Anands's books) as he is the receiver of goods and Anand's Account will be credited (in Sanjay's books) as he is the giver of goods. When Sanjay's makes the payment for these goods, Anand's Account will be debited in Sanjay's books as he is the receiver of cash and Sanjay's Account will be given credit in Anand's books as he is the giver of cash. So, the rule is : Debit the receiver and credit the giver.

2. **Real Accounts :** These are the accounts of assets. Asset entering the business is given debit and asset leaving the business is given credit. For example, when goods are sold for cash, Cash Account will be given debit as cash comes in and Goods Account will be credited as goods go out. So, the rule is : debit what comes in and credit what goes out.

3. **Nominal Accounts :** These accounts deal with expenses, incomes, profits and losses. Accounts of expenses and losses are debited and accounts of incomes and gains are credited. For example, when rent is paid to the landlord, Rent account will be debited as it is an expense and Cash Account (real account) will be credited as it goes out. Similarly when commission is received, Cash Account will be debited as cash is received and Commission Account will be credited as it is an income. Thus, the rule is : debit all expenses and losses and credit all incomes and gain.

The rules of double entry system are shown in the following chart :

Rules of Double Entry

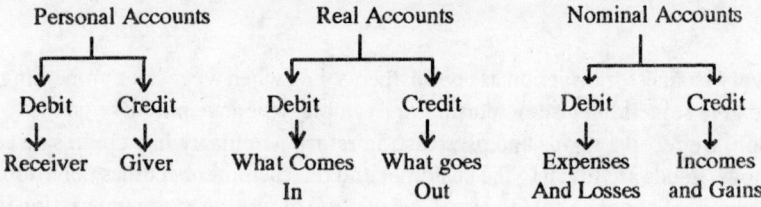

ANALYSIS OF TRANSACTIONS

To make a correct record of the transactions, each transaction must be analysed. The following questions may be asked in this respect :

1. What are the two accounts involved in the transaction to be recorded ?
2. Whether the two accounts involved in the transaction are personal, real or nominal ?
3. What rules of debit and credit are applicable to the accounts involved ?
4. Which account should be debited or credit ?

The above method will make the recording of transactions more simple and easy. The chart explains the procedure of analysing the transactions.

To have a clear understanding of the Double Entry System, it is necessary to keep in mind the following which are common to every business :

(1) The business has to enter into business dealings with a number of persons or firms. So, an account of each person or firm, with whom the business has business dealings, is opened. Such accounts are known as Personal Accounts.

(2) The business must necessarily have some assets such as stock, cash, furniture etc., with the help of which the business may be carried on.

Therefore, an account of each asset in the business is opened. Such accounts are classed as Real or Property Accounts.

(3) There must be certain sources from which the income of the business is derived. Similarly, certain expense must be incurred to earn the income. There, an account of each expense and income is opened in the books. Such accounts are known as Nominal or Fictitious Accounts.

Thus, three types of accounts, namely, Personal Accounts, Real or Property Accounts and Nominal or Fictitious Accounts are opened to keep a complete record of all the financial transaction of the business.

ADVANTAGES OF DOUBLE ENTRY SYSTEM

The following are the main advantages which can be derived from the use of this system :

1. It provides a complete record of every transaction whether it relates to the personal or impersonal accounts.
2. It provides an arithmetical check on the records as the total of debit entries must be equal to the total credit of all entries.
3. The amount owing to outsiders and the amount due to the business can be ascertained with the help of personal accounts.
4. The profit and loss account can be prepared with the help of nominal accounts which is helpful to the business to ascertain the operating results of the business.
5. It helps to prepare the balance sheet of the business which is helpful to ascertain the financial position of the business on a particular day.
6. It helps to reduce the occurrence of the errors and frauds and when occurred can be deducted easily. It can work well with the help of internal check system.

DISADVANTAGES OF DOUBLE ENTRY SYSTEM

The following are the main disadvantages of this system :

1. This system requires the maintenance of a number of books of accounts which is not practical in small concerns.
2. The system is costly because a number of records are to be maintained.
3. There is no guarantee of absolute accuracy of the books of account inspite of agreement of the trial balance.

ACCOUNTING CYCLE

It refers to a complete sequence of accounting procedures which are required to be repeated in the same order during each accounting period. Accounting cycle includes :

1. **Recording** : First, all transactions should be recorded in the Journal or Books of Original Entry known as subsidiary books as and when they take place.

2. **Classifying :** All entries in the Journal or Books of Original Entry should be posted to the appropriate ledger accounts to find out at a glance the total effect of all such transactions in a particular account.

3. **Summarising :** Last stage is to prepare the trial balance and final accounts with a view to ascertaining the profit or loss made during a trading period and the financial position of the business on a particular date.

BASIC TERMS

1. **Business Transactions :** Any exchange of money or money's worth as goods and services between two parties is called a business transaction. It may relate to purchase and sale of goods, receipt and payment of cash and rendering of service by one entry to another.

2. **Debtor :** A debtor is a person who owes money. The amount due from him is called debt. The amount due from a person as per the books of account is called a book debt.

3. **Creditor :** A person to whom money is owing or payable is called a creditor.

4. **Capital :** This is the owner's financial interest or holding in the business and is represented by the value of net assets (i.e., total assets less liabilities).

5. **Goods :** This includes all articles, commodities or merchandise in which the business deals. Thus, cloth would be goods for a dealer in cloth, furniture would be goods for a dealer in furniture and so on.

6. **Assets :** Any physical thing or right owned that has a money value is an asset. In other words, an asset is that expenditure which results in acquiring of some property or benefit of a lasting nature.

7. **Equity :** A claim which can be enforced against the assets of the firm is called equity. In other words, the rights to properties are called equities. Equities are two types : the right of creditors and the right of owners. The equities of creditors represent debts of the business and are called liabilities. The equity of the owners is called capital, proprietorship or owner's equity. Thus,

   Assets = Liabilities + Capital

8. **Income :** It is the favourable change in owner's equity which results from business operations. In other words, income is an inflow of assets which results in an increase in the owner's equity.

9. **Expenditure :** An expenditure takes place when asset or service is acquired.

10. **Expense :** It means an expenditure whose benefit is finished or enjoyed immediately such as salaries, rent, etc.

    The purchase of goods is an expenditure whereas cost of goods sold is an expense. Similarly, if an asset is acquired during the year, it is an expenditure, if it is consumed during the same year, it is also an expense of the year.

11. **Drawings :** Any amount of goods withdrawn by the owner of a business for personal use is called drawings.

12. **Loss :** A loss is an expenditure without any benefit to the concern. On the other hand, expense is incurred to result in some benefit.

13. **Voucher :** Any written document in support of a business transaction is called a voucher.

14. **Turnover :** It means total trading income from cash sales and credit sales.

ACCOUTING EQUATION

American accountants have derived the rules of debit and credit through accounting equation which is given below :

Assets = Equities

The equation is based on the principle that accounting deals with property and rights to property and the sum of the properties owned is equal to the sum of the rights to the properties. The properties owned by a business are called assets and the rights to properties are known as liabilities or equities of the business.

Equities may be divided into equities of creditors representing debts of the business known as liabilities and equity of the owners known as capital. Keeping a view the two types of equities the equation given below can be stated as below :

Assets = Liabilities + Capital

RULES OF ACCOUNTING EQUATION

1. **Regarding Assets :** Increases in assets are debits and decreases in assets are credits.

2. **Regarding Liabilities :** Increases in liabilities are credits and decreases in liabilities are debits.

3. **Regarding Capital :** Increases in capital are credits and decreases are debits.

4. **Regarding Expenses :** Increases in expenses are debits ; decreases are credits.

5. **Regarding Incomes or Profits :** Increases in incomes or profits are credits, decreases are debits.

24

BOOK KEEPING

Book-keeping is the science and art of correctly recording in books of accounts all those business transaction that result in the trasfer of money or money's worth. Book-keeping is recording of the financial transactions of a business in a methodical manner so that information on any point in relation to them may be quickly obtained. A book-keeper may be responsible for keeping all the financial records of a business or only a minor segment such as maintenance of the customers' accounts in a department store. Much of the work of a book-keeper is clerical in nature and can be accomplished through the use of mechanical and electronic equipment. Thus, book-keeping is more of a routine work.

On the other hand, Accounting is primarily concerned with the design of the system of records, the preparation of reports based on the recorded data, the interpretation of the reports and finally communicating the results of the interpretation to persons who are interested in such results. Accountants often direct and review the work of book-keepers. The work of accountants at the beginning may include some book-keeping but accountants must possess a much higher level of knowledge, conceptual understanding and analytical skill than is required of the book-keepers.

SUBSIDIARY BOOKS

All transactions are first entered in the Journal in the order in which they occur and from the Journal they are posted to the respective accounts in the ledger. But this would involve a tremendous amount of work because each transaction requires a separate debit to the receiving account and a credit to the giving account to bring into record the two fold aspect of each transaction. A considerable saving of clerical labour can be brought about if transactions of similar nature are recorded in separate journals so as to permit the sub-divisions of the Journal. This would facilitate not only the division of the journal but it would also make easier the job of posting in the ledger, as the posting can then be made in the form of totals being transactions of similar nature. These sub-divisions of the Journals into various books recording transactions of similar nature are called subsidiary books. These subsidiary books are also known as books of original entry because transactions are first recorded in these books to be subsequently transferred to their respective accounts in the ledger.

REASONS FOR MAINTAINING THE SUBSIDIARY BOOKS

The various reasons for maintaining the subsidiary books are given as under:

1. **Economy in Labour :** If the transactions are recorded in the books of accounts directly, it will consume less time than if the transaction is recorded in the journal and then posted to the ledger.

2. **More Accuracy :** There will be more accuracy in the books of accounts as entries are made in total only and that too once in a month.

3. **Statistical Records :** Additional information can be collected while maintaining a subsidiary book. For example, sales book can collect the information relating to the sales of different areas or of different salesmen.

4. **Maintenance of Accounts :** If specialised books are kept, it may be possible to avoid maintenance of some accounts books. For example, the date of payment cheque no. etc. noted in the purchases book will obviate the need of maintaining the creditors account.

The various books in which the Journal may be subdivided are as follows :

1. Cash Book to record cash receipts and payments.

2. Purchases Book or Bought Book or Invoice Book for recording credit purchase of goods.

3. Sales Book or Day Book for recording all goods sold on credit.

4. Purchases Returns Book or Returns Outwards Book for recording all purchases returned to creditors.

5. Sales Returns Book or Returns Inwards Book for recording all sales returned by customers.

6. Bills Receivable Book to keep a record of bills received from customers.

7. Bills Payable Book to keep a record of bills payable to creditors.

8. Journal Proper to keep a record of those transactions for which there is no separate book.

CASH BOOK

The object of the Cash Book is to keep a daily record of the transactions relating to receipts and payments of cash. The number of transactions relating to cash are usually large because most of the business dealings ultimately resolve themselves into cash transactions, so it is necessary to keep a separate book for cash transactions. If every cash transaction were recorded in the Journal, a tremendous amount of work will be involved in debiting or crediting Cash Account every time cash is received or paid. If the cash book is maintained, the botheration of posting every item of receipt or payment of cash individually to Cash Account in the ledger is avoided.

Cash Book plays dual role as a book of original entry as well as a ledger. It is a subsidiary book because all cash transactions are first recorded in the Cash Book and then from cash Book posted to various accounts in the ledger. The recording of transactions in the Cash Book takes the shape of a Ledger Account. As receipts of cash are entered on the debit side and payments of cash on the credit side, so there is no need of Cash Account in the ledger. Therefore, Cash Book serves the purpose of a ledger account.

From the above, it is clear, that Cash Book fulfils the functions of a subsidiary book and ledger both.

The following are the three types of Cash Book :

1. Simple Cash Book.
2. Cash Book with Discount columns.
3. Cash Book with Bank and Discount columns.

SIMPLE CASH BOOK

This type of Cash Book makes a record of all the receipts and payments of cash. All cash received in the form of coin, notes, cheques, postal orders, bank drafts or treasury notes will be recorded on the debit side and payments on the credit side. The ruling of this type of Cash Book is as follows :

When cash is received, it is earned on the debit side of the Cash Book in the amount column alongwith the name of the party paying the cash in the particulars column. Receipt number with which cash has been received by the cashier is also written in the R.N. (Receipt No.) column. Similarly, cash paid is entered on the credit side of the Cash Book. Each payment must be supported by a voucher number is entered in the V.N. (Voucher No.) column.

At regular periodic intervals, preferably daily, Cash Book should be balanced like other ledger accounts and the balance shown by it should be equal to cash in hand, if no mistake or fraud has been committed. The Cash Book should always show a debit balance (i.e. cash in hand) because total cash paid can never exceed the opening balance plus cash received.

Simple Cash Book

Receipts   Payments

Date	Particulars	R.N.	L.F.	Amount	Date	Particulars	V.N.	L.F.	Amount
				Rs.					Rs.

POSTING OF SIMPLE CASH BOOK

Opening balance appearing on the debit side of the Cash Book is not posted to any account in the ledger as it comes in the Cash Book from the opening entry recorded in the journal proper. The other transactions recorded on the debit side of the Cash Book are posted to the credit of the respective accounts in the ledger to complete the second aspect of the entry as the first aspect of the transactions has been covered by giving debit to Cash Account in the Cash Book itself. Similarly, the entries appearing on the credit side of the Cash Book are posted to the debit of the respective accounts in the ledger.

CASH BOOK WITH DISCOUNT COLUMNS OR TWO COLUMN CASH BOOK

When an additional column for discount alongwith cash column is provided on each side of the Cash Book, it is known as Two Column Cash Book. Discount column on the debit side represents cash discount allowed to customers and the credit side of this column indicates cash discount received from creditors.

Cash columns are balanced like other ledger accounts but discount columns are not balanced but totalled.

POSTING OF TWO COLUMN CASH BOOK

The posting of cash columns will be the same as we have described in case of simple Cash Book. Each item of discount allowed appearing on the debit side of the Cash Book will be posted to the credit of respective personal account and total of discount column should be posted to the debit side of Discount Account with the words "To Sundry Accounts" or "Amount as per Cash Book". Similarly, each item of discount received appearing on the credit side of the Cash Book in the discount column will be posted to the debit of respective personal account and total of discount received column should be posted to the credit of Discount Account with the words "By Sundry Accounts" or "By Amount as per Cash Book".

Example 1 : Enter the following transaction in a Two Column Cash Book and post them into the ledger.

1992			Rs.
March	1	Cash in hand	9,000
"	3	Bought goods for cash	4,200
"	5	Paid for wages	4,100
"	7	Withdrew from bank for expenses	7,500
"	7	Cash paid to Nirmala	1960
		discount allowed	140
"	10	Cash sales	13,500
"	13	Received cash from Madan Bhatia	3,900
		allowed him discount	110
"	15	Purchased stationery from Shaheen on credit	190

March	16	Paid for postage stamps	150
"	18	Amount introduced as capital	5,000
"	21	Received cash from Mukesh	7,840
		allowed him discount	150
"	24	Paid cash for travelling expenses	130
"	26	Amount paid into bank	2,500
"	27	Cash paid to V. Kumar	975
		discount allowed by him	25
"	28	Credit purchases from Ashok Jain	3,810
"	30	Cash Purchases	1,490
"	30	Paid salaries	2,795
"	30	Deposited into bank all cash in excess of	2,005

CASH BOOK WITH BANK AND DISCOUNT COLUMNS OR THREE COLUMN CASH BOOK

With the development in the banking industry, many payments are made and received through cheques. In such a case, the Cash Book should have a bank column in addition to the cash and discount columns to have a record of Bank Account in the Cash Book. Such type of Cash Book is known as Three Column Cash Book.

In such a Cash Book, the cash columns and the bank columns represent Cash Account and Bank Account respectively, but the discount columns are only memorandum columns and do not stand for Discount Account. So, Cash Account and Bank Account will not be opened in the ledger. The following points need consideration in the preparation of Three Column Cash Book :

1. **Cash Paid into Bank :** When cash is paid into the bank, it should be debited to Bank Account by entering the amount in the bank column on the debit side of the Cash Book as "To Cash" and credited to Cash Account by entering the amount in the cash column on the credit side of the Cash Book as "By Bank" to record the fact of cash having gone out of the business. This transaction needs no posting in the ledger as both accounts (i.e. Cash Account and Bank Account) involved appear in the Cash Book, so letter "C" is written in the L.F. column against this entry on each side of the Cash Book to indicate that the contra effect of this transaction is recorded on the opposite side. Such type of entry appearing on both sides of the Cash Book is known as Contra Entry.

2. **Cash withdrawn from bank :** Similarly, when cash is withdrawn from the bank for office use, the entry should be to debit Cash Account by entering the amount in the cash column on the receipts side of the Cash Book as "To Bank" and to credit the bank column as "By Cash". No posting in the ledger is required for this transaction as both accounts (Cash Account and bank Account) involved appear in the Cash Book.

3. **Receipt of Cheque :** If a cheque is received and kept in the cash box (i.e. not sent to the Bank for collection), it should be debited in the cash

SOLUTION 1 :

TWO COLUMN CASH BOOK

Receipts

Date	Particulars	R.N.	L.F.	Discount	Cash
1993				Rs.	Rs.
Mar.1	To Balance b/d				9,000
" 7	To Bank Account				7,500
" 10	To Sales Account				13,500
" 13	To Madan Bhatia			110	3,900
" 18	To Capital Account				5,000
" 21	To Mukesh			150	7,840
				260	46,640
July 1	To Balance b/d				2,000

Payments

Date	Particular	R.N.	L.F.	Discount	Cash
1992				Rs.	Rs.
Mar. 3	By Purchases Account				4,200
" 5	By Wages Account				4,100
" 7	By Nirmala			40	1,960
" 16	By Postage Account				150
" 24	By Travelling Exp. A/c				
" 26	By Bank Account			130	2,500
" 27	By V. Kumar				975
" 30	By Purchases Account			25	1,490
" 30	By Salaries Account				2,700
" 30	By Bank Account (Amount deposited in excess of Rs. 2005)				26,245
" 30	By Balance c/d				2,000
				75	46,640

Note : Stationery purchased on credit and credit purchases have not been recorded in the Cash Book as these transactions do not involve any receipt or payment of cash.

column ; but if it is immediately sent to the bank for collection, the debit should be given in the bank column. Later on when cheque kept in the cash book is sent to the bank for collection, contra entry will be recorced in the Cash Book by giving debit to bank column recording the fact of cheque coming to the bank and credit to cash column indicating that cheque has gone out of office.

4. **Payment by Cheque :** Such payments should be credited in the bank column of the Cash Book.

5. **Dishonoured Cheque :** If a cheque sent to the bank for collection is dishonoured, it should be credited in the bank column of the Cash book to cancel the previous debit given to the bank column when the cheque was deposited in the bank.

6. Bank charges and payments made by the bank on behalf of the customer. These entries should be entered in the bank column on the credit side of the Cash Book as they reduce the balance at bank.

POSTING OF THREE COLUMN CASH BOOK

1. Opening balances of cash and bank columns are not posted to any account as they come in the Cash Book from the opening entry in the journal.

2. Contra entries are not posted to any account as the dual-aspect in respect of them has been complied in the Cash Book itself.

3. Remaining items appearing in the Cash Book and totals of discount columns are posted in the same way as we have described in case of Two Column Cash Book.

Examples 2 : Enter the following transactions in a Three Column Cash Book:
1993
Apr. 1 Cash in hand Rs. 6,374; Balance at Bank Rs. 6,490
    " 3 Cash Sales Rs. 5,400
    " 5 Paid Rs. 4,000 into bank.
    " 6 Received a cheque for Rs. 700 from Mamta
    " 8 Paid into bank Sneh's cheque for Rs. 700.
    " 10 Paid to Anuradha by cheque Rs. 980 and discount allowed by him Rs. 20.
    " 12 Cash Purchases Rs. 2,500
    " 14 Withdrew from bank for office use Rs. 4,000.
    " 15 Received cheque for Rs. 950 from Lucky & Co., allowed him discount Rs. 50.
    " 18 Cash sales Rs. 8,500.
    " 19 Paid into bank Luck's & Co.'s cheque for Rs. 950 and Cash Rs. 3,000.
    " 21 Cash paid for stationery Rs. 120.
    " 23 Paid commission to Rakesh by cheque Rs. 500.
    " 25 Received cheque for Rs. 2,000 from Om Prakash and paid the same into bank.
    " 27 Lucky & Co.'s cheque dishonoured.
    " 29 Draw a cheque for Rs. 800 for personal use.
    " 31 Paid salaries by cheque Rs. 1,200 and by cash Rs. 500.
    " 31 Bank charges Rs. 20 and insurance premium Rs. 820 as shown in Pass Book.

SOLUTION 2 :

CASH BOOK

Receipt							Payments						
Date	Particulars	V.N.	L.F.	Dis-count	Cash	Bank	Date	Particulars	V.N.	L.F.	Dis-count	Cash	Bank
				Rs.	Rs.	Rs.					Rs.	Rs.	Rs.
1993							1993						
Apr. 1	To Balance b/d				6,374	16,490	Apr. 5	By Bank Account		C		7,000	
" 3	To Sales Account		C		5,400		" 8	By Bank Account		C		700	
" 5	To Cash Account		C			7,000	" 10	By Anuradha			20		980
" 6	To Mamta (cheque received)				700		" 12	By Purchases Account				2,500	
" 8	To Cash Account		C			7,00	" 14	By Cash Account		C			5,000
" 14	To Bank Account		C		4,000		" 19	By Bank Account		C		4,950	
" 15	To Lucky & Co. (cheque received)		C	50	950		" 21	By Stationery Account				120	
" 18	To Sales Account				8,500		" 23	By Commission Account					500
" 19	To Cash Account (Cheque 950+ Cash 3,000)		C			3,950	" 27	By Lucky & Co.			50		950
" 25	To Om Prakash					2,000	" 29	By Drawings Account					800
							" 31	By Salaries Account				500	1,200
							" 31	By Bank Charges Account				20	
							" 31	By Insurance Prem, A/c					820
							" 31	By Balance b/d				10,154	18,870
				50	25,924	25,140					70	25,924	29,140
	To Balance c/d				10,154	18,870							

PETTY CASH BOOK

It is undesirable to burden the main Cash Book with numerous small payments on accounts of expenses like carriage, cartage, coolie hire, postage, refreshment to customers etc., so a separate book, called "Petty Cash Book" is usually maintained. The person maintaining the Petty Cash Book is known as petty cashier. All small payments to be made by cash are recorded in the Petty Cash Book.

The best method of recording petty cash payments is to enter them in a Petty Cash Book maintained in a columnar form. In such a Petty Cash Book, a separate column for each usual head of expenditure and for the total small cash payments is provided. The advantage of a Columnar Petty Cash Book is that it saves unnecessary labour used in posting each item of petty cash payment separately in the ledger ; only totals of various columns are to be posted in the ledger. This book is also known as Analytical Petty Cash Book because the various small cash payments get automatically analysed when they are entered in their respective columns.

The Petty Cash Book is just like the Cash Book. The amounts received by the petty cashier from the main cashier are entered on the debit side of the Petty Cash Book and payments on the credit side of the Petty Cash Book. Every small payment is entered twice on the credit side - one in the total payments column and second in one of the analytical amount columns. The periodic total of each column is posted to the expenses accounts concerned, while the total of payments columns serves to find out the balance of cash with the petty cashier.

IMPREST SYSTEM OF PETTY CASH BOOK

Under this system, a round sum necessary for the possible needs of the business to meet petty cash expenses for the week of month is drawn by the cheque and handed over to the pettry cashier. The petty cashier finds out the amount spent during the period and gets a cheque for the exact amount expended by him so that he may start the next period with the same amount as in the beginning of the last period. For example, Rs. 500 are given to the petty cashier on June 1 and he has spent Rs. 460 during the month, he will be paid Rs. 460 so that he may again start the next month with Rs. 500.

Example 3 : Prepare Columnar Petty Cash Book on imprest system from the following particulars and post it to the ledger :

1994			
June	1	Received for petty cash payments	500
"	2	Paid for postage	40
"	5	Paid for stationery	25
"	8	Paid for advertisement	50
"	12	Paid for wages	20

June	16	Paid for carriage	15
"	20	Paid for conveyance	22
"	25	Paid for travelling expenses	80
"	27	Paid for postage	50
"	28	Wages to office cleaner	10
"	30	Paid for telegrams	25
"	30	Sent registered notice to landlord	3

PURCHASE BOOK

This book is kept to record all credit purchases of goods for resale. To be eligible for being recorded in the Purchases Book, the goods purchased on credit must be those in which the firm normally deals. Cash Purchases of goods are entered in the Cash Book, so these are not recorded in the Purchases Book. This book is also known as Invoice Book. The ruling of the Purchases Book is as follows :

Date	Particulars	Invoice No.	L.F.	Details	Amolunt
				Rs.	Rs.

In particulars column, name of the party and particulars of the goods purchases are written.

POSTING OF PURCHASES BOOK

Each supplier's account is individually credited in the ledger with the amount of goods purchased from him because he is the giver of goods. The periodical total of the Purchases Book is posted to the debit of Purchases Account with the words "To Sundries as per Purchases Book".

SALES BOOK

Sales Book, also known as Day Book, is used to record all credit sales of goods in which the firm normally deals. The sale of any asset is not recorded in it. Similarly, cash sales are not entered in it because these are entered in the Cash Book. The ruling of the Sales Book is the same as that of the Purchases Book.

POSTING OF SALES BOOK

Each customer's account is individually debited in the ledger with the amount of goods sold to him as he is the receiver of goods. The periodical total of the Sales Book is posted to the credit of Sales Account with the words "To Sundries as per Sales Book".

PURCHASES RETURNS BOOK

This book keeps a record of the returns outwards, that is, return of goods bought. The person returning the goods sends a debit note to the supplier

SOLUTION 3 :

PETTY CASH BOOK

Cash Received	Date	Particulars	L.F.	Total payment	Analysis of Payments						
					Postage & Telegrams	Cartage & Carriage	Printing & Advertisement	Travel Expenses	Wages	Stationery	Sundries
Rs.	1984			Rs.	Rs.	Rs.	Rs.	Rs.	Rs.	Rs.	Rs.
500	Jun. 1	To Cash									
	" 2	By Postage		40	40						
	" 5	By Stationery		25						25	
	" 8	By Advertisement		50			50				
	" 12	By Wages		20					20		
	" 16	By Carriage		15		15					
	" 20	By Conveyance		22							22
	" 25	By Travelling Expenses		80				80			
	" 27	By Postage		50	50						
	" 28	By Wages		10					10		
	" 30	By Telegrams		20	20						
	" 30	By Registered Notice to landlord		3	3						
				335	113	15	50	80	30	25	22
	" 30	By Balance c/d		165							
500				500							
165	July 1	To Balance b/d									
335	" 1	To Cash Account									

Note : There is no separate column for conveyanced, so it is shown in the Sundries Column.

informing him that he is debiting the latter's account with amount of goods returned. This book is also known as Returns Outwards Book.

POSTING OF PURCHASES RETURNS BOOK

Each supplier's account is individually debited with the value of goods returned to him and the periodical total of this book is credited to Returns Outwards Account or Purchases Returns Account as the goods go out.

SALES RETURNS BOOK

Sales Returns Book, also known as Returns Inwards Book, is kept for recording returns inwards, that is, returns of goods sold by us. The trader sends a credit note to the customer informing him that he has credited the latter's account with the value of goods returned.

POSTING OF SALES RETURNS BOOK

Each customer's account is credited with the value of goods returned by him. The periodical total of the book is debited to Returns Inwards Account or Sales Returns Account as returned goods enter the business.

JOURNAL PROPER

Journal proper is used for recording only those transactions as cannot be recorded in any of the other subsidiary books. Examples of such transactions are :

1. Opening entries.
2. Transfer entries (transfer from one account to another)
3. Adjusting entries.
4. Closing entries.
5. Entries relating to rectification of errors.
6. Entries relating to dishonour of bills or promissory notes.
7. Withdrawal of goods by the proprietor for personal use of loss of goods by theft, fire, etc.
8. Credit purchase or sale of assets.
9. Bad debts.

25

LEDGERS

When all the accounts are kept in one ledger, a trial balance can be extracted as a test of the arithmetical accuracy of the accounts though certrain errors may not be revealed by such trial balance. If the trial balance total disagrees, the number of entries for a small business being relatively few, the books can easily and quickly be checked so as to locate the errors. However, when the firm has grown and the accounting work has been so sub-divided that there are several or many ledgers, a trial balance, the totals of which do not agree, can result in a great deal of unnecessary checking before the errors are found. What is required, in fact, is a type of trial balance for each ledger or a section of the groups of ledgers and this requirement is met by self balancing ledgers or sectional balancing.

LEDGERS

The important ledgers maintained by Financial as well as Costing Departments are as :

FINANCIAL LEDGERS

The three important financial ledgers are :
  (1) **General Ledger :** It contains
      (i) all real, nominal and personal accounts except these of trade debtors and trade creditors.
      (ii) a total account, termed as "Cost Ledger Control Account". It records all items of expenditure and income which relate to cost accounts. This account is a memorandum account only.
  (2) **Sale or Debtors' Ledger :** It contains personal accounts of all trade debtors from whom goods are sold on credit.
  (3) **Purchases or Bought or Creditors' Ledger :** It contains personal account of all trade creditors from whom goods are bought on credit.

General ledger is usually in the charge of an accountant whereas purchases and sales ledger (known as trade or subsidiary ledgers) are placed in the charge of an accounts clerk. When there are a large number of customers and suppliers, purchases and sales ledgers may further be subdivided into sections - (a) alphabetically as A-G, H-L, M-R, S-Z ; (b) departmentally as A Deptt., B Department, Hosiery Department, Drapery Department ; or (c) geographically, as local, provincial, national, international.

Costing Ledgers

(1) **Stores Ledgers :** This ledger contains all stores accounts. A separate account is opened for each item of store.

(2) **Work-in-progress or Job Ledger :** This ledger records production during a period and the costs incurred. A separate account is opened for each job, product etc. in process.

(3) **Finished Goods or Stock Ledger :** The ledger records details of finished goods. A separate account is opened for each finished or completed product or job.

(4) **Cost Ledger :** It is the principal ledger of cost department. It contains:

(i) **Cost Control Accounts :** These accounts are maintained for the purpose of exercising control over the three Subsidiary ledgers discussed above and also to complete double entry in cost accounts. They summarise masses of detailed information contained in the subsidiary ledgers and thus provide immense help to management in policy formulation. They also facilitate reconciliation of cost and financial accounts.

The important cost control accounts are as follows :

(a) **Stores Ledger Control Account :** The purpose of stores ledger is to maintain item-wise record of raw materials and other stores. In cost ledger, a Stores Ledger Control Account is opened pertaining to this subsidiary ledger. The total materials received in stores (which can be found by looking at Purchases Journal) is shown on the debit side of Stores Ledger Control Account and the total materials issued out of Stores (which can be found by looking at Materials Abstract) is credited in the Account. The balance of this account shall tally with the total of the balances of the individual stores accounts in the Stores Ledger. Sometimes, separate ledgers are maintained for raw materials and other stores. In that case, there will be two separate control accounts namely Materials Ledger Control Account and Stores Ledger Control Account.

(b) **Work-in-progress Ledger Control Account :** For every job, product or process, cost of materials, labour and factory expenses are incurred. All such costs are debited in different accounts relating to different jobs. These accounts are kept in a job or work-in-progress ledger. A Work-in-progress Ledger Control Account is opened in the Cost Ledger. The cost of production of completed jobs will be credited to this account and the total expenses incurred on all the jobs debited so as to show the total work-in-progress at any time. The balance of this account must be equal to the total of individual balances of Job or Process accounts in the Job Ledger. The Work-in-progress Ledger Control account is referred to as Work-in-progress Account also.

(c) **Finished Goods Ledger Control Account :** In Finished Goods Ledger, a separate account is opened for recording the quantity and price of each and every finished products manufactured. In Cost Ledger, a Finished Goods Ledger Control Account is maintained. It represents the total value of finished goods in stock at a particular time.

(d) **General Ledger Adjustment Account :** In Cost Ledger, a General Ledger Adjustment Account is opened to record all items of income and expenditure. This account is also referred as Cost Ledger Control Account (in costing books). Personal Accounts are shown in financial accounts and not in cost accounts. The General Ledger Adjustment Account completes the double entry in the cost ledger and hence all such accounts which pertain to fixed assets or cash or outsiders are posted to this account. All expenditures are shown on the credit side of this account and the result of such expenditure in the form of sales is shown on the debit side of this account. The balance represents the value of stores, stock-in-hand and the amount of work-in-progress.

(e) **Cost Ledger Control Account (in financial books) :** Since the Costing Department is not distinct entity from the Financial Department and all the purchases and sales are recorded through financial books, a Cost Ledger Control Account must be opened in the financial books. This is only a memorandum account. In this account all the items of revenue and expenditure affecting Cost Accounts are recorded. This account is just the reverse or contra of the General Ledger Adjustment Account in the Cost Ledger and, therefore, the balance of this account should tally with the balance of its counterpart in the Cost Ledger.

(ii) **Other Accounts :** They include all other impersonal accounts (real as well as nominal) which affect costs, e.g., wages control account, factory overhead account, administration overhead account, selling and distribution overhead account, cost of sales account, etc. Sometimes, following additional accounts are also opened :

(a) **Overheads Suspense Account :** Sometimes, while valuing semi-finished jobs, works overheads are not included. Similarly while valuing closing stock of finished goods, office overheads are not charged. In such cases normally, at the end of an accounting period, the estimated amount of such overheads is debited to Works or Office Overheads Accounts, as the case may be. In the beginning of next accounting period, the entries are reserved to close the suspense accounts.

(b) **Capital Orders :** For each item of capital work to be performed in the factory itself, e.g., producing tools and equipments, certain expenditures shall be incurred in the form of materials, wages and other expenses. Such expenditures should be recorded in Capital Order Account and later on capitalised.

(c) **Service Orders :** If repairs and maintenance works are done in the factory, the cost is debited to Repairs and Maintenance Account and later transferred to various overheads accounts, because the expenditure might have been incurred on Production, Administration and Selling and Distribution Departments.

No separate account is maintained for Direct Expenses since they are directly charged to work-in-progress account.

When the finished goods are sold, they are transferred to Cost of Sales Account. In the last, a Costing Profit and Loss Account can be prepared with the help of all the above accounts.

PROCEDURE OF SELF-BALANCING

It is quite evident from the division of ledger that none of the ledgers contain all the information required for the preparation of a trial balance. For example, from the sales book the items are posted to the debit of the customer's concerned account in the sales ledger. The total of the sales book is posted to the credit of the sales account and being a nominal account is opened in the General Ledger. Thus sales ledger will be having all debit entries with the result neither of them is complete in itself for the preparation of a trial balance. Similarly, from the purchases book, the items are posted to the credit of suppliers accounts in the purchase ledger and total of purchases is posted to the debit of purchases account and being a nominal account, it will be opened in the general ledger. Thus purchase ledger contains credit entry while the general ledger contains the debit entry. These examples clearly show that none of the three ledgers contains in itself all the data for the preparation of a trial balance independently.

In order to make each ledger self balancing it is necessary that the ledger which contains debit entry should be provided with a credit entry and the one which contains debit entry should be provided with the credit entry. This is achieved by opening an extra account called General Ledger Adjustment Account in each of the sales and purchases ledger adjustment account in the general ledger. Contra entries of that are already recorded in one ledger will be posted to the adjustment accounts in each ledger. Such contra entries are made in monthly or periodical totals in order to save the clerical labour. As every entry in the ledger has its contra posting (in total) in the Adjustment Account which is opened at the end of each ledger, the double entry of every transaction is recorded in the same ledger. A separate trial balance can be prepared from each ledger in which balance on adjustment account opened at the end of the ledger is included and such trial balance must agree provided all the transactions are recorded correctly.

In order to make the ledgers self balancing, relevant changes will have to be made in the subsidiary books. Analysis columns will be added to the cash book, journal and to all other books of original entry.

The information required for the preparation of accounts under self-balancing system is obtained from the following subsidiary books :

1. **Cash Book :** Cash received from sundry debtors, cash paid to sundry creditors, discount received from creditors.

2. **Purchases Book :** Amount of credit purchases during a specified period.

3. **Sales Book :** Amount of credit sales made during a specified period.

4. **Purchases Returns Book :** Amount of purchases returns during a specified period.

5. **Sales Returns Book :** Amount of sales returns during a specified period.

6. **Bills Receivable Book :** Total amount of bills received from sundry debtors during a specified period.

7. **Bills Payable Book :** Total amount of bills accepted and given to creditors during a specified period.

8. **Journal :** Opening balances, bad and doubtful debts, interest, dishonour of bills, etc.

JOURNAL ENTRIES FOR SELF-BALANCING SALES LEDGER

All debtors accounts are opened in the Sales ledger and entries are made on the debit side of these accounts from the sales book. In order to make this ledger self balancing, a general ledger adjustment account is opened in sales ledger and all entries in totals appearing on the debit side of various debtors accounts will be shown on the credit side of this account and all credit entries of various debtors accounts on the debit side of this account.

In order to make the general ledger self-balancing a sales ledger adjustment account is opened in the general ledger. It will contain all entries of general ledger adjustment account (in sales ledger) but on reverse sides i.e. all entries appearing on the debit side of various debtors accounts are debited to sales ledger adjustment account (in general ledger) and all credit entries in the various debtors accounts are credited to sales ledger adjustment account (in general ledger).

The following journal entries are passed to make the sales ledger self-balancing :

(i) For credit sales, bills receivable dishonoured, interest and expenses charged to debtors during the period.

Sales Ledger Adjustment A/c   Dr.
    (in General Ledger)

    To General Ledger Adjustment A/c
    (in Sales Ledger)

(ii) For total of cash received from debtors, discount allowed to them, bills received, sales returns and bad debts written off.

General Ledger Adjustment A/c
    (in Sales Ledger)

    To Sales Ledger Adjustment A/c
    (in General Ledger)

JOURNAL ENTRIES FOR SELF-BALANCING PURCHASES LEDGER

All creditors accounts are opened in the purchases ledger and entries are made on the credit side of these accounts from the purchase book. In order to made this ledger self balancing, a general ledger adjustment account is opened in the purchases ledger and all entries in total appearing on the credit side of the various creditors will be shown on the debit side of this account and all debit entries of various creditors accounts on the credit of this account are shown.

In order to make the general ledger self balancing, a purchase ledger adjustment account is opened in the general ledger. It will contain all entries of general ledger adjustment account (in purchases ledger) but on the reverse side i.e. all entries appearing on the credit side of various creditors accounts are credited to purchases ledger adjustment (in general ledger) and all debit entries in the various creditors accounts are debited to purchases ledger adjustment account (in general ledger).

The following journal entries are passed to make the purchases ledger self balancing :

(i) For credit purchases, bills payable dishonoured, interest and expenses charged by creditors.
General Ledger Adjustment A/c
(in Purchase Ledger)
To Purchases Ledger Adjustment A/c
(in General Ledger)

(ii) For total cash paid to creditors, discount received, bills accepted and purchases returns :
Purchases Ledger Adjustment A/c
     (in General Ledger)
To General Ledger Adjustment A/c
     (in Purchases Ledger)

TRANSFER FROM ONE LEDGER TO ANOTHER

Sometimes goods are purchased from and sold to the same person but his personal account will be kept both in purchases and sales ledger. Settlement of such person's account will be made by deducting one account from the other and paying or being paid the balance. The same person cannot be a debtor and creditor of the firm, so his smaller account must be transferred to the greater, either from the purchases ledger to sales ledger or from sales ledger to the purchases ledger, as the case may be. Transfer entries must be made through the journal in order to avoid omission of such cases from the accounts. Suppose Hitesh's Account in purchases ledger shows a balance of Rs. 3,000 and in sales ledger a balance of Rs. 5,000. The former will, therefore, be transferred to the latter. The following entries are passed for this purpose :

Hitesh (in Purchases Ledger)   Dr. 3,000
          To Hitesh (in Sales Ledger)   3,000
(For transfer of balance from Hitesh's Account in purchases ledger to his account in sales ledger)
The following adjustment entries will also be made :

(i)   Purchases Ledger Adjustment A/c   Dr. 3,000
         (in General Ledger)
      To General Ledger Adjustment A/c   3,000
         (in Purchases Ledger)
      (For amount transferred from purchases ledger to sales ledger)

(ii) General Ledger Adjustment A/c   Dr. 3,000
         (in Sales Ledger)
      To Sales Ledger Adjustment A/c   3,000
         (in General Ledger)

26

TRIAL BALANCE

We know that the fundamental principle of Double Entry System of Accounting is that for every debit, there must be a corresponding credit. Thus, for every debit or a series of debits given to one or several accounts, there is a corresponding credit or a series of credits of an equal amount given to some other account or accounts and vice versa. It follows, therefore, that the sum total of debit amounts should equal the credit amounts of the ledger at any date. But if the various accounts in the ledger are balanced, then the total of all debit balances must be equal to the total of all credit balances if the books of accounts are arithmetically accurate.

Thus, at the end of the financial year or at any other time, the balances of all the ledger accounts are extracted and are written up in a statement known as Trial Balance and finally totalled up to see if the total of debit balances is equal to the total of credit balances. A Trial Balance may thus be defined as a statement of debit and credit totals or balances extracted from the various accounts in the ledger with a view to test the arithmetical accuracy of the books.

The agreement of the Trial Balance reveals that both the aspects of each transaction have been recorded and that the books are arithmetically accurate. If the Trial Balance does not agree, it shows that there are some errors which must be detected and rectified if the correct final accounts are to be prepared. Thus, Trial Balance forms a connecting link between the ledger accounts and the final accounts. The following are the main objectives of preparing the trial balance:

1. To have balances of all the accounts of the ledger in order to avoid the necessity of going through the pages of the ledger to find it out.
2. To have a proof that the double entry of each transaction has been recorded because of its agreement.
3. To have arithmetic accuracy of the books of accounts because of the agreement of the trial balance.

4. To have material for preparing the profit and loss account and balance sheet of the business.

LIMITATIONS OF TRIAL BALANCE

The following are the main limitations of the trial balance:

1. Trial Balance can be prepared only in whose concerns where double entry system of accounting is adopted. This system is very costly and cannot be adopted by the small concerns.

2 Though trial balance gives arithmetic accuracy of the books of accounts but there are certain errors which are not disclosed by the trial balance. That is why it is said that trial balance is not a conclusive proof of the accuracy of the books of accounts.

3. If trial balance is not prepared correctly then the final accounts prepared will not reflect the true and fair view of the state of affairs of the business. Whatever conclusions and decisions are made by the various groups of persons will not be correct and will mislead such persons.

PREPARATION OF TRIAL BALANCE

A trial balance can be prepared by the following two methods:

1. **Total Method :** In this method, the debit and credit totals of each account are shown in the two amount columns (one for the debit total and the other for the credit total) against it.

2. **Balance Method :** In this method, the difference of each amount is extracted. If debit side of an account is bigger in amount than the credit side, the difference is put in the debit column of the Trial Balance and if the credit side is bigger, the difference is written in the credit column of the Trial Balance.

Trial Balance can be prepared on a loose sheet having four columns. A specimen is given as follows:

TRIAL BALANCE OF ....

As on ....

Serial No.	Name of the Account	Dr. Balance (or Total) Rs.	Cr. Balance (or Total) Rs.

Of the two methods of preparation, the second is usually used in practice because it facilitates the preparation of the final accounts.

Example 1. The following Trial Balance has been prepared wrongly. You are asked to prepare the Trial Balance correctly.

Name of Accounts	Debit Balance Rs.	Credit Balance Rs.
Cash in hand		2,000
Purchases Returns	4,000	
Wages	8,000	
Establishment Expenses	12,000	
Sales Returns		8,000
Capital	22,000	
Carriage Outward		2,000
Discount Received	1,200	
Commission Earned	800	
Machinery		20,000
Stock		10,000
Debtors	8,000	
Creditors		12,000
Sales		44,000
Purchases	28,000	
bank Overdraft	14,000	
Manufacturing Expenses		14,000
Loan from Ashok	14,000	
Carriage Inward	1,000	
Interest on Investments		1,000
	1,13,000	1,13,000

SOLUTION

CORRECT TRIAL BALANCE

as at ......

Name of Accounts	Debit Balance Rs.	Credit Balance Rs.
Cash in hand	2,000	
Purchases Returns		4,000
Wages	9,000	
Establishment Expenses	12,000	
Sales Returns	8,000	
Capital		22,000
Carriage Outward	2,000	
Discount Received		1,200
Commission Earned		800
Machinery	20,000	
Stock	10,000	
Debtors	8,000	
Creditors		12,000
Sales		44,000
Purchases	28,000	
Bank Overdraft		14,000
Manufacturing Expenses	14,000	
Loan from Ashok		14,000
Carriage Inward	1,000	
Interest on Investments		1,000
	1,13,000	1,13,000

ERRORS

The agreement of a Trial Balance is not a conclusive proof as to the absolute accuracy of the books. It only gives an indication of the arithmetical accuracy.

The Trial Balance may agree and yet there may be some errors of the following types remaining undisclosed :

1. **Omission of an Entry in a Subsidiary Books :** If an entry has not been recorded in a subsidiary book, both the debit and credit of that transaction would be omitted and the agreement of the Trial Balance will not be affected in any way.

2. **A Wrong Entry in a Subsidiary Book :** If a credit purchase of Rs.465 from Anno is wrongly written as Rs.564 in the Purchase Book, such an error will not be disclosed by the Trial Balance. As the posting on both the debit side of Purchases Account and credit side of Annu's Account will be with the wrong amount of Rs.564, so the Trial Balance will agree.

3. **Posting an Item to the Correct Side but in the Wrong Account :** If a purchase of Rs.500 from Ravi Kant has been credited to Man Mohan instead of Ravi Kant, it will not affect the agreement of the Trial Balance, so the Trial Balance will not detect such an error.

4. **Compensating Errors :** These are errors which compensate themselves in the net result i.e., over-debits or under-debits of various accounts being neutralized by the over-credits or under-credits to the same extent of some other accounts. For example, under-posting of Rs.500 on the debit side of a certain account would be compensated by underposting of Rs.100 on the credit side of another account and an omission of credit posting of Rs.400 to a third account. It is quite possible that this error may also be neutralised by overposting of Rs.500 on the debit side in some other account or accounts.

5. **Errors of Principle :** These errors will not affect the agreement of the Trial Balance as they arise from the debiting or crediting of wrong heads of accounts as would be inconsistent with the fundamental principles of double entry accounting. For example,Rs.6,550 spent on extension of building wrongly debited to Repairs Accounts instead of Building Account will not affect the agreement of the Trial Balance. Thus, such errors arise whenever an asset is treated as an expense or vice versa or a liability is treated as an income or vice versa.

The disagreement of the Trial Balance will disclose the following classes of errors:

1. **An Item Omitted to be Posted from a Subsidiary Book into the Ledger:** i.e. A purchase of Rs. 1,000 from Navin omitted to be credited to his account. As a result of this error, the figure of sundry creditors to be shown in the Trial Balance will reduce by Rs. 1,000 and the total of credit side of the Trial Balance will be Rs. 1,000 less as compared to the debit side of the Trial Balance.

2. **Posting of Wrong Amount to a Ledger Account :** i.e. credit sale of Rs. 2,000 to Arti wrongly posted to her account as Rs. 200. The effect of this

error will be that the figure of sundry debtors will be reduced by Rs. 1,800 and the total of the debit side of the Trial Balance will be Rs. 1,800 less than the total of the credit side of the Trial Balance.

3. **Posting an Amount to the Wrong Side of the Ledger Account :** i.e. Rs. 50 discount allowed to a customer wrongly posted to the credit instead of the debit of the Discount Account. As a result of this error, the credit side of the Trial Balance will exceed by Rs. 100 (double the amount of the error).

4. **Wrong Additions or Balancing of Ledger Accounts :** i.e. while balancing Capital Account at the end of the financial year, credit balance of Rs. 89,000 wrongly taken as Rs. 79,000. As a result of this error, the credit total of the Trial Balance will be Rs. 10,000 too short.

5. **Wrong Totaling of Subsidiary Books :** i.e. Sales Book is overcast by Rs. 10. As a result of this error, credit side of the Trial Balance will be Rs. 10 too much because Sales Account will appear at a higher figure on the credit side of the Trial Balance.

6. **An Item in the Subsidiary Book Posted Twice to a Ledger Account:** i.e., a payment of Rs. 1,000 to a creditor twice to his account.

7. Omission of a balance of an account in the Trial Balance, i.e. cash and bank balances may have been omitted to be included in the Trial Balance.

8. Balance of some account wrongly entered in Trial balance, i.e. a balance of Rs. 513 in Stationery Account wrongly entered as Rs. 315 in the Trial Balance.

9. Balance of some account written to the wrong side of the Trial Balance, i.e., balance of Commission Earned Account wrongly shown to the debit side instead of the credit side of the Trial Balance.

10. An error in the totalling of the Trial Balance will bring the disagreement of the Trial Balance.

Example 2. A book-keeper, taking out a trial balance as on 30th May, 1991 found that it did not agree. He proceeded to check the entries and discovered the following errors :

1. A credit sale of Rs. 1,000 to Ajay had been correctly entered in the Sales Book but Ashok's Account had been debited with Rs. 100 only.

2. The total of the Bills Payable Book, Rs. 5,000 had been posted to the credit of Bills Receivable Account.

3. Rs. 2,500 paid to Sohan had been wrongly posted to Madan.

4. Rs. 100 owing by a customer had been omitted from the list of debtors.

5. The discount column of the Cash Book representing discount allowed to customer has been over-added by Rs. 10.

6. Goods worth Rs. 100 taken by the proprietor omitted to be recorded in the books.

7. Depreciation on furniture, Rs. 100, had not been posted to Depreciation Account.

8. The total of Sales Book had been added Rs. 1,000 short.

Which of the above errors caused the totals of the Trial Balance to disagree and by how much did the totals differ ?

SOLUTION

The effect of the above noted errors on the Trial Balance will be as follows:

1. Ashok's Account has been given less debit for Rs. 9000, so the debit side of the Trial Balance would be short by Rs. 900.

2. This error will not affect the agreement of the Trial Balance because the posting of the Bills Payable Book has been made to the correct side but in the wrong Account. The credit given to Bills Received Account instead of Bills Payable Account does not affect the agreement of the Trial Balance.

3. This error will not affect the agreement of the Trial Balance because the amount paid has been posted to right side though to a wrong account.

4. Sundry debtors have been shown in the Trial Balance with a less amount of Rs. 100, so debit side of the Trial Balance is short by Rs. 100.

5. Discount Account has been given an excess debit of Rs. 10 so debit side of the Trial Balance exceeds by Rs. 10.

6. This error will have no affect on the agreement of the Trial Balance because the dual aspect of the entry has been omitted i.e., neither of the two accounts involved in this transaction has been given debit or credit.

7. Depreciation of furniture has not been debited to Depreciation Account, so debit side of the Trial Balance will be Rs. 100 too short.

8. Sales Account has been given less credit for Rs. 1,000, so credit side of the Trial Balance would be short by Rs. 1,000.

The combined affect of all the errors is that the credit side of the Trial Balance would exceed the debit side by Rs. 90.

LOCATION OF ERRORS

Whenever a Trial Balance disagrees, the following steps should be taken to locate the causes of the difference :

1. Re-check the totals of the Trial Balance and ascertain the exact amount difference in the Trial Balance.

2. Divide the difference of the Trial Balance by two and find out if there is any balance of the same amount in the Trial Balance. It may be that such a balance might have been recorded on the wrong side of the Trial Balance, thus causing a difference of double the amount.

3. If the mistake is not located by the above steps, the difference in the Trial Balance should be divided by 9. If the difference is evenly divisible by 9, the error may be due to transposition or transplacement of figures. A transposition occurs when 57 is written as 75, 197 as 791 and so on. A transplacement takes place when the digits of the numbers are moved to the left or right, e.g. when Rs. 5,694 is written as Rs. 56.94 or Rs. 569-40. If there is a transposition or transplacement of figures, the search can be narrowed down to numbers where these errors might have been made.

4. See that the balances of all accounts including cash and bank balances have been included in the Trial Balance.

5. See that the opening balances have been correctly brought forward in the current year's books.

6. If the difference is of a large amount, compare the Trial Balance of the current year with that of the previous year and see that the figures under similar head of accounts are very near the same as those of the previous year and whether their balance fall on the same side of the Trial Balance. If the difference between the previous year figures and the current year figures is large one, establish the cause of difference.

7. If the above listed steps fail to detect the errors, check your work as follows ;

    (a) Check the totals of the subsidiary books paying particular attention to 'carry forwards'.

    (b) Check the posting made from the Journal or subsidiary books in the ledger.

    (c) Re-check the balances extracted from ledger.

    (d) Re-cast the list of balances.

If all these efforts fail to locate the errors, all the books of prime entry (subsidiary books) must be cast, and, if necessary, the postings to the ledger should be re-checked.

27

PROFIT AND LOSS ACCOUNT

This account is prepared to calculate the net profit of the business. There are certain items of incomes and expenses of the business which must be taken into consideration for calculating net profit of the business. These are of indirect nature, i.e. concerning the whole business and relating to various activities which are done by the business for the purpose of making the goods available to the consumers. Indirect expenses may be selling and distribution expenses, management expenses, financial expenses, extraordinary losses and expenses to maintain the assets into working order. This account is prepared from nominal accounts and its balance is transferred to capital account as the whole profit or loss will be that of owner and it will increase or decrease his capital. The specimen proforma of this account is given below:

PROFIT AND LOSS A/c
For the year ended 31st December, 1991

	Rs.		Rs.
To Gross Loss b/d		By Gross Profit b/d	
To selling and Distribution		" Interest Received	
Expenses :		" Discount	
Advertisement		" Commission	
Travellers' Salaries, Expenses		" Rent from Tenants	
& Commission		" Income from Investments	
Bad Debts		" Apprenticeship Premium	
Godown Rent		" Interest on Debentures	
Export Expenses		" Income from any other Source	
Carriage Outwards		" Miscellaneous Revenue Receipts	
Bank Charges		" By Net Loss transferred to	
		Capital A/c	
To Management Expenses :			
Rent, Rates and Taxes			
Heating and Lighting			
Office Salaries			
Printing & Stationery			
Postage & Telegrams			

Telephone Charges			
Legal Charges			
Audit Fees			
Insurance			
General Expenses			
To Depreciation and Maintenance :			
Depreciation			
Repairs & Maintenance			
To Financial Expenses :			
Discount Allowed			
Interest on Capital			
Interest on Loans			
Discount on Bills			
To Extraordinary Expenses :			
Loss by fire (not covered by			
Insurance)			
Cash defalcations			
To Net profit transferred to			
Capital A/c			

Important Points in Profit and Loss Account

1. **Salaries :** These include salaries paid to office, godown and warehouse staff and should be shown in Profit and Loss Account being indirect expenses. Salaries to partners must be debited separately. Salaries and wages are treated as unproductive and shown in Profit and Loss Account. If salaries are paid after deduction of Income tax or Provident Fund then these should be added back to the salaries in order to have gross figure of salaries to be shown in Profit and Loss Account.

   If salaries are paid in kind by providing certain facilities to the employees such as house free of rent, meals or cloth or washing facility free charge, e.g. in hospitals, hotels, farms, etc., then the value of such facilities should be regarded as salaries.

2. **Rent, Rates and Taxes :** These include offices and warehouse rent, municipal rates and taxes. Factory rent, rates and taxes should be debited to Trading Account and others to Profit and Loss Account. If any rent is received on sub-letting of the building, the same should be shown separately on the credit side of the Profit and Loss A/c. If rent is paid after deduction of some taxes, then these should be added back to know the correct amount of rent payable.

3. **Interest :** Interest paid on loans, overdrafts and bills overdue is an expense and is taken to the debit of Profit and Loss Account. Interest received on loans advances by the firm, on deposits and on securities is a gain and is shown on the credit side of Profit and Loss Account A/c. Interest on capital should be shown separately on the debit side and interest on drawings on the credit side of Profit and Loss Account.

4. **Commission :** Commission received for doing the work of other firms may be credited to profit and loss as a gain and commission payable to the agents employed to sell the firm's goods debited as an expense.

5. **Repairs :** Repairs and small renewals or replacements relating to the plant and machinery, fixtures, fittings and utensils, etc. are generally included under this heading and such expenditure, being as expense, is debited to profit and loss account.

6. **Depreciation :** It is an expense due to wear and tear, lapse of time and exhaustion of assets used in business. This is loss sustained by fixed assets and should be charged to Profit and Loss Account.

7. **Stable Expenses :** These are incurred for the fodder of the horse and wages paid to persons looking after stable. Being indirect expenses these should debited to profit and loss account.

8. **Trade Expenses :** These are expenses of a varied nature for which it is not worthy to open separate accounts. They are amalgamated under trade or general or sundry or petty expenses. These are debited to profit and loss account being miscellaneous business expenses.

9. **Samples :** Samples of the goods manufactured by the business concerns are often distributed free of charge to push up sales. Being indirect expenses these are debited to profit and loss account.

10. **Advertisement :** All sums spent on advertising should be charged to Profit and Loss Account. If a large amount is paid under a contract covering two or three years, proportionate part should be shared to Profit and Loss Account and the balance appears as an asset in the Balance Sheet.

11. **Apprentice Premium :** This is the amount charged from a person to whom training is given by the business. It is a gain and should be credited to Profit and Loss Account. If some amount of apprentice premium has been received in advance, due adjustment must be done in order to calculate the correct amount of income.

Expenses not to be shown in Profit and Loss A/c

1. **Domestic and Household Expenses :** These expenses are not shown in Profit and Loss Account, as these are personal expenses of the proprietor and should be treated as drawings.

2. **Income Tax :** It should be treated as a personal expense of the proprietor and added to drawings. It should not be shown as an expense in Profit and Loss A/c.

3. **Life Insurance Premium :** Premium paid on the life policy of proprietary should be charged to the Drawings Account.

Closing Entries for Profit and Loss A/c

1. For transfer of various expenses to Profit & Loss A/c

Profit and Loss A/c

    To Various Expenses A/c Dr.

2. For transfer of various incomes and gains to Profit & Loss A/c.

    Various Income & Gains A/c Dr.

        To Profit & Loss A/c

3. (a) For Net Profit   (b) For Net Loss

    Profit & Loss A/c   Capital A/c   Dr.

        To Capital A/c   To Profit & Loss A/c

Example 1. From the following balances extracted at the close of year ended 31 December 1989, prepare Profit and Loss Account as at that date :

	Rs.		Rs.
Gross Profit	51,000	Discount (Dr.)	500
Carriage Outward	2,500	Discount (Dr.)	1,500
Salaries	5,500	Printing & Stationery	250
Rent	1,100	Rates & Taxes	350
Fire Insurance Premium	900	Travelling Expenses	200
Bad Debts	2,100	Sundry Trade Expenses	300
Commission Received	1,000	Discount allowed by Creditors	800

Profit & Loss Account of M/s. ......

For the year ended 31st December, 1991

	Rs.		Rs.
To Carriage Outward	2,500	By Gross Profit b/d	51,000
Salaries	5,500	Apprentice Premium	1,500
Rent	1,100	Discount by Creditors	800
Fire Insurance Premium	900	Commission	1,000
Bad Debts	2,100		
Discount	500		
Printing & Stationery	250		
Rent & Taxes	350		
Travelling Expenses	200		
Sundry Trade Expenses	300		
To Net Profit transferred to			
Capital A/c	40,600		
	54,300		54,300

Requirements as to 'Profit & Loss A/c' :

The requirement as to profit and loss account can be put into two categories:

1. General Requirements ; and

2. Special Requirements as per Schedule-VI Part II

1. **General Requirements** : These basically relate to three matters :

    (i) **Heading** : In case of companies, it is not necessary to split the profit and loss account into three sections, viz. Trading Account, Profit and Loss Account and Profit & Loss Appropriation Account. Of course splitting up of the account into three sections is not forbidden and should be done to give a better view about the profit earned and distributed by the company during particular period. The Profit & Loss Account can be prepared under two headings :

(a) Profit & Loss Account giving details regarding the Gross Profit and the Net Profit earned by the company during a particular period.

(b) Profit & Loss Appropriation Account giving details regarding the balance of Profit & loss A/c brought forward from the last year, the Net Profit (or loss) earned (or made) during the year and appropriations made during the year.

Items which are shown in the Profit & Loss Account are popularly terms as items appearing - "above the line". While the items which are shown in the Profit & Loss Appropriation Account are popularly termed as items appearing "below the line".

(ii) **Provision for Taxation :** Companies are charged income tax at a high rate. Usually the tax rate is about 50% or more of the taxable profits. Though provisions for taxation is an appropriation of profits, yet the common practice is to show it above the line, i.e. in Profit & Loss Section and not in Profit & Loss Appropriation Section. In other words profit after tax is taken from "Profit & Loss Account" to "Profit & Loss Appropriation Account".

(iii) **Accounting Year :** Though the Companies Act permits a company to select any period of 12 months as its accounting year. However, on account of tax laws it has become almost obligatory for every company to close its books of accounts on 31st March, every year.

2. **Special Requirements as per Schedule VI : Part II :** The Profit & Loss Account of a company must be prepared in accordance with the requirement of Part II of Schedule VI of the Companies Act, 1956. These requirements are summarised as follows :

(a) The Profit & Loss Account should clearly disclose the result of the working of the company during the period covered by the account. It should disclose separately incomes and expenses of a non-recurring nature and exceptional transactions. The Profit & Loss Account should particularly disclose information in respect of the following items :

(i) The turn-over of the company

(ii) Commission paid to sole-selling agents

(iii) Commission paid to other selling agents

(iv) Brokerage and discount on sales other than the usual trade discount

(v) Opening and closing of goods, purchases made or cost of goods manufactured or value of services rendered during the period covered by the account.

- (vi) Interest on company's debentures and other fixed loans

- (vii) Amount charged to income tax

- (viii) Remuneration payable to the managerial personnel

- (ix) Amount paid to auditors for services rendered as - (a) auditor and (b) as advisor in any other capacity, viz. taxation matters, company law matters, management services, etc.

- (x) The details of licensed, installed and actual capacity utilized.

- (xi) Value or imports, earnings in foreign exchange and amounts remitted during the year in foreign currencies on account of dividends.

28

BALANCE SHEET

A Balance Sheet is a statement prepared with a view to measure the financial position of a business on a certain fixed dated. The financial position of a concern is indicated by its assets on a given date and its liabilities on that date. Excess of assets over liabilities represent the capital and is indicative of the financial soundness of a company. A Balance Sheet is also described as a 'statement showing the sources and application of capital'. It is a statement and not an account and prepared from real and personal accounts. The left hand side of the balance sheet may be viewed as a description of the sources from which the business has obtained the capital with which it currently operates and the right hand side as a description of the form in which that capital is invested on a specified date.

On the left hand side of the balance sheet, the several liability items describe how much capital was obtained from trade creditors, from banks, from bill holders and other outside parties. The owner's equity section shows the capital supplied by the owner.

Capital obtained from various sources has been invested according to managements, best judgement of the optimum mix or combination of assets for the business. A certain fraction is invested in buildings, another fraction in stock, another fraction is retained as cash for current need of the business and so on. The assets side of the balance sheet, therefore, shows the result of these management judgements as on the date of the balance sheet.

A properly drawn up balance sheet gives information relating to (1) the nature and value of assets, (2) the nature and extent of liabilities, (3) whether the firm is solvent, (4) whether the firm is overtrading.

If assets exceed the liabilities, the firm is solvent, i.e., able to pay its debts in full. A business is, therefore, sovlent by the amount of ownership capital in it, as it is the excess of assets over liabilities. The last point, i.e. (4) concerns the stability of the business. If the total of the debts due to creditors (including bank, overdraft) is greater than the liquid assets (i.e., cash, investment, bills, etc.) the position of the firm may be financially unsound. Where the debts are being incurred without sufficient means of payment, the firm is said to be overtrading. For the position to be quite sound, there should be some working capital, i.e., some spare liquid assets available for current expenditure. It is not a wise policy to lock up the capital in fixed assets. The concern may be solvent without being sound.

Classification of Assets and Liabilities

Assets : Assets are property and possession of a business. Stock, land and buildings, book debts, cash, bills receivables are some examples of assets. The classification of assets depends on their nature. The various types of assets are :

1. **Fixed Assets :** Those assets which are acquired and held permanently in the business and are used for the purpose of earning profits are called fixed assets. Land and buildings, machinery, furniture and fixtures are some examples of these assets.

2. **Current Assets :** Those assets such as cash, debtors and stock that can be realised and readily available to discharge liabilities are called current assets.

3. **Tangible Assets :** These are definite assets which can be seen, touched and have volume such as machinery, cash, stock, etc.

4. **Fictitious Assets :** These assets are fictitious in nature, i.e., they are virtually not assets. These are either the past accumulated losses or expenses which are incurred once in the life of a business and are capitalized for the time being. Profit and loss account (debit balance), organisation expenses, discount on the issue of shares, advertisement expenses capitalized for the time being are examples of such assets.

5. **Intangible Assets :** Those assets which cannot be seen, touched and have no volume but have value are called intangible assets. Goodwill, patents and trade marks are examples of such assets but quite valuable to undertaking. An intangible asset may not be fictitious. If on account of the past goodwill purchased along with an existing concern, sales are readily effected and profit is readily earned, the asset is certainly not fictitious though it is intangible. However, if the amount of goodwill was paid in respect of a losing concern, the asset would be fictitious.

6. **Wasting Assets :** Those assets as mines, quarries etc. that become exhausted or reduce in value by their working are called wasting assets.

7. **Liquid Assets :** These are cash or such items as marketable securities which can be converted into cash quickly.

8. **Contingent Assets :** It is an asset the existence, value and ownership of which is dependent on the occurrence or non-occurrence of a specified act. Suppose a firm has filed a suit for some specified property now in

possession of someone else. If the suit is decided in firm's favour, the firm will get the property. At the moment it is contingent asset. Similar would be the position of a patent applied for arising of a firm's own research effort. Contingent liability in respect of a contract for capital expenditure already entered into will give rise to an asset on payment, at present it is only a contingent asset.

Liabilities : A liability is an amount which a busines is legally bound to pay. It is a claim by an outsider on the assets of a business. Liabilities may be classified into four categories :

1. **Fixed Liabilities :** These are those liabilities which are payable only on the termination of the business such as capital which is a liability to the owner.

2. **Long Term Liabilities :** Those liabilities which are not payable within the next accounting period but will be payable within next five to ten years are called long term liabilities such as debentures.

3. **Current Liabilities :** Those liabilities which are payable out of current assets within the next accounting period usually year or already due are called current liabilities. Sundry creditors, bills payable, and short term bank overdraft are examples of such liabilities.

4. **Contingent Liabilities :** A contingent liability is one which is not an actual liability but which will become an actual one on the happening of some event which is uncertain. Thus such liabilities have two characteristics : (a) uncertainty as to whether the amount will be payable at all, and (b) uncertainty about the amount involved. It is sufficient if the amount of such liability is stated on the face of the Balance Sheet by way of a note unless there is a probability that a loss will materialise. In that event it is no more a contingent liability and a specific provision should be made therefore. Examples of such liabilities are :

   (a) Claims against the companies not acknowledged as debts.
   (b) Uncalled liability on partly paid up shares.
   (c) Arrears of fixed cumulative dividend.
   (d) Estimated amount of contracts remaining to be executed on capital account and not provided for.
   (e) Liability of a case pending in the court.
   (f) Bills of exchange, guarantees given against a particular firm or person.

Grouping and Marshalling of Assets & Liabilities

The arrangement of assets and liabilities in certain groups and in a particular order is called Grouping and Marshalling of the Balance Sheet of a business. Assets and liabilities can be arranged in the Balance Sheet into two ways :

1. In order of liquidity
2. In order of permanence

1. **In order of Liquidity :** When assets and liabilities are arranged according to their realisability and payment preferences, such an order is called liquidity order. Such arrangement is given in Balance Sheet (I).

2. **In order of Permanence :** When the order is reversed from that what is followed in case of liquidity, it is called order of permanence. This order is followed in case of joint stock companies compulsorily but can be followed in other concerns also. Fixed assets and liabilities are shown first on the assumption that these will be sold or paid only on the insolvency of a business. This order of Balance Sheet is given in Balance Sheet (II).

Balance Sheet (I)

Liabilities	Rs.	Assets	Rs.
Current Liabilities :		Liquid Assets :	
Bills Payable		Cash in Hand	
Sundry Creditors		Cash at Bank	
Bank Overdraft		Floating Assets :	
Long Term Liabilities :		Sundry Debtors	
Loan from Bank		Investments	
Debentures		Bills Receivable	
Fixed Liabilities :		Stock in Trade	
Capital		Prepaid Expenses	
		Fixed Assets :	
		Machinery	
		Building	
		Furniture & Fixtures	
		Motor Car	
		Fictitious Assets :	
		Advertisement	
		Misc. Expenses	
		Profit & Loss A/c	
		Intangible Assets	
		Goodwill	
		Patents	
		Copyright	
Total	_____	Total	_____

Note : For contingent liabilities, if any.

Balance Sheet (II)

Liabilities	Rs.	Assets	Rs.
1. Fixed Liabilities		1. Intangible Assets	
2. Long Term Liabilities		2. Fictitious Assets	
3. Current Liabilities		3. Fixed Assets	
		4. Floating Assets	
		5.. Liquid Assets	

According to Section 210 of the Companies Act, a company is required to prepare a balance sheet at the end of each trading period. Section 211 requires the balance sheet to be set up in the prescribed form. This provision is not applicable to banking, insurance, electricity and other companies governed by special Acts. The Central Government has also the power to exempt any class of companies from compliance with the requirements of the prescribed form if it deems to be in public interest. The object of prescribing the form is to elicit proper information from the company so as to give a 'true and fair' view of the state of the company's affairs. As a matter of fact both window dressing and creating secret reserves will be considered against the provision of Section 211.

Schedule VI Part-I gives the prescribed form of a company's balance sheet. Notes and instructions regarding various items have been given in brackets below each item. It may be noted that if information required to be given under any of the items or sub-items in the prescribed form cannot be conveniently given on account of lack of space, it may be given in a separate schedule or schedules. Such schedules will be annexed to and from part of the balance sheet.

Schedule VI, Part I permits presentation of balance sheet both in horizontal as well as vertical forms.

Notes :

1. Paise can also be given in addition to rupees, if desired.

2. Dividends declared by subsidiary companies after the date of the balance sheet should not be included unless they are in respect of a period which closed on or before the date of the balance sheet.

3. Any reference to benefits expected from contracts to the extent not executed shall not be made in the balance sheet but shall be made in the Board's report.

4. Particulars of any redeemed debentures which the company has power to issues should be given.

5. Where any of the company's debentures are held by a nominee or a trustee for the company, the nominal amount of the debentures and the amount at which they are stated in the books of the company shall be stated.

6. A statement of investments (whether shown under "investment" or under "current assets" as stock-in-trade) separately classifying trade investments and other investments should be annexed to the balance-sheet, showing the names of the bodies corporate (including separately the names of the bodies corporate under the same management) in whose shares or debentures, investments have been made (including all investments whether existing or not, made subsequent to the date as at which the previous balance-sheet was made out) and the nature and

extent of the investments so made in each such body corporate; provided that in the case of an investment company, that is to say, a company whose principal business is the acquisition of shares, stock, debentures or other securities, it shall be sufficient if the statment shows only the investments existing on the date as at which the balance-sheet has been made out. In regard to the investments in the capital of partership firms, the names of the firm (with the names of all their partners, total capital and the shares of each partner) shall be given in the statement.

7. If, in the opinion of the Board, any of the current assets, loans and advances have not a value on realisation in the ordinary course of business at least equal to the amount at which they are stated, the fact that the Board is of that opinion shall be stated.

8. Except in the case of the first balance sheet laid before the company after the commencement of the Act, the corresponding amount of the immediately preceding financing year for all items shown in the balance sheet shall be also given in the balance sheet. The requirements in this behalf shall, in case of companies preparing quarterly or half-yearly accounts, etc., relate to the balance sheet for the corresponding date in the previous year.

9. Current accounts with Directors and Managers, whether they are credit or debit, shall be shown separately.

10. The information required to be given under any of the items or sub-items in the form, if it cannot be conveniently included in the balance sheet itself, shall be furnished in a separate schedule or schedules to be annexed to and forming part of the balance sheet. This is recommended when items are numerous.

11. Where the original cost (of fixed assets) and additions and deductions thereto, relate to any fixed assets which has been acquired from a country outside India, and in consequence of a change in the rate of exchange at any time after the acquisition of such assets, there has been an increase or reduction in the liability of the company, as expressed in Indian currency, for making payment towards the whole or a part of the cost of the asset, or for repayment of the whole or a part of monies borrowed by the company from any person, directly or indirectly, in any foreign currency specifically for the purpose of acquiring the asset (being in either cases the liability existing immediately before the date on which the change in the rate of exchange takes effect), the amount by which the liability is so increased or reduced during the year, shall be added to, or as the case may be, deducted from the cost, and the amount arrived at after such addition or deduction shall be taken to be the cost of the fixed assets.

29

FINANCIAL STATEMENTS ANALYSIS

MEANING OF FINANCIAL STATEMENTS

Financial statements at least refer to the two statements which are prepared by a business concern at the end of the year. These are : (i) Income statement of trading and profit and loss account which is prepared by a business concern in order to know the profit earned and loss sustained during a specified period; (ii) Position statement or Balance Sheet which is prepared by a business concern on a particular date in order to know its financial position. To these statements are added the statement of Retained Earnings and some other statements (as funds flow statement, cash flow statement, etc.) and schedules of fixed assets (as Investments, Equipments) and Debtors, etc. to give a full view of the financial affairs. All these statements are collectively called as package of financial statements. Statement of earnings (when prepared separately) or Profit and Loss Appropriation Account shows the utilisation of profits of the company i.e., dividend declared, amount transferred to general reserve or any other reserve as shown in this account. Funds flow statements summarises the changes in working capital in a specified period and indicates the various sources and applications of funds. Cash flow statement gives the various items of inflow and outflow of cash. Various schedules of fixed assets are prepared by companies to show as to how the figure shown in the balance sheet has been arrived at.

NATURE OF FINANCIAL STATEMENTS

Financial statements are prepared for the purpose of presenting a periodical review or report by the management and deal with the state of investment in business and result achieved during the period under review. They reflect a combination of recorded facts, accounting conventions and personal judge-ments and conventions applied affect them materially. From this it is clear that financial statements are affected by these things, i.e. recorded facts, accounting conventions and personal judgements. Only those facts which are recorded in the business books will be reflected in the financial statements. For example, fixed assets are recorded in the books at cost price and shown in the balance sheet at cost price irrespective of their market or realisable price. Again, financial statements are prepared by following certain principles which are in use from a long time. All anticipated losses are to be provided whereas anticipated profits are not to be taken into account while preparing financial statements. Such convention wil not reflect the true position of the business as the actual position of the business will definitely be better as compared to the position depicted from the financial statements. Personal judgement of the accountant again will reflect the preparation of financial statements. For example, the choice of the method of depreciation or which expenditure is to be capitalised or not will also affect the preparation of the financial statements.

The following points reflect truely the nature of financial statements of business entities :

(i) These are reports or summarised reviews about the performance, achievements and weakness of the business.

(ii) These are prepared at the end of the accounting period so that various parties may take decisions of their future actions in respect of the relationship with the business.

(iii) The reliability of financial statements depends on the reliability of accounting data. These statements cannot be said to be true and fair representatives of the strength or profitability of the concern if there are numerous frauds and defalcations in the accounts.

(iv) The figures in the financial statements are a combination of recorded facts. There may be certain developments and factors which may be very important for the business are not taken into account as these are not recorded in the routine of accounting. Moreover, fixed assets are recorded at historical value without taking into consideration the changes in their values due to price level fluctuations.

(v) These statements are prepared as per accounting concepts and conventions.

(vi) These statements are influenced by the personal judgement of the accountant though he is expected to be more objective in his approach. These judgements may relate to valuation of inventory, depreciation of fixed assets and while making distinction between capital and revenue.

IMPORTANCE OF FINANCIAL STATEMENTS

The information given in the financial statements is very useful to a number of parties. These are the following :

1. **Owners :** The owners provide funds for the operations of a business and they want to know whether their funds are being properly utilised or not.

The financial statements prepared from time to time satisfy their curiosity.

2. **Creditors :** Creditors (i.e., suppliers of goods and services on credit, bankers and other lender of money) want to know the financial position of a concern before giving loans or granting credit. The financial statements help them in judging such position.

3. **Investors :** Prospective investors, who want to invest money in a firm, would like to make an analysis of the financial statements of that firm to know how safe the proposed investment will be.

4. **Employees :** Employees are interested in the financial position of a concern they serve, particularly when payment of bonus depends upon the size of the profits earned. They would like to know that the bonus being paid to them is correct; so they become interested in the preparation of correct Profit and Loss Account.

5. **Government :** Central and State Governments are interested in the financial statements because they reflect the earnings for a particular period for purposes of taxation. Moreover, these financial statements are used for compiling statistics concerning business which, in turn, help in compiling notional accounts.

6. **Research Scholars :** The financial statements, being a mirror of the financial position of a firm, are of immense value to the research scholar who wants to make a study into financial operations of a particular firm.

7. **Consumers :** Consumers are interested in the establishment of good accounting control so that cost of production may be reduced with the resultant reduction of the prices of goods they buy.

8. **Managers :** Management is the art of getting things done through others. This requires that the subordinates are doing work properly. Financial statements are an aid in this respect because they serve the manager in appraising the performance of the subordinates. Actual results achieved by the employees can be measured against the budegeted performanced they are expected to achieve and remedial action can be taken if the performance is not upto the mark.

LIMITATIONS OF FINANCIAL STATEMENTS

The following are the main limitations of the financial statements :

(i) **Interim and not final reports :** Financial statements do not depict the exact position and are essential interim reports. The exact position can be only known if the business is closed.

(ii) **Lack of precision and definiteness :** Financial statements may not be realistic because these are prepared by following certain basic concepts and conventions. For example, going concern concept gives us an idea that business will continue and assets are to be recorded at cost but the book value at which the asset is shown may not be actually realisable.

Similarly, by following the principle of conservatism the financial statements will not reflect the true position of the business.

(iii) **Lack of objective judgement :** Financial statements are influenced by the personal judgement of the accountant. He may select any method for depreciation, valuation of stock, amortisation of fixed assets and treatment of deferred revenue expenditure. Such judgement if based on integrity and competency of the accontant will definitely affect the preparation of the financial statements.

(iv) **Records only monetary facts :** Financial statements disclose only monetary facts, i.e., those transactions are recorded in the books of accounts which can be measured in monetary terms. Those transactions which cannot be measured in monetary terms such as, conflict between production manager and marketing manager may be very important for a business concern but not recorded in the business books.

(v) **Historical in nature :** These statements are drawn after the actual happening of the events. They attempt to present a view of the past performance and have nothing to do with the accounting for the future. Modern management is forward looking but these statements do not directly help them in making future estimates and taking decisions for the future.

(vi) **Artificial view :** These statements do not give a real and correct report about the worth of the assets and their loss of value as these are shown on historical cost basis. Thus, these statements provide artificial view as market or replacement value and the effect of the changes in the price level are completely ignored.

(vii) **Scope of manipulations :** These statements are sometimes prepared according to the needs of the situation or the whims of the management. A highly efficient concern may conceal its real profitability by disclosing loss or minimum profit whereas an inefficient concern may declare dividend by wrongly showing profit in the profit and loss account. For this under or over valuation of inventory, over or under charge of depreciation, excessive or inadequate provision for anticipated losses and other such manipulations may be resorted to. Window dressing may also be resorted to in order to show better financial position of a concern than its real position.

(viii) **Inadequate Information :** There are many parties who are interested in the information given in the financial statements but their objectives and requirements differ. The financial statements fail to meet the needs of all. These are mainly prepared to safeguard the interest of shareholders.

The above limitations of financial statements must be taken into consideration before making an analysis of financial statements.

MEANING OF ANALYSIS OF FINANCIAL STATEMENTS

Analysis is the process of critically examining in detail accounting information given in the financial statements. For the purpose of analysis, individual items are studied, their interrelationship with other related figures established, the data is sometimes rearranged to have better understanding of the information with the help of different techniques or tools for the purpose. Analysing financial statements is a process of evaluating relationship between component parts of financial statements to obtain a better understanding of firm's position and performance. In the words of Myer, "Financial Statements Analysis is largely a study of relationship among the various financial factors in a business as disclosed by a single set of statements and a study of the trend of these factors as shown in a series of statements". The analysis of financial statements thus refer to the treatment of the information contained in the financial statement in a way so as to afford a full diagnosis of the profitability and financial position of the firm concerned. For this purpose financial statements are classified methodically, analysed and compared with the figures of previous years or other similar firms.

OBJECTIVES (OR USES) OF FINANCIAL ANALYSIS

Financial analysis is helpful in assessing the financial position and profitability of a concern. This is done through comparison by ratio for the same concern against the industry as a whole ; or for one concern against the predetermined standards ; or for one department of a concern against other departments of the same concern. Accounting ratios calculated for a number of years show the trend of the change of position, i.e., whether the trend is upward or downward or static. The ascertainment of trend helps us in making estimates for the future. For example, ratios of gross profit to sales for the last five years indicate a rising trend, we can safely estimate that ratio of gross profit to sales for the next year will also rise. Keeping in view the importance of accounting ratio the accountant should calculate the ratios in appropriate form, as early as possible, for presentation to management for managerial control.

In short, the main objectives of analysis of financial statements are to assess :

- (i) the present and future earning capacity or profitability of the concern,
- (ii) the operational efficiency of the concern as a whole and of its various parts or departments.
- (iii) the short-term and long-term solvency of the concern for the benefit of the debenture holders and trade creditors.
- (iv) the comparative study in regard to one firm with another firm or one department with another department.
- (v) the possibility of developments in the future by making forecasts and preparing budgets.

(vi) the financial stability of a business concern

(vii) the real meaning and significance of financial data, and

(viii) the long-term liquidity of its funds.

METHODICAL ANALYSIS

The data given in the financial statements are to be suitably arranged. The objective to be achieved should be kept in mind at all times while arranging the data of financial statements properly. The statements are usually prepared in single vertical column or 'T' form statements by adding or subtracting the significant figures of financial records. This also helps to show the information side by side for comparison purposes of number of firms or number of years.

The vertical presentation of financial statements facilitates comparison of figures with that of previous year and also help us to calculate ratios which interpret the position of the company in a better way. This presentation brings out many additional facts like cost of goods sold, gross profit, operating profit etc. in case of Profit and Loss Account and shareholder's funds, capital employed, working capital, etc. in case of Balance Sheet.

In addition to the analysis, interpretation also requires comparison to draw meaningful results. Mere examination of the various components of financial statements like current assets, current liabilities, long-term liabilities, shareholder's fund, working capital, gross profit, operating profit, cost of goods sold, etc. will not lead to definite conclusion in regard to the financial status of a business. Comparison of related components like current assets with current liabilities, long-term liabilities with shareholder's fund, gross profit with sales, etc. is required to draw meaningful conclusions about the position of a company. So, to interpret the position of a company, it is necessary not only to separate the totals given in its financial statements into various components of like nature but also to make comparisons of the related components.

TYPES OF FINANCIAL STATEMENTS ANALYSIS

Different types of financial statements analysis can be made on the basis of

(i) the nature of the analyst and the material used by him,

(ii) the objective of the analysis, and

(iii) the modus operandi of the analysis.

(i) **According to the nature of the analyst and the material used by him:** On this basis, the financial analysis can be external and internal analysis:

(a) **External Analysis :** It is made by those persons who are not connected with the enterprise. They do not have access to the enterprise. They do not have access to the detailed record of the company and have to depend mostly on published statements. Such type of analysis is made by investors, credit agencies, governmental agencies and research scholars.

(b) **Internal Analysis :** The internal analysis is made by those persons who have access to the books of accounts. They are members of the organisation. Analysis of financial statements or other financial data for managerial purposes is the internal type of analysis. The internal analyst can give more reliable result than the external analyst because every types of information is at his disposal.

(ii) **According to the objectives of the analysis :** On this basis the analysis can be long-term and short-term analysis.

(a) **Long-term Analysis :** This analysis is made in order to study the long-term financial stability, solvency and liquidity as well as profitability and earning capital city of a business concern. The purpose of making such types of analysis is to know whether in the long-run the concern will be able to earn a minimum amount which will be sufficient to maintain a reasonable rate of return on the investment so as to provide the funds required for modernisation, growth and development of the business and to meet its costs of capital. This type of analysis helps the long-term financial planning which is essential for the continued success of a business.

(b) **Short-term Analysis :** This is made to determine the short-term solvency, stability and liquidity as well as earning capacity of the business. The purpose of this analysis is to know whether in the short run a business concern will have adequate funds readily available to meet its short-term requirements and sufficient borrowing capacity to meet contingencies in the near future. This analysis is made with reference to items of current assets and current liabilities (working capital analysis) to have fairly sufficient knowledge about the company's current position which may be helpful for short-term financial planning and long-term planning.

(iii) **According to the modus operandi of the analysis :** On this basis, the analysis may be horizontal analysis and vertical analysis.

(a) **Horizontal (or Dynamic) Analysis :** This analysis is made to review and analyse financial statements of a number of years and therefore based on financial data taken from several years. This is very useful for long-term trend analysis and planning. Comparative financial statement is an example of this types of analysis.

(b) **Vertical (or Static) Analysis :** This analysis is made to review and analyse the financial statements of one particular year only. Ratio analysis of the financial year relating to a particular accounting year is an example of this type of analysis.

TECHNIQUES (TOOLS OR METHODS) OF ANALYSIS AND INTERPRETATION

The following techniques can be used in connection with analysis and interpretation of financial statements.

1. Comparative Financial Statements (or Analysis)
2. Common Measurement Statements (or Analysis)
3. Trends Percentages Analysis
4. Fund Flow Statement (or Analysis)
5. Net Working Capital Analysis
6. Cash Flow Statement (or Analysis)
7. Ratio Analysis.

1. **Comparative Financial Statements (or Analysis) :** These statements are prepared in a way so as to provide time perspective to the consideration of various elements of financial position embodied in such statements. This is done to make the financial data more meaningful. The statements of two or more years are prepared to show absolute data of two or more years, increases or decreases in absolute data in value and in terms of percentages. Comparative statements can be prepared for both income statement as well as position statement or balance sheet.

(i) **Comparative Income Statement :** This statement discloses the net profit or net loss resulting from the operation of business. Such statement shows the operating results for a number of accounting periods so that changes in absolute data from one period to another period may be stated in terms of absolute change or in terms of percentage. This statement helps in deriving meaningful conclusions as it is very easy to ascertain the changes in sales volume, administrative expenses, selling and distribution expenses, cost of sales, etc.

(ii) **Comparative Balance Sheet :** This statement prepared on two or more different dates can be used for comparing assets and liabilities and to find out any increase or decrease in these items. This facilitates the comparison of figures of two or more periods and provide necessary information which may be useful in forming an opinion regarding the financial condition as well as progressive outlook of the concern.

2. **Common Measurement (size) Statement (Common Measurement Analysis) :** This statement indicates the relationship of various items with some common items (expressed as percentage of the common item).

In the income statement the sale figure is taken as base and all other figures are expressed as percentage of sales. Similarly in the Balance Sheet the total of assets and liabilities is taken as base and all other figures are expressed as a percentage to this total. The percentages so calculated can be easily compared with the corresponding percentages in other periods and meaningful conclusions can be drawn.

3. **Trend Percentages Analysis :** This analysis is an important tool of horizontal financial analysis. This methods is immensely helpful in making a comparative study of the financial statements of several years. Under this methods trend percentages are calculated for each item of the financial statements taking the figure of base year as 100. The starting year is usually taken as the base year. The trend percentages show the relationship of each item with its preceding year's percentages. These percentages can also be presented in the form of Index Numbers showing relative change in the financial data of certain period. This will exhibit the direction (i.e., upward or downward trend) to which the concern is proceeding. These trend ratios may be compared with industry in order to know the strong or weak points of a concern. These are calculated only for major items instead of calculating for all items in the financial statements.

4. **Funds Flow Statement (or Analysis) :** This statement is prepared to reveal clearly the various sources wherefrom the funds are produced to finance the activities of a business concern during the accounting period and also brings to highlight the uses to which these funds are put during the said period.

5. **Cash Flow Statement (or Analysis) :** This statement is prepared to know clearly the various items of inflow and outflow of cash. It is an essential tool for short-term financial analysis and is very helpful in the evaluation of current liquidity of a business concern. It helps the business executives of a business in the efficient cash management and internal financial management.

6. **Statement of changes in Working Capital (or Net Working Capital Analysis) :** This statement is prepared to know the net change in Working Capital of a business between two specified dates. It is prepared from current assets and current liabilities of the said dates to show the net increase or decrease in Working Capital.

7. **Ratio analysis :** It is done to develop meaningful relationship between individual items or group of items usually shown in the periodical financial statements published by the concern. An accounting ratio shows the relationship between the two inter-related accounting figures as gross profit to sales, current assets to current liabilities, loaned capital to owned capital, etc. Ratio should not be calculated between the two unrelated figures as sales and discount on issue of shares, operating cost and equity capital, etc. as it will not serve any useful purpose.

Absolute figures are valuable but they alone convey no meaning unless compared with another. Accounting ratios show inter-relationships which exist among various accounting data. When relationships among various accounting data supplied by financial statements are worked out,they are known as accounting ratios.

Accounting ratios can be expressed in various ways such as:

   (i) a pure ratio say ratio of current assets to current liabilities is 2:1 or

  (ii) a rate say current assets are two times of current liabilities or

 (iii) a percentage say current assets are 200% of current liabilities.

Each method of expression has a distinct advantage over the other. The analyst will select that mode which will best suit his convenience and purpose.

IMPORTANCE OR ADVANTAGES OF RATIO ANALYSIS

Ratio Analysis stands for the process of determining and presenting the relationship of items and groups of items in the financial statements. It is an important technique of financial analysis. It is a way by which financial stability and health of a concern can be judged. The following are the main points of importance of ratio analysis:

   (i) **Useful in financial position analysis :** Accounting ratios reveal the financial position of the concern. This helps the banks, insurance companies and other financial institutions in lending and making investment decisions.

  (ii) **Useful in simplifying accounting figures :** Accounting ratios simplify, summarise and systematise the accounting figures in order to make them more understandable and in lucid form. They highlight the inter-relationship which exists between various segments of the business as expressed by accounting statements. Often the figures standing alone cannot help them convey any meaning and ratios help them to relate with other figures.

 (iii) **Useful in assessing the operational efficiency :** Accounting ratios help to have an idea of the working of a concern. The efficiency of the firm becomes evident when analysis is based on accounting ratios. They diagnose the financial help by evaluating liquidity, solvency, profitability, etc. This helps the management to assess financial requirements and the capabilities of various business units.

 (iv) **Useful forecasting purposes :** If accounting ratios are calculated for a number of years, then a trend is established. This trend helps in setting up future plans and forecasting. For example, expenses as a percentage of sales can be easily forecasted on the basis of sales and expenses of the past years.

  (v) **Useful in locating the weak spots of the business :** Accounting ratios are of great assistance in locating the weak spots in the business even though the overall performance may be efficient. Weakness in financial structure due to incorrect policies in the past or present are revealed through accounting ratios. For example, if a firm finds that increase in distribution expenses is more than proportionate to the results expected or achieved, it can take remedial steps to overcome this adverse situation.

(vi) **Useful in comparison of performance :** Through accounting ratios comparison can be made between one department of a firm with another of the same firm in order to evaluate the performance of the various departments in the firm. Manager is naturally interested in such comparison in order to know the proper and smooth functioning of such departments. Ratios also help him to make any change in the organisation structure.

Limitations of Accounting Ratios

Ratio analysis is very important in revealing the financial position and soundness of the business. But, inspite of its advantages, it has some limitations which restricted its use. These limitations should be kept in mind while making use of ratio analysis for interpreting the financial statements. The following are the limitations of accounting ratios:

1. **False results, if based on incorrect accounting data :** Accounting ratios can be correct only if the data (on which they are based) are correct. Sometimes, the information given in the financial statements is affected by window dressing, i.e. showing position better than what actually is. For example, if inventory values are inflated or depreciation is not charged on fixed assets, not only will one have an optimistic view of profitability of the concern but also of its financial position. So the analyst must always be on the look-out for signs of window dressing, if any.

2. **No idea of probable happenings in future :** Ratios are an attempt to make an analysis of the past financial statements; so they are historical documents. Now-a-days keeping in view the complexities of the business, it is important to have an idea of the probable happenings in future.

3. **Variation in accounting methods :** The two firms' results are comparable with the help of accounting ratios only if they follow the same accounting methods or bases. Comparison will become difficult if the two concerns follow the different methods of providing depreciation or valuing stock. Similarly, if the two firms are following two different standards and methods, an analysis by reference to the ratios would be misleading. Moreover, utilisation of inbuilt facilities, availability of facilities and scale of operation would affect financial statements of different firms. Comparison of financial statements of such firms by means of ratios is bound to be misleading.

4. **Price level changes :** Changes in price levels make comparison for various years difficult. For example, the ratio of sales to total assets in 1990 would be much higher than in 1976 due to rising prices, fixed assets being shown at cost and not at market price.

5. **Only one method of analysis :** Ratio analysis is only a beginning and gives just a fraction of information needed for decision-making. So, to have a comprehensive analysis of financial statements, ratios should be used along with other methods of analysis.

6. **No common standards :** It is very difficult to lay down a common standard for comparison because circumstances differ from concern to concern and the nature of each industry is different. For example, a business with current ratio of more than 2:1 might not be in a position to pay current liabilities in time because of an unfavourable distribution of current assets in relation to liquidity. On the other hand, another business with a current ratio of even less than 2:1 might not be experiencing any difficulty in making the payment of current liabilities in time because of its favourable distribution of current assets in relation to liquidity.

7. **Different meaning assigned to the same term :** Different firms, in order to calculate ratio may assign different meanings. For example, profit for the purpose of calculating a ratio may be taken as profit after tax and interest. This may affect the calculation of ratio in different firms and such ratio when used for comparison may lead to wrong conclusion.

8. **Ignores qualification factor :** Accounting ratios are tools of quantitative analysis only. But sometimes qualification factors may surmount the quantitative aspects. The calculations derived from the ratio analysis under such circumstances may get distorted. For example, though credit may be granted to a customer on the basis of information regarding his financial position, yet the grant of credit ultimately depends on debtor's character, honestly, past record and his managerial ability.

9. **No use if ratios are worked out for insignificant and unrelated figures :** Accounting ratios may be worked for any two insignificant and unrelated figures as ratio of sales and investment in government securities. Such ratios may be misleading. Ratios should be calculated on the basis of cause and effect relationship. One should be clear as to what is cause and what is effect before calculating a ratio between two figures.

Classification of Ratios

Ratios may be classified in a number of ways keeping in view the particular purpose. Ratios indicating profitability are calculated on the basis of profit and loss account; those indicating financial position are computed on the basis of balance sheet and those which show operating efficiency or productivity of effective use of resources are calculated on the basis of figures in the profit and loss account and the balance sheet. This classification is rather crude and unsuitable to determine the profitability and financial position of the business. To achieve this purpose effectively, ratios may be classified as:

(i) Profitability ratios

(ii) Turnover ratios

(iii) Financial ratios

(iv) Leverage ratios.

1. **Profitability Ratios :** Profitability ratios are of utmost importance for a concern. These ratios are calculated to enlighten the end results of business activities which is the sole criterion of the overall efficiency of a business concern. The following are the important profitability ratios :

(A) **Gross Profit Ratio :** This ratio tells gross margin on trading and is calculated as under :

$$\text{Gross Profit Ratio} = \frac{\text{Gross Profit}}{\text{Net Sales}} \times 100$$

For example, if gross profit is Rs. 42,000 and net sales are Rs. 3,00,000, the Gross Profit Ratio will be 14% (i.e.,42,000/3,00,000 ×100).

(B) **Operating Ratio :** This ratio indicates the proportion that the cost of sales bears to sales. Cost of sales includes direct cost of goods sold as well as other operating expenses,administration,selling and distribution expenses which have matching relationship with sales. It excludes income and expenses which have no bearing on production and sales,i.e.,non-operating incomes and expenses as interest and dividend received on investment,interest paid on long-term loans and debentures,profit or loss on sale fixed assets or long-term investments. It is calculated as follows :

$$\frac{\text{Cost of Goods Sold} + \text{Operating Expenses}}{\text{Net Sales}} \times 100$$

Here,

Cost of Goods Sold = Opening Stock + Purchases + Direct Expenses + Manufacturing Expenses - Closing Stock or Sales - Gross Profit

Operating Expenses = Administration Expenses + Selling and Distribution Expenses

For example, if cost of goods sold = Rs. 1,40,000, operating expenses Rs. 2,00,000 and net sales Rs. 6,80,000 are given, then operating ratio will be 50%, (i.e., Rs. 1,40,000 + Rs. 2,00,000 + Rs. 6,00,000 x 100).

Lower the ratio, the better is it. Higher the ratio, the less favourable it is because it would have a smaller margin of operating profit or the payment of dividends and the creation of reserves. This ratio should be analysed further to throw light on the levels of efficiency prevailing in different elements of totals cost :

C. **Expenses Ratios :** These are calculated to ascertain the relationship that exists between operating expenses and volume of sales. The following ratios will help in analysing operating ratio :

(i) Material Consumed Ratio

$$= \frac{\text{Material Consumed}}{\text{Net Sales}} \times 100$$

(ii) Conversion Cost Ratio

$$= \frac{\text{Labour Expenses} + \text{Manufacturing Expenses}}{\text{Net Sales}} \times 100$$

(iii) Administrative Expenses Ratio

$$= \frac{\text{Administrative Expenses}}{\text{Net Sales}} \times 100$$

(iv) Selling and Distribution Expenses Ratio

$$= \frac{\text{Selling and Distribution Expenses}}{\text{Net Sales}} \times 100$$

The total of these four ratios will be equal to operating ratio.

D. **Operating Profit Ratio :** This ratio establishes the relationship between operating profit and sales and is calculated as follows :

$$\text{Operating Profit Ratio} = \frac{\text{Operating Profit}}{\text{Net Sales}} \times 100$$

Where Operating Profit = Net Profit + Non-operating Expenses
                     - Non-operating Income

or

= Gross Profit - Operating expenses

Operating profit ratio can also be calculated with the help of operating ratio as follows :

Operating Profit Ratio = 100 - Operating Ratio.

This ratio indicates the portion remaining out of every rupee worth of sales after all operating costs and expenses have been met. Higher the ratio, the better it is.

E. **Net Profit Ratio :** This ratio is very useful to the proprietors and prospective investors because it reveals the overall profitability of the concern.

This is the ratio of net profit after taxes to net sales and is calculated as follows :

$$\text{Net Profit Ratio} = \frac{\text{Net Profit}}{\text{Net Sales}} \times 100$$

This ratio differs from the operating profit ratio in as much as it is calculated after deducting non-operating expenses, such as loss on sale of fixed assets, etc. from operating profit and adding non-operating income like interest or dividends on investments, profit on sale of investments or fixed assets, etc. to such profit. Higher the ratio, the better it is because it gives idea of improved efficiency of the concern.

F. **Return on Capital Employed :** This ratio is an indicator of the earning capacity of the capital employed in the business. By capital employed, we mean not only the equity share capital, but also in addition to that the various fixed liabilities representing borrowed amount as also capital reserves, revenue reserves and undistributed profit as reduced by the fictitious assets. This ratio is calculated as follows :

$$\text{Return on Capital Employed} = \frac{\text{Net Profit}}{\text{Capital Employed}} \times 100$$

Here,

Net Profit = Net trading profit after depreciation but before interest on long-term liabilities (representing borrowed amount), dividend on shares and taxation. Some people take profits after taxation.

Capital Employed = Equity Share Capital + Preference Share Capital + Undistributed Profit + Reserves and Surplus Long-term Liabilities - Fictitious Assets.

Alternatively : Tangible Fixed and Intangible Assets + Current Assets - Current Liabilities.

This ratio is considered to be the most important ratio because it reflects the overall efficiency with which capital is used. This ratio is a helpful too for making capital budgeting decision ; a project yielding higher return is favoured. For example, if the capital employed is Rs. 1,00,000 and net profit before interest, tax and dividend is Rs. 15,000, the return on capital employed will be 15% (i.e., 15,000 x 100 / 1,00,000).

G. **Return on Shareholders' Investment (or Owners' Net Capital) Ratio :** The ratio, also called return on proprietors' funds, is a measure of the percentage of not profit to shareholders' funds. The ratio is expressed as follows :

Return on Shareholders' Investment Ratio

$$= \frac{\text{Net Profit after tax, Interest and Preference Dividend}}{\text{Equity Shareholders' Funds}} \times 100$$

Here,

Equity Shareholders' Funds = Equity Share Capital + Capital Reserves + Revenue Reserves + Balance of Profit and Loss Ac count - Fictitious Assets.

Suppose profit after interest, taxes and preference dividend is Rs. 5,00,00 and equity shareholders' funds is Rs. 25,00,000. Then return on shareholders' investment will be 20% (i.e., (Rs. 5,00,000 x 100 / Rs. 25,00,000).

The ratio of net profit to shareholders' funds shows the extent to which profitability objective is being achieved. Higher the ratio, the better it is.

H. **Return on Total Assets :** This ratio is calculated to measure the profit after tax against the amount invested in total assets to ascertain whether assets are being utilized properly or not. It is calculated as under :

$$\text{Return on Total Assets} = \frac{\text{Net Profit after tax}}{\text{Total Assets}} \times 100$$

Suppose net profit after tax is Rs. 20,000 and total assets are Rs. 1,00,000. Return on total asses will be 20% (i.e., Rs. 20,000 x 100 / Rs. 1,0,000). The higher the ratio, the better it is for the concern.

I. **Debt Service Ratio (or Fixed Charges Cover) :** This ratio is important from lender's point of view and indicates whether the business can earn sufficient profits to pay periodically the interest charges on fixed or long-term loans or debentures. It is calculated as follows :

$$\text{Debt Service Ratio} = \frac{\text{Net profit before interest and tax}}{\text{Interest on long-term liabilities}}$$

Suppose the net profit before interest and tax is Rs. 2,00,000 and interest on long-term liabilities is Rs. 20,000. Then debt service ratio will be 10 times (i.e., Rs. 2,00,000 / Rs. 20,000). The more the ratio, the more is the margin of safety for the lenders. If the ratio is one (i.e., profits are just equal to interest), it will show a bad position of the company as nothing will be left for shareholders and will be unsafe for the lenders also.

J. **Earning per share :** It is calculated as follows :

$$\text{Earning per share} = \frac{\text{Net Profit — Preference Dividend}}{\text{Number of Equity Shares}}$$

If there are both preference and equity share capital, then out of net income first of all preference dividends should be deducted in order to find out the net income available for equity shareholders. The performance and prospects of the company are affected by earning per share. If earning per share increases, there is a possibility that the company may pay more dividend or issue bonus shares. In short the market price of the share of a company will be effected by all these factors.

Though the earning per share is the most widely published data, yet it should be used cautiously as earning per share cannot represent the various financial operations of the business. Moreover, the financial data collected in respect of different companies may be affected by different practices followed by the companies relating to stock in trade, depreciation, etc. This ultimately will affect the calculation of earning per share and that is why earning per share should be used with precaution while comparing the performance and prospects of two companies.

K. **Price Earning Ratio :** This is computed by the following formula:

$$\text{Price Earning Ratio} = \frac{\text{Market Price per Equity Share}}{\text{Earning per Share}}$$

For example, if the company's share price is Rs. 40 and the earning per share is Rs. 10, then price earning ratio is 4 (i.e., 40/10). Or, it means that the market value of every rupee of earning is four times. It is a very important ratio in order to know whether the shares of the company are undervalued or in predicting the future market price. This can be done by comparing the price earning ratios of two companies. For example, if earning per share in Delhi Ltd. is Rs. 10 and the market price of its equity share is Rs. 40 while price earning ratio of other companies is 5, then it can be concluded that the equity share of Delhi Ltd. is undervalued by Rs. 10. This ratio helps the shareholders to decide whether shares should be purchased or not in a company. If the shares are to be purchase then it indicates the possibility of capital appreciation.

L. **Payout Ratio :** This is determined as follows :

$$\text{Payment Ratio} = \frac{\text{Dividend per equity share}}{\text{Earning per share}}$$

This ratio indicates as to what proportion of earning per share has been used for paying dividend and what has been retained for ploughing back. This ratio is very important from shareholder's point of view as it tell him that if a company has used whole or substantially the whole of its earnings for paying dividend and retained nothing for future growth and expansion purposes, then there will be very dim chances of capital appreciation in the price of share of such company. In other words, an investor who is more interested in capital appreciation must look for a company having low payout ratio.

M. **Dividend Yield Ratio :** This is computed as under :

$$\text{Dividend Yield Ratio} = \frac{\text{Dividend per share}}{\text{Market price per share}} \times 100$$

This ratio is important for those investors who are interested in the dividend income. As the shareholder purchases the shares in the open market, so his yield (rate of return) is not equal to the dividend declared by the company. In fact, he calculates dividend per share by dividing the rate of dividend by paid-up value of share. Then he calculates yield by dividing dividend per share by the market price of share. For example, if a company declares 15% dividend and its share is of Rs. 6 paid-up and the market price of which is Rs. 9 then the yield will be calculated as under :

$$\text{Dividend per share} = \frac{15}{100} \times \text{Re. } 0.90$$

$$\text{Dividend Yield Ratio} = \frac{\text{Dividend per share}}{\text{Market price per share}} \times 100$$

$$= \frac{0.90}{9.00} \times 100 = 10\%$$

Thus, in the above case, the effective earning rate to the investor in equity share is 10% and not 15% as declared by the company.

30

BUDGETING

A budget is a detailed plan of operations for some specific future period. It is an estimate prepared in advance of the period to which it applies. It acts as a business barometer as it is complete programme of activities of the business for the period covered. It is defined as "a financial and/or quantitative statement, prepared prior to a defined period of time, of the policy to be pursued during that period for the purpose of attaining a given objective". Thus, the essentials of a budget are :

(a) it is prepared in advance and is based on a future plan of actions;
(b) it relates to a future period and is based on objective to be attained;
(c) it is a statement expressed in monetary and/or physical units prepared for the implementation of policy formulated by the management.

Different types of budgets are prepared by an industrial concern for different purposes. A Sales Budget is prepared for the purpose of forecasting sales for a future period. A Manufacturing Cost Budget is prepared for forecasting the manufacturing costs. The Master Budget embodies forecasts-for sales and other incomes, for manufacturing, marketing and other expenses, for cash and capital requirements besides forecasting the figure of profit or loss.

MEANING OF BUDGETARY CONTROL

Budgetary is defined as "the establishment of budgets relating to the responsibilities of executives to the requirements of a policy, and the continuous comparison of actual with budgeted results, either to secure by individual action the objective of that policy or to provide a basis for its revision. It is the system of management control and accounting in which all operations are forecasted and planned so far as possible ahead, and the actual results with the forecasted and planned ones. Thus, budgetary control involves :

(a) establishment of budgets;
(b) continuous comparison of actual with budgets for achievement of

targets and placing the responsibility for failure to achieve the budget figures;

(c) revision of budgets in the right of changed circumstances.

The difference between budget, budgeting and budgetary control has been stated thus : "Budgets are the individual objectives of a department, etc., whereas Budgeting may be said to be the act of building budgets. Budgetary control embraces all this and in addition includes the science of planning the budgets themselves and the utilisation of such budgets to effect an overall management tool for the business planning and control.

ADVANTAGES OF BUDGETING

Budgeting offers may advantages. It may be conceived as one of the supreme examples of rationality in management. It is a useful management tool for comparing the current items with pre-planned items with a view to attain equilibrium between ends and means, output and effort. It corrects the deviations from preplanned path through the media of observation, research, planning, control and decision making and thus helps in performance of future activities in an orderly way. It uncovers uneconomies in operations, weaknesses in the organisational structure and minimises wasteful spending. It acts as a friend, philosopher and guide to the management. Its advantages can be summarised as follows :

1. It brings efficiency and economy in the working of the business enterprise. Even though a monetary reward is not offered, the budget becomes a game - a goal to achieve or a target to shoot at - and hence it is more likely to be achieved or hit than if there was no predetermined goal or target. The budget is an impersonal policeman that maintains ordered effort and brings about efficiency in result.

2. It establishes divisional and departmental responsibility. It thus prevents alibis and "buck-passing" when the budget figures are not met.

3. It co-ordinates the various division of a business, namely, the production, marketing, financial and administrative divisions. It forces executives to think, and think as a group. This results in smoother operation of the entire plant.

4. It guards against undue optimum leading to over-expansion because the targets are fixed by the executives after cool and careful thought.

5. It acts as a safety signal for the management. It shows when to proceed cautiously and when manufacturing or merchandising expansion can be safely undertaken. It serves as an automatic check on the judgment of the executives as losses are revealed in time which is a caution to the management to stop wastages.

6. Uniform policy without the disadvantages of a military type of business organisation can be pursued by all divisions of the business by means of centralisation of budgetary control.

7. Seasonal variations in production can be reduced by developing new

"fill in" products. This results in decreasing the cost of production by increasing volume of output.

8. The use of budget figures as measures of operating performance and financial position makes possible the adoption of the standard cost principle in divisions other than the production division.

9. It helps management in obtaining the most profitable combination of different factors of production. This results in a more economical use of capital.

10. Management which have developed a well-ordered budget plan and which operate accordingly, receive greater favour from Credit Agencies.

11. It is the only means of predetermining when and to what extent financing will be necessary avoiding the possibility of both over and under-capitalisation.

LIMITATIONS TO BUDGETING

The budgeting's system is not a perfect tool. It has its own limitations which are as follows :

1. **Opposition against the very spirit of budgeting :** There will be always active and passive resistance to budgetary control as it points out at the efficiency or inefficiency of individuals. The opposition is also due to human nature - the tendency to resist change. Moreover, any system of budgetary control cannot be successful unless it has the full support of the top management.

2. **Budgeting and changing economy :** The preparation of a budget which gives a realistic position of the firm's affairs under inflationary pressure and changing Government policies is really difficult. Thus, the accurate position of the business cannot be estimated.

3. **Time factor :** Accuracy in budgeting comes through experience. Management must not expect too much during the development period.

4. **Not a substitute for management :** Budget is only a management tool. It cannot substitute management. Besides that no budgetary programme can be successful unless adequate arrangements are made for supervision and administration.

5. **Co-operation required :** The success of the budgetary control depends upon willing co-operation and teamwork. Budget officer must get co-operation from all departmental managers. These managers must feel the responsibility for achieving or bettering departmental goals laid down in the budget.

Inspite of these limitations it can be safely said that the technique of budgetary control is a must for each business enterprise. It leaves sufficient time for the top management for overall policy and planning consideration. Much success can be achieved if the top management devotes attention chiefly to unusual or exceptional items that appear in daily, weekly and monthly statements and reports. The success of budgetary control must depend on the adequacy and reliability of records, the past and the present performances, on the interest of all executives and subordinates in the purposes of such control, proper departmentalisation and sub-division of factory activities, a close classification and proper division and analysis of the expenditure, and the most suitable system of cost and financial accounts.

STEPS IN BUDGETARY CONTROL

Budgetary control requires the following steps to be taken :

Organisation for Budgeting

The setting up of a definite plan of organisation is the first step to be taken prior to beginning the real work of installing budgetary control. The responsibility of each executive must be clearly defined. There should be no uncertainty regarding the point where the jurisdiction of one executive ends and that of another begins.

Budget Manual

The budget manual is a written document or booklet which specifies the objectives of the budgeting organisation and procedures. It is a document which sets out, *inter alia*, the responsibilities of the persons engaged in, the routine of, and the forms and records required for, budgetary control. Following are some of the important matters covered in a budget manual :

1. A statement regarding the objectives of the organisation and how they can be achieved through budgetary control.
2. A statement regarding the functions and responsibilities of each executive by designation both regarding preparation and execution of budgets.
3. Procedures to be followed for obtaining the necessary approval of budgets. The authority of granting approval should be stated in explicit terms. Whether one, two or more signatures are to be required on each document should also be clearly stated.
4. Time-tables for all stages of budgeting.
5. Reports, statements, forms and other records to be maintained.
6. The accounts classification to be employed. It is necessary that the framework within which the costs, revenues and other financial amounts are classified must be identical both in the accounts and the budget departments. There are many advantages attaching to the use of budget manual. It is a formal record defining the functions and responsibilities of each executive. The methods and procedures of budgetary control are standardised. There is synchronisation of the efforts of all which result in maximisation of the profits of the organisation.

Responsibility for Budgeting
Budget controller

Of course, the chief executive is ultimately responsible for the budget programme but it will be better if the large part of the supervisory responsibility is delegated to an official designated as Budget Controller or Director. The Budget Controller or Director should have knowledge of the technical side of the business and should report direct to the President.

Budget committee

The Budget Controller will be assisted in his work by the Budget Committee. The Budget Committee will consist of Heads of the various Departments such as Production, Sales, Finance etc. with Budget Controller as its Chairman. It will be the duty of the Budget Committee to submit, discuss and finally approve the budget figures. Each Head of the Department will have his own sub-committee with executives working under him as its members.

Fixation of the budget period

"Budget period" means the period for which a budget is prepared and employed. The budget period will depend upon (i) the nature of the business and (ii) the costing techniques to be applies. For example, in case of continuous or mass production industries it is necessary to compare continuously the actual with budgets, and, therefore, the budget period should be a short one. Similar is the case of of a garment manufacturer as his business depends on the vagaries of taste and fashion. But in case of structural or heavy engineering works a longer budget period will be suitable.

Budget Procedure

After the establishment of budget organisation and fixation of the budget period the actual work of budgetary control begins. The procedure followed in designing and operating a budgetary control system largely depends upon the nature of the business.

Determination of key factor

Key factor is that factor the extent of whose influence must first be assessed in order to ensure that functional budgets (relating to different functions of a business e.g. sales, production, purchases, cash, etc.) are reasonably capable of fulfillment. This is also termed as 'Principal Budget' or 'Limiting' or 'Governing' factor. It is essential to consider this factor before preparing the budgets. In some concerns the key factor might be sales; while in others it might be production, materials, labour, machinery or capital. This most important factor which governs the whole process of preparation of budgets should be predetermined. The budget relating to that particular factor should be prepared first and the other budgets should be based upon it. A co-ordinated plan should then be finally approved.

The examples of key factor, which can be one or even more than one in a particular concern, are as under :

Firstly, sales may be the key factor and if it is so, it would be because of the restricted demand in the market or limited efforts for sales promotion. Management might be another important key factor because of deficiency of capable managers or limited funds at the disposal of executives. Thirdly, materials may be the limiting factor on account of inadequate availability of supply, fixed quotas license restrictions, etc. Labour is yet another key factor because there might be death of workers in general or in certain grades. Lastly, plant may be the governing factor, plant capacity might be limited due to shortage in supply or lack of capital or space.

These factors are not of a permanent nature and they can be overcome by the management in the long run if an effort is made in this direction by selecting optimum level of production, dealing more profitable products, introducing new methods, changing material mix, working overtime or extra shifts, providing incentives to workers, hiring new machinery etc.

Making of forecasts

Forecast means an estimate about the probability at a given period of time. It differs from a budget. Budget is an operating and financial plan of a business enterprise. It is sort of commitment or a target which the management seeks to attain on the basis of the forecasts made. Forecasts are made regarding sales, production cost and financial requirements of the business. Physical quantities as well as monetary values are estimated separately.

Consideration of alternative combination of forecasts

Alternative combinations of forecasts are considered with a view to obtain the most efficient overall plan so as to maximise profits. When the large-profit combination of forecasts is selected, the forecasts should be regarded as being finalised.

Preparation of budgets

On finalisation of the forecasts the budgets will be prepared. Production budget will be prepared on the basis of sales budget and also after taking into consideration the available productive capacities. Different costs of production budgets will also be prepared on the basis of the production budget. Financial budget will be prepared on the basis of sales forecast and production budget. All these budgets will be combines and co-ordinated into one Master Budget. These budgets may be revised from time to time taking into account the current developments.

TYPES OF BUDGETS

There are various types of budgets. Some of the important ones have been discussed below.

Sales Budget

The Sales Budget, generally, forms the fundamental basis on which all the other budgets are built up. The budget is essentially a forecast of sales to be achieved in a budget period. The Sales Manager should be made directly responsible for the preparation and execution of this budget. He should take into consideration the following factors while preparing the sales budget :

  (a) **Past sales figures and trend :** The record of previous experience forms the most reliable guided as to future sales as the past performance is related to actual business conditions. However, the other factors such as seasonal fluctuations, growth of market, trade cycles, etc., should not be lost sight of.

(b) **Salesmen's estimate :** Salesmen are in a position to estimate the potential demand of the customers more accurately because they come in direct contact with the customers. However, proper discount should be made for over optimistic or too conservative estimates of the salesmen depending upon their temperament.

(c) **Plant capacity :** It should be the endeavor of the business to ensure proper utilisation of plant facilities and that the sale budget provides an economic and balanced production in the factory.

(d) **General trade prospects :** The general trade prospects considerably affect the sales. Valuable information can be gathered in this connection from trade papers and magazines.

(e) **Orders on hand :** In case of industries where production is quite a lengthy process, orders on hand also have a considerable influence on the amount of sales.

(f) **Proposed expansion or discontinuance of products :** It affects sales and, therefore, it should also be considered.

(g) **Seasonal fluctuations :** Past experience will be the best guide in this respect. However, efforts should be made to minimise the effects of seasonal fluctuations by giving special concessions or off-season discounts thus increasing the volume of sales.

(h) **Potential market :** Market research should be carried out for ascertaining the potential market for the company's products. Such an estimate is made on the basis of expected population growth, purchasing power of consumers and buying habits of the people.

(i) **Availability of material and supply :** Adequate supply of raw materials and other supplies must be ensured before drafting the sales programme.

(j) **Financial aspect :** Expansion of sales usually require increase in capital outlay also, therefore, sales budget must be kept within the bounds of financial capacity.

(k) **Other factors :**

　(i) The nature and degree of competition within the industry :

　(ii) Cost of distributing goods;

　(iii) Government controls, rules and regulations related to the industry; and

　(iv) Political situation - national and international - as it may have an influence upon the market.

The Sales Manager, after taking into consideration all these factors, will prepare the Sales Budget in terms of quantities and money, distinguishing between products, periods and areas of sale.

Production Budget

This budget provides an estimate of the total volume of production product wise with the scheduling of operations by days, weeks and months and a forecast of the closing finished product inventory. Generally the production budget is upon the sales budget but in case of companies which find it difficult to forecast sales on account of frequent changes in style and fashions, it is based upon past experience. The responsibility of the Total Production Budget lies with Works Manager and that of Department Production Budgets lies with Departmental Works Managers.

The production budget may be expressed in quantitative or financial units or both. The objects of its preparation are :

1. To answer the following questions :
   (a) What is to be produced ?
   (b) When is it to be produced ?
   (c) How is it to be produced ?
   (d) Where is it to be produced ?
2. To chalk down and organise the production programme for achieving the sales target.
3. To serve as a basis for preparation of production cost budgets, for example, material cost budget, labour cost budget, etc.
4. To prepare a cash forecast : There are two problems connected with the production budget : (i) determining the annual production required and (ii) pro-rating it throughout the year. The planning of production programme is essential to have sufficient stock for sales to keep inventories within reasonable limits and to manufacture goods most economically. To achieve it the following factors should be taken into consideration.
   (i) **Inventory policies** : Inventory standards should be predetermines so that neither there is a shortage nor over-stocking of goods.
   (ii) **Sales requirements** : The quantity of goods to be sold would decide to a greater extent how much is to be produced. Therefore, this budget depends upon the sales budget.
   (iii) **Production stability** : For reduction of costs, stability in employment and better utilisation of plant facilities, the production should be evenly distributed throughout the year in case of seasonal industries, since it is not possible to have stable levels of production or inventory, an effort should be made to have the optimum balance between the two.
   (iv) **Plant capacity** : How much can be produced depends upon the available plant capacity. There must be sufficient capacity to produce the annual requirements and also to meet seasonal high demands.
   (v) **Availability of materials and labour** : Adequate and timely supply of raw materials and labour force should have an important effect on the planning of production.

(vi) **Time taken in production process :** The production should commence well in time keeping in view how much time it would take in the factory to translate the raw materials into finished goods.

The Sales and the Production Budgets are interdependent and must be prepared in co-operation with both the Sales and the Production Departments.

Cost of Production Budget

After determining the volume of production, it is necessary to determine the cost of procuring this output. Cost of production includes materials, labour and overheads and, therefore, separate budgets for each of these items will be prepared.

Materials Budget

Materials may be direct or indirect. The materials budget generally deals only with the direct materials. Indirect materials are generally included in the works overhead budget. The preparation of materials budget includes the following :

(a) the preparation of estimates of raw materials requirements.

(b) the scheduling of purchases in required quantities at the required time.

(c) the controlling of raw material inventories.

Material requirements are estimated regarding each class of products by multiplying the exact material requirement for each class of product by the number of unit of that class. The total quantity required for the budget period is first estimated and then is further broken down by component time period (months and quarters) in the materials budget. The break-up and length of the period should be in uniformity with the production budget.

In case of concerns whose raw material requirements can be standardised, the materials budget can be prepared very exactly on this basis. In case it is not possible, the percentage of raw materials to total cost of products should be calculated on the basis of the historical data. On the basis of this information a rough estimate can be made regarding the raw materials required for the budgeted period. The figure should further be adjusted taking into account the current price trends and the normal wastage of materials in the course of production.

The Buying Department should proceed to find the most profitable means of procuring the requisite quantity and quality of raw materials. Consideration must also be given to the amount of stock to be carried forward.

The materials budget can be classified into two categories (i) materials requirement budget (ii) materials procurement or purchase budget. The former tells about the total quantity of materials required during the budget period; while the latter tells about the materials to be acquired from the market during the budget period. Materials to be acquired are estimated after taking into account the closing inventory and the opening inventory of the materials for which orders have already been placed.

Direct Labour Budget

The direct labour budget tells about the estimates of direct labour requirements essential for carrying out the budgeted output. In preparation of this budget previous records of the percentage labour cost in the total cost of each product, group or department will be considerably helpful. The budget may give details regarding direct labour costs only, or both direct labour hours and cost. In the former case the cost can be calculated by making an estimate of cost per unit of production. The cost per unit multiplied by the budgeted units will give the estimated cost of direct labour. In the latter case estimates will have to be made about (i) direct labour hours and (ii) average wage rate. Internal factors such as the method of wage payment, the type of production process and the available costing records will determine whether and how it is possible to express production in terms of direct labour hours. The average wage rate payable for a particular product or department, will be calculated on the basis of the historical ratio between wages paid and direct labour hours worked in the department or for the product after taking into account the current conditions.

Direct Labour Budget (like Direct Materials Budget) may be divided into two categories : (i) Direct Labour Requirement Budget (ii) Direct Labour Procurement Budget. The former tells about the total direct labour required in terms of quantity or/and value while the latter will state the additional direct workers to be recruited.

Factory Overhead Budget

Manufacturing or Factory overheads include the cost of indirect labour, indirect material and indirect expenses. The manufacturing overheads can be classified into three categories (i) Fixed i.e. which tend to remain constant irrespective of change in the volume of output (ii) Variable i.e. which tend to vary with the output and (iii) Semi-variable i.e. which are partly variable and partly fixed. The manufacturing overheads budget will provide an estimate of all these overheads to be incurred in the budget period.

Fixed manufacturing overheads can be estimated without much difficulty on the basis of the past information and knowledge of any changes which may occur during the ensuing budget period. Variable overheads are estimated after considering the scheduled production and operating conditions in the budget period.

Administrative Overhead Budget

The budget covers expenses of all administrative offices, and of management salaries. A careful analysis of the needs of all administrative departments of the enterprise is very necessary. The minimum requirements for the efficient operation of each department can be estimated on the basis of costs for prior years, and after a study of the plans and responsibilities of each administrative department for the budget period. The budget for the entire administrative division will be prepared by totalling the separate budgets of all administrative departments.

Selling and Distribution Overhead Budget

The budget includes all expenses relating to selling, advertising, delivery of goods to customer, etc. It is better if such costs are analysed according to products, types of customers, territories, and the sales departments in the organisation itself. The responsibility for the preparation of this budget rests with the executives of the sales departments. There must be a co-ordination of selling expenses with the volume of sales expected and an effort should be made to control the costs of distribution. The preparation of the budget would depend on the analysis of the market situations by the management, advertising policies, research programmes and the fixed and variable elements.

Capital Expenditure Budget

The budget provides a guidance as to the amount of capital that may be needed for procurement of capital asset during the budget period. The budget is prepared after taking into account the available productive capacities, probable reallocation of existing assets and possible improvement in production techniques. If necessary separate budget may be prepared for each item of assets, such as a building budget, a plant and equipment budget, etc.

Cash Budget

A cash budget is a forecast of the cash position by time periods for a specific duration of time. Cash forecast may be made for a short period or a long duration. The cash budget forms an important part in co-ordinating efficient working of the company. It tells about the working capital required and available at different periods. The budget is prepared by the Chief Accountant.

The main objectives of preparing cash budget are as under :

(i) The probable cash position as a result of planned operations is indicated, and thus the excess or shortages of cash is known. This helps in arranging short-term borrowings in advance to meet the situation of shortage of cash or making investments in times of excess of cash.

(ii) Cash can be co-ordinated in relation to total working capital, sales, investment and debt.

(iii) A sound basis for credit and for current control of cash position is established.

The cash budget can be prepared by any of the following methods :

(i) Receipts and payments method,
(ii) The adjusted profit and loss method,
(iii) The balance sheet method.

(i) **Receipt and payments method :** In case of this method the cash receipts from various sources and the cash payments to various agencies are estimated. In the opening balance of cash, estimated cash receipts are added and from the total, the total of estimated cash payments are deducted to find out the closing balance. If monthly/quarterly cash budgets are to be prepared, first of all the closing balance of first month/quarter will be computed which will be the opening balance for the next month/quarter. Similarly the closing balance for 2nd month/quarter can be known and so on. The estimated receipts may be from cash sales, credit collections, interest, dividend, miscellaneous receipts, issue of share capital, loans, etc. Estimated diburements may be regarding materials, labour, overheads, granting loan or repayment of loan, payment of advance tax, purchase of assets, etc.

(ii) **Adjusted profit and loss method :** In case of this method the cash budget is prepared on the basis of opening cash and bank balances, projected profit and loss account and the balances of the various assets and liabilities. Cash from operations is not that figure of profit which is shown by the profit and loss account, but is the figure of profit as adjusted in the light of non-cash items such as depreciation, loss on sale of capital assets, preliminary expenses written off from P. & L. a/c., etc. Since these items do not affect cash position though they have been charged to the profit and loss account, they are added back to the profit or deducted from loss, as the case may be. Likely issue of new shares, realisation from sale of fixed assets or raising long term loans are taken as other sources of cash. Similarly, likely redemption of preference shares (in case of redeemable preference shares), payment of long-term loans, purchase of fixed assets, payment of dividends, etc. are taken as applications of cash. Moreover, increase in current liabilities such as creditors, bills payable will mean less cash payment or decrease in current assets such as debtors, stock, bills receivables, prepaid expenses, etc. will mean less investment in these assets; therefore, they will be all taken as sources of cash. Increase in current assets and decrease in current liabilities, on the same basis, will mean decrease in cash resources.

(iii) **Balance Sheet Method :** With the help of budgeted balances at the end except cash and bank balances, a budgeted balance sheet can be prepared and the balancing figure would be the estimated closing cash/bank balance. Thus, under this method, closing balances other than cash/bank will have to be found out first to be put in the budgeted balance sheet. This can be done by adjusting the anticipated transactions of the year in the opening balances.

Research and Development Budget

Research and development costs are to be incurred so that the products or the methods of the concern do not become out of date. The research and development budget is a forecast of all such expenses.

The Final or Master Budget

The Master Budget is a summary of the budget schedules in capsule form made for the purpose of presenting, in one report, the highlights of the budget forecast. The Chartered Institute of Management Accountants, England defines it as "the summary budget, incorporating its component functional budgets, which is finally approved, adopted and employed". Thus, it is a summary budget which incorporates all other budgets. It sets, out the plan of operations for all departments in considerable detail for the budget period. The budget may take the form of a Profit and Loss Account and a Balance Sheet as at the end of the budget period.

The Master Budget requires the approval of the Budget Committee before it is put into operation. It may happen, sometimes, that a number of master budgtets have to be prepared before the final one is agreed upon. The budget generally contains details regarding sales (net), production costs, cash position and key account balances (e.g. debtors, stock, fixed assets, bills payable, etc.). It also shows the gross and the net profits, and the important accounting ratios.

FIXED AND FLEXIBLE BUDGETING

Fixed Budget

A budget prepared on the basis of a standard or fixed level of activity is known as a fixed budget. It does not change with the change in the level of activity. Therefore, it becomes an unrealistic measuring yard in case the level of activity (volume of production or sales) actually attained does not conform to the one assumed for budgeting purposes. The management will not be in a position to assess the performance of different departmental heads on the basis of budgets prepared by them because they can serve as measuring sticks only when the actual level of activity corresponds to the budgeted level of activity. On account of these defects of fixed budgeting, it has become a common practice in case of concerns where sales and production cannot be estimated accurately to give up the concepts of fixed budgeting as it does not provide for automatic adjustments with volume changes.

Flexible Budget

A budget prepared in a manner so as to give the budgeted cost for any level of activity is known as a flexible budget. Such a budget is prepared after considering the fixed and variable elements of cost and the changes that may be expected for each item at various levels of operation. Flexible budgeting is desirable in the following cases :

(i) Where on account of typical nature of the business the sales are unpredictable, e.g. in luxury or semi-luxury trades.

(ii) Where the venture is a new one and, therefore, it is almost impossible to foresee the public demand, e.g. novelties in the fashion.

(iii) Where the business is subject to the vagaries of nature such as soft drinks, etc.

(iv) Where the progress depends on adequate supply of labour and the business is an area which is already suffering from shortage of labour.

INDEX